COVID-19

Editors

MICHELLE NG GONG
GREGORY S. MARTIN

CRITICAL CARE CLINICS

www.criticalcare.theclinics.com

Consulting Editor
GREGORY S. MARTIN

July 2022 • Volume 38 • Number 3

ELSEVIER

1600 John F. Kennedy Boulevard • Suite 1800 • Philadelphia, Pennsylvania, 19103-2899

http://www.theclinics.com

CRITICAL CARE CLINICS Volume 38, Number 3
July 2022 ISSN 0749-0704, ISBN-13: 978-0-323-98777-6

Editor: Joanna Collett
Developmental Editor: Hannah Almira Lopez

Critical Care Clinics (ISSN: 0749-0704) is published quarterly by Elsevier Inc., 360 Park Avenue South, New York, NY 10010-1710. Months of issue are January, April, July, and October. Business and Editorial Offices: 1600 John F. Kennedy Blvd., Suite 1800, Philadelphia, PA 19103-2899. Customer Service Office: 6277 Sea Harbor Drive, Orlando, FL 32887-4800. Periodicals postage paid at New York, NY and additional mailing offices. Subscription prices are $266.00 per year for US individuals, $921.00 per year for US institutions, $100.00 per year for US students and residents, $296.00 per year for Canadian individuals, $953.00 per year for Canadian institutions, $338.00 per year for international individuals, $953.00 per year for international institutions, $100.00 per year for Canadian students/residents, and $150.00 per year for foreign students/residents. To receive student/resident rate, orders must be accompanied by name of affiliated institution, date of term, and the signature of program/residency coordinator on institution letterhead. Orders will be billed at individual rate until proof of status is received. Foreign air speed delivery is included in all *Clinics* subscription prices. All prices are subject to change without notice. POSTMASTER: Send address changes to *Critical Care Clinics*, Elsevier Periodicals Customer Service, 11830 Westline Industrial Drive, St. Louis, MO 63146. **Customer Service: 1-800-654-2452 (US). From outside of the US, call 1-314-447-8871. Fax: 1-314-447-8029. E-mail: journalscustomerservice-usa@elsevier.com (for print support) or journalsonlinesupport-usa@elsevier.com (for online support).**

Reprints. For copies of 100 or more of articles in this publication, please contact the Commercial Reprints Department, Elsevier Inc., 360 Park Avenue South, New York, NY 10010-1710. Tel.: 212-633-3874; Fax: 212-633-3820; E-mail: reprints@elsevier.com.

Critical Care Clinics is also published in Spanish by Editorial Inter-Medica, Junin 917, 1er A, 1113, Buenos Aires, Argentina.

Critical Care Clinics is covered in *MEDLINE/PubMed (Index Medicus)*, *EMBASE/Excerpta Medica*, *Current Concepts/Clinical Medicine*, *ISI/BIOMED*, and *Chemical Abstracts*.

Contributors

CONSULTING EDITOR

GREGORY S. MARTIN, MD, MSC
Professor, Division of Pulmonary, Allergy, Critical Care and Sleep Medicine, Research Director, Emory Critical Care Center, Director, Emory/Georgia Tech Predictive Health Institute, Co-Director, Atlanta Center for Microsystems Engineered Point-of-Care Technologies (ACME POCT), President, Society of Critical Care Medicine, Atlanta, Georgia, USA

EDITORS

MICHELLE NG GONG, MD, MS
Chief, Division of Critical Care Medicine, Jay B. Langner Critical Care Service, Professor of Medicine, Professor of Epidemiology and Population Health, Albert Einstein College of Medicine, Chief, Division of Pulmonary Medicine, Director of Critical Care Research, Department of Medicine, Montefiore Medical Center, Bronx, New York, USA

GREGORY S. MARTIN, MD, MSc
Professor, Division of Pulmonary, Allergy, Critical Care and Sleep Medicine, Research Director, Emory Critical Care Center, Director, Emory/Georgia Tech Predictive Health Institute, Co-Director, Atlanta Center for Microsystems Engineered Point-of-Care Technologies (ACME POCT), President, Society of Critical Care Medicine, Atlanta, Georgia, USA

AUTHORS

HASAN M. AL-DORZI, MD
College of Medicine, King Saud bin Abdulaziz University for Health Sciences, King Abdullah International Medical Research Center and Intensive Care Department, King Abdulaziz Medical City, Ministry of National Guard Health Affairs, Riyadh, Saudi Arabia

YASEEN M. ARABI, MD, FCCP, FCCM
College of Medicine, King Saud bin Abdulaziz University for Health Sciences, King Abdullah International Medical Research Center and Intensive Care Department, King Abdulaziz Medical City, Ministry of National Guard Health Affairs, Riyadh, Saudi Arabia

ALLISON M. BLATZ, MD
Department of Pediatrics, Division of Infectious Diseases, Children's Hospital of Philadelphia, Philadelphia, Pennsylvania, USA

NAOMI BOYER, BSc, MBBS
Department of Critical Care, SPACeR Group (Surrey Peri-Operative, Anaesthesia and Critical Care Collaborative Research Group), Royal Surrey Hospital, Guildford, Surrey, United Kingdom

JEN-TING CHEN, MD, MS
Assistant Professor, Division of Critical Care Medicine, Department of Medicine, Montefiore Medical Center, Albert Einstein College of Medicine, Bronx, New York, USA

J. PERREN COBB, MD, FACS, FCCM
Director, Surgical Critical Care, Professor and Clinical Scholar, Departments of Surgery and Anesthesiology, Critical Care Institute, Keck School of Medicine of USC, Health Care Consultation Center, Los Angeles, California, USA

MAI COLVIN, MD
Assistant Professor of Medicine, Division of Critical Care Medicine, Montefiore Medical Center, Albert Einstein College of Medicine, Bronx, New York, USA

CRAIG M. COOPERSMITH, MD
Professor, Department of Surgery, Director, Emory Critical Care Center, Emory University, Vice Chair of Research, Department of Surgery, Program Director, Surgical Critical Care Fellowship, Department of Surgery, Emory University School of Medicine, Director, Surgical/Transplant Intensive Care Unit, Emory University Hospital, Atlanta, Georgia, USA

NEHA S. DANGAYACH, MD, MSCR, FAAN, FNCS
Assistant Professor, Neurocritical Care Division, Departments of Neurosurgery and Neurology, Icahn School of Medicine at Mount Sinai, New York, New York, USA

LEWIS A. EISEN, MD
Director of Clinical Affairs, Division of Critical Care, Department of Medicine, Montefiore Medical Center, Albert Einstein College of Medicine, Bronx, New York, USA

SUSANNAH EMPSON, MD
Department of Anesthesiology, Perioperative, and Pain Medicine, Stanford, California, USA

LAURA EVANS, MD, FCCM
Adult Guidelines Co-Chair Associate Professor, Pulmonary, Critical Care and Sleep Medicine, University of Washington, Director of Critical Care/Associate Medical Director, University of Washington Medical Center, Seattle, Washington, USA

EDDY FAN, PhD
Department of Medicine, Division of Respirology, Sinai Health System and University Health Network, Institute of Health Policy, Management and Evaluation, Dalla Lana School of Public Health, Toronto General Hospital Research Institute, Interdepartmental Division of Critical Care Medicine, University of Toronto, Toronto, Ontario, Canada

BRUNO L. FERREYRO, MD
Department of Medicine, Division of Respirology, Sinai Health System and University Health Network, Institute of Health Policy, Management and Evaluation, Dalla Lana School of Public Health, University of Toronto, Toronto, Ontario, Canada

LUI G. FORNI, BSc, PhD, MBBS, MRCPI, AFICM, JFCMI
Department of Critical Care, SPACeR Group (Surrey Peri-Operative, Anaesthesia and Critical Care Collaborative Research Group), Royal Surrey Hospital, Guildford, Surrey, United Kingdom; Department of Clinical and Experimental Medicine, Faculty of Health Sciences, University of Surrey, Stag Hill, Guildford, United Kingdom

DEREK V. GIBBS, MD
Internal Medicine Resident Physician, Division of General Internal Medicine, Department of Medicine, University of Cincinnati School of Medicine, Cincinnati, Ohio, USA

JAMES HILTON, MBBS, MRCP
Department of Critical Care, SPACeR Group (Surrey Peri-Operative, Anaesthesia and Critical Care Collaborative Research Group), Royal Surrey Hospital, Guildford, Surrey, United Kingdom

KRISTIN M. HUDOCK, MD, MSTR
Assistant Professor of Medicine, Assistant Professor of Pediatrics, Division of Pulmonary, Critical Care and Sleep Medicine, Department of Medicine, University of Cincinnati School of Medicine, Division of Pulmonary Biology, Cincinnati Children's Hospital Medical Center, Cincinnati, Ohio, USA

JOHN A. KELLUM, MD, MCCM
Center for Critical Care Nephrology, University of Pittsburgh, Pittsburgh, Pennsylvania, USA

JOHN KRESS, MD
Professor of Medicine, Section of Pulmonary and Critical Care, Director, Medical ICU, University of Chicago, Chicago, Illinois, USA

MATTHEW LEVITUS, MD
Assistant Professor of Medicine, Division of Critical Care Medicine, Associate Medical Director, Cardiothoracic and Surgical ICU, Jack D. Weiler Hospital, Montefiore Medical Center, Albert Einstein College of Medicine, Bronx, New York, USA

MITRA K. NADIM, MD, FASN
Division of Nephrology and Hypertension, Department of Medicine, Keck School of Medicine of USC, University of Southern California, Los Angeles, California, USA

VIRGINIA NEWCOMBE, MD, PhD
Associate Professor, University Division of Anaesthesia, Department of Medicine, University of Cambridge, Cambridge, United Kingdom

MARLIES OSTERMANN, MD, PhD
Department of Critical Care, King's College London, Guy's & St Thomas' NHS Foundation Hospital, London, United Kingdom

NIDA QADIR, MD
Associate Clinical Professor, David Geffen School of Medicine, University of California, Los Angeles, Los Angeles, California, USA

ADRIENNE G. RANDOLPH, MD, MS
Department of Anesthesiology, Critical Care and Pain Medicine, Division of Critical Care, Boston Children's Hospital, Boston, Massachusetts, USA

SAMUEL REDNOR, DO
Director of Wellness, Division of Critical Care Medicine, Assistant Professor of Clinical Medicine, Albert Einstein College of Medicine, Attending Physician, Division of Critical Care Medicine, Jack D. Weiler Hospital, Bronx, New York, USA

ANGELA J. ROGERS, MD
Department of Pulmonary, Allergy and Critical Care Medicine, Stanford, California, USA

KRISTIN SCHWAB, MD
Assistant Clinical Professor, David Geffen School of Medicine, University of California, Los Angeles, Los Angeles, California, USA

EMILY SCHWITZER, MD
Fellow Physician, David Geffen School of Medicine, University of California, Los Angeles, Los Angeles, California, USA

SCOTT A. SHAINKER, DO, MS
The Annie and Chase Koch Chair in Obstetrics and Gynecology, Director, New England Center for Placental Disorders, Department of Obstetrics and Gynecology, Beth Israel Deaconess Medical Center, Assistant Professor of Obstetrics, Gynecology, and Reproductive Biology, Harvard Medical School, Boston, Massachusetts, USA

SATYA S. SHREENIVAS, MD, MBA
Interventional Cardiology Attending Physician, Division of Cardiology, The Christ Hospital, Cincinnati, Ohio, USA

ROMAIN SONNENVILLE, MD, PhD
Associate Professor, Department of Intensive Care Medicine, AP-HP, Hôpital Bichat-Claude Bernard, Université de Paris, Paris, Paris, France

MANUEL TISMINETZKY, MD
Department of Medicine, Division of Respirology, Sinai Health System and University Health Network, Toronto, Ontario, Canada

JENNIFER G. WILSON, MD, MS
Department of Emergency Medicine, Stanford, California, USA

Contents

With an ever-increasing number of COVID-19 survivors, providers are tasked with addressing the longer lasting symptoms of COVID-19, or post-acute sequelae of SARS-CoV-2 infection (PASC). For critically ill patients, existing knowledge about postintensive care syndrome (PICS) represents a useful structure for understanding PASC. Post-ICU clinics leverage a multidisciplinary team to evaluate and treat the physical, cognitive, and psychological sequelae central to both PICS and PASC in critically ill patients. While management through both pharmacologic and nonpharmacologic modalities can be used, further research into both the optimal treatment and prevention of PASC represents a key public health imperative.

Initial reporting suggested that kidney involvement following COVID-19 infection was uncommon but this is now known not to be the case. Acute kidney injury (AKI) may arise through several mechanisms and complicate up to a quarter of patients hospitalized with COVID-19 infection being associated with an increased risk for both morbidity and death. Mechanisms of injury include direct kidney damage predominantly through tubular injury, although glomerular injury has been reported; the consequences of the treatment of patients with severe hypoxic respiratory failure; secondary infection; and exposure to nephrotoxic drugs. The mainstay of treatment remains the prevention of worsening kidney damage and in some cases they need for renal replacement therapies (RRT). Although the use of other blood purification techniques has been proposed as potential treatments, results to-date have not been definitive.

Patients with severe acute respiratory syndrome coronavirus 2 (SARS-CoV-2) are prone to venous, cerebrovascular, and coronary thrombi, particularly those with severe coronavirus disease 2019 (COVID-19). The pathogenesis is multifactorial and likely involves proinflammatory cascades, development of coagulopathy, and neutrophil extracellular traps, although further investigations are needed. Elevated levels of D-dimers are common in patients with COVID-19 and cannot be used in isolation to predict venous thromboembolism in people with SARS-CoV-2. If given early in hospital admission, therapeutic-dose heparin improves clinical outcomes in patients with moderate COVID-19. To date, antithrombotics have not improved outcomes in patients with severe COVID-19.

Acute respiratory distress syndrome (ARDS) is a heterogeneous syndrome arising from multiple causes with a range of clinical severity. In recent years, the potential for prognostic and predictive enrichment of clinical trials has been increased with identification of more biologically homogeneous subgroups or phenotypes within ARDS. COVID-19 ARDS also exhibits significant clinical heterogeneity despite a single causative agent. In this review the authors summarize the existing literature on COVID-19 ARDS phenotypes, including physiologic, clinical, and biological subgroups as well as the implications for improving both prognostication and precision therapy.

Pregnant women are at increased risk for severe coronavirus disease 2019 (COVID-19) and COVID-19-related complications. Their increased risk in conjuncture with the normal physiologic changes in pregnancy poses unique challenges for the management of the critically ill pregnant patient. This article will review the initial management of pregnant patients who develop acute hypoxic respiratory failure and subsequent treatment of those that deteriorate to acute respiratory distress syndrome and require advanced therapies. Moreover, fetal monitoring and timing of delivery will be reviewed.

Extracorporeal membrane oxygenation (ECMO) is an intervention for severe acute respiratory distress syndrome (ARDS). Although COVID-19-related ARDS has some distinct features, its overall clinical presentation resembles ARDS from other etiologies. Thus, similar evidence-based practices for its management should be applied. These include lung-protective ventilation, prone positioning, and adjuvant strategies, such as ECMO, when appropriate. Current evidence suggests that ECMO in COVID-19-related ARDS has similar efficacy and safety profile as for non-COVID-19 ARDS. The high number of severe COVID-19 cases and demand for therapies, such as ECMO, poses a unique opportunity to increase the understanding on how to optimize this intervention.

Neurologic complications can be seen in mild to severe COVID-19 with a higher risk in patients with severe COVID-19. These can occur as a direct consequence of viral infection or consequences of treatments. The spectrum ranges from non-life-threatening, like headache, fatigue, malaise, anosmia, dysgeusia, to life-threatening complications, like stroke, encephalitis, coma, Guillain-Barre syndrome. A high index of suspicion can aid in early recognition and treatment. Outcomes depend on severity of underlying COVID-19, patient age, comorbidities, and severity of the complication. Postacute sequelae of COVID-19 range from fatigue, headache, dysosmia, brain fog, anxiety, depression to an overlap with postintensive care syndrome.

were better positioned to adapt to the demands of the pandemic, due to their established standardization of care and integration of critical care within the larger structure of the hospital or health care system. CCOs should continue to make changes, based on the real experience of COVID-19 that would lead to improved care during the ongoing pandemic, and beyond.

CRITICAL CARE CLINICS

SERIES OF RELATED INTEREST

Emergency Medicine Clinics
https://www.emed.theclinics.com/
Clinics in Chest Medicine
https://www.chestmed.theclinics.com/

THE CLINICS ARE AVAILABLE ONLINE!
Access your subscription at:
www.theclinics.com

Preface

Critical Care Response to COVID-19 Pandemic: Building on the Past to Bridge to the Future

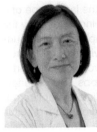 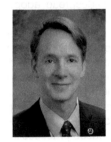

Michelle Ng Gong, MD, MS   Gregory S. Martin, MD, MSc
Editors

At the end of 2021, the COVID-19 pandemic led to more than 286 million cases and over 5.4 million deaths worldwide. COVID-19 is now the deadliest pandemic in the history of the United States. As we reflect on the last 2 years, it is also clear that the pandemic was a pivotal moment for critical care medicine. Never before have the availability and delivery of intensive care medicine been so crucial in a health care crisis. Common critical care issues like acute respiratory distress syndrome (ARDS), ventilators, proning, dialysis, sepsis, and respiratory failure were commonly discussed in the press and social media. There were also much anxiety, fear, and conjecture on the best way to manage this new disease. Two years into the pandemic with the benefit of hindsight, perspective, and evidence to guide care, the pandemic has proven to be reaffirming, challenging, and ultimately promising for the future of critical care medicine.

Although there was much speculation in the beginning of the pandemic that COVID-19 is fundamentally different from pneumonia and ARDS, Empson and colleagues demonstrated that there have always been different ARDS phenotypes and that general evidence-based ARDS management remains the key to caring for COVID-19 patients with ARDS. The management of acute kidney injury (Hilton and colleagues) and respiratory failure with noninvasive ventilation and high-flow nasal cannula (Al-Dorzi HM and colleagues) did not differ greatly from before, but the need for such organ support certainly expanded during the pandemic. Special populations like children (Blatz and colleagues) and pregnant women (Levitcus M and colleagues) became critically ill in large numbers, requiring noncritical care clinicians to rapidly acquire fundamental critical care skills and knowledge and adapt it to COVID-19. Use of extracorporeal membrane oxygenation (Tisminetzky and

Crit Care Clin 38 (2022) xiii–xv
https://doi.org/10.1016/j.ccc.2022.03.001
0749-0704/22/© 2022 Published by Elsevier Inc.

colleagues) expanded, although the optimal timing and patient selection remain unclear during the pandemic. Rednor and colleagues highlight how the growing entity of critical care organizations in many medical systems was leveraged to facilitate and streamline a centralized response during the pandemic and what we can learn for future health care crisis and disasters.

Among the biggest challenges in ARDS was the lack of any effective pharmacologic therapy. Prior to the pandemic, randomized controlled trials in ARDS and sepsis were often negative because of the heterogenous nature of the condition and the difficulty in enrolling large number of patients. Even when beneficial management is demonstrated, it often takes years for widespread adoption (low-tidal-volume ventilation and proning, for examples). The COVID-19 pandemic changed the landscape of clinical trials in critical care. With a large number of patients developing respiratory failure from one etiology and the use of pragmatic platform trials, an unprecedented number of patients were enrolled into clinical trials that were completed within months and that yielded a number of beneficial interventions, including corticosteroids, interleukin-6 inhibitors, and anticoagulation (Chen JT and colleagues and Gibbs and colleagues). Meta-analysis of randomized controlled trials and updates to clinical practice guidelines, which often take years to complete, took weeks during the pandemic, resulting in the rapid adoption of evidence-based practices in critical care. However, similar to many critical illnesses, interventions for COVID-19 seem to work best when used early to prevent progression to organ failure and mechanical ventilation. Interventions in patients with established organ failure have been less effective. It may be that critical care trials need to shift upstream to the prevention of organ failure rather than its treatment after acute injury or illness. In addition, some of these interventions effective in COVID-19 like corticosteroids have reopened questions about its potential benefit in special populations of non-COVID-19–related ARDS.

It is clear that future clinical trials in critical care medicine will be fundamentally different from before the pandemic. There will be more platform trials with adaptive designs and more careful phenotyping of patients either at the beginning of the trial or within the trial to better understand which patient population may most benefit. However, tragic the COVID-19 pandemic has been, this issue of *Critical Care Clinics* has reaffirmed how our prior research and experience were vital foundations on which critical care was able to respond to and manage the patients in the pandemic. But it is also hopeful in that it demonstrates how much advancement could be made even in a crisis and how critical care research can be most productive in the future.

Michelle Ng Gong, MD, MS
Division of Critical Care Medicine
Jay B. Langner Critical Care Service
Albert Einstein College of Medicine
Division of Pulmonary Medicine
Department of Medicine
Montefiore Medical Center
111 East 210th Street
Gold Zone (Main Floor)
Bronx, NY 10467, USA

Gregory S. Martin, MD, MSc
Division of Pulmonary, Allergy
Critical Care and Sleep Medicine
Emory Critical Care Center
Emory/Georgia Tech Predictive
Health Institute
49 Jesse Hill Jr Drive SE
Atlanta, GA 30303, USA

E-mail addresses:
mgong@montefiore.org (M.N. Gong)
greg.martin@emory.edu (G.S. Martin)

Postacute Sequelae of COVID-19 Critical Illness

Kristin Schwab, MD*, Emily Schwitzer, MD, Nida Qadir, MD

KEYWORDS

- Postacute sequelae of SARS-CoV-2 • Postintensive care syndrome
- Post–acute COVID-19 syndrome • Post-COVID-19 programs • Long COVID

KEY POINTS

- Many survivors of COVID-19 critical illness will experience long-term impairments in physical, mental, cognitive, social, and financial health
- The sequelae of COVID-19 critical illness overlap considerably with postintensive care syndrome; existing knowledge of postintensive care syndrome can serve as a useful framework for approaching patients with COVID-19 recovering from critical illness
- Evaluation and management of postintensive care syndrome and postacute sequelae of COVID-19 critical illness require a multidisciplinary approach
- Post-ICU clinics offer opportunities for quality improvement and research that may improve the care of patients while they are in the ICU

INTRODUCTION

Coronavirus disease 2019 (COVID-19) has claimed over 4 million deaths worldwide[1] and has created an unprecedented burden on intensive care units globally.[2] Much of the dialogue surrounding the pandemic has centered on mortality, which has been as high as 50% in critically ill patients.[3] However, most patients will survive acute illness from COVID-19, and survival, despite being a desired outcome, is also fraught with challenges. Initial reports from Italy, France, and the United States suggest that 66% to 87% of hospitalized patients with COVID-19 have symptoms that persist after hospital discharge.[4–6] The term "long COVID" has helped to raise awareness of the postacute sequelae of SARS-CoV-2 infection (PASC) and the potentially long-lasting health consequences that can stem from acute illness. Particularly in patients surviving COVID-19 critical illness, survival will not equate to recovery, and understanding and addressing the long-term needs of survivors is a societal imperative. While PASC has been reported even among patients who were not critically ill or hospitalized, this review focuses on PASC in patients surviving COVID-19 critical illness.

David Geffen School of Medicine, University of California Los Angeles, 10833 Le Conte Avenue, Room 43-229 CHS, Los Angeles, CA 90095, USA
* Corresponding author. David Geffen School of Medicine at UCLA, 10833 Le Conte Avenue, Room 43-229 CHS, Los Angeles, CA 90095.
E-mail address: kschwab@mednet.ucla.edu

Crit Care Clin 38 (2022) 455–472
https://doi.org/10.1016/j.ccc.2022.01.001
0749-0704/22/© 2022 Elsevier Inc. All rights reserved.

Postintensive care syndrome (PICS), defined as new or worsening impairments in mental, cognitive, or physical health following critical illness,[7] affects nearly all ICU survivors at the time of hospital discharge, and continues to impact more than half of these patients 1 year after discharge.[8] This syndrome has been studied and described for over a decade and can serve as a useful framework for approaching patients surviving COVID-19 critical illness who continue to have impairments in the postacute setting. In this review, we describe PICS—and what this can tell us about PASC in the critically ill.

CLINICAL MANIFESTATIONS OF POSTINTENSIVE CARE SYNDROME AND POSTACUTE SEQUELAE OF SARS-CoV-2 INFECTION IN THE CRITICALLY ILL

Due to medical, scientific, and technological advances in the last several decades, survival rates of patients with ICU have increased dramatically.[9,10] This rise in survivorship coupled with an aging population have created a growing cohort of patients suffering from varied long-term consequences of critical care.[11,12] In recent years, there has been a growing body of literature outlining the long-term sequelae of an intensive care unit (ICU) stay (**Fig. 1**).[13] While the 3 major components of PICS—deficits in mental, cognitive, or physical health—are illustrated individually, a complex relationship exists between each domain, with a single impairment in any one domain influencing the others,[8,14–16] and often coexisting with the others.[17,18] The clinical manifestations, incidence, and risk factors for each component are first described, and then compared with our existing knowledge about these symptoms in PASC.

Cognitive Impairment

In terms of cognitive functioning, critical illness can lead to new and clinically important cognitive impairments regardless of age, coexisting disease, and preexisting conditions, often mirroring the degree of impairment seen in Alzheimer's dementia.[19,20] Patients who have experienced delirium in the ICU are at particularly high risk for long-term cognitive impairment.[19] The areas of cognition most commonly affected include attention, concentration, mental processing speed, memory, and executive function, with dysfunction in the latter 2 prevalent in 35% of ICU survivors at 3 months.[21,22] In turn, this places patients

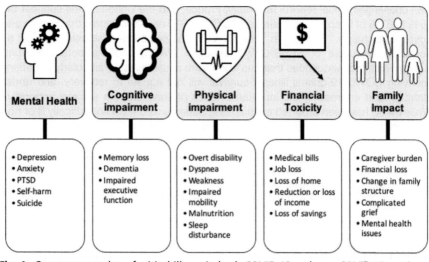

Fig. 1. Common sequelae of critical illness in both COVID-19 and non–COVID-19 survivors.

at higher risk for disruptions in medication adherence and appropriate follow-up, and acts as a major obstacle in returning to premorbid levels of socioeconomic functioning.[12,22,23] A number of factors unique to COVID-19 ICU survivors increases their risk for cognitive impairment. Frequently, they are mechanically ventilated and on high amounts of sedation.[24] Additionally, they have experienced critical illness with the added burdens of social isolation due to infection control measures; lack of family visitation has been identified as an independent risk factor for ICU delirum.[25] Consequently, cognitive deficits have been described as some of the most common and debilitating long-term sequelae in patients with PASC, with decreased concentration, memory concerns, and cognitive impairment reported in a median of 24%, 19%, and 17% of patients, respectively.[26]

Physical Impairment

The spectrum of physical impairment in patients with PICS is wide, with up to 80% of patients experiencing a new physical dysfunction at the time of discharge.[27,28] These include critical illness neuropathy (CIN), critical illness myopathy (CIM), cachexia, fatigue, dyspnea, impaired pulmonary function, decreased exercise tolerance, sexual dysfunction, and respiratory failure.[29–31] Functionally, patients are believed to lose as much as a kilogram of lean body mass (LBM) per day, which predisposes to muscle weakness and related physical impairments that can persist for months to years.[11,32,33] ICU-acquired weakness, defined as neuromuscular dysfunction with no plausible cause other than critical illness and its treatments, is thought to originate from CIN, CIM, or a combination of the two.[31,34] While the prevalence varies widely based on patient population, risk factors, and methods used for diagnosis, it is believed that 43% of patients in the ICU suffer from this complication, which is associated with both hospital mortality and long-term mortality, with decreased survival seen in patients up to 5 years later.[35,36] Consequently, patients have difficulties performing their daily activities with persistently lower health-related quality of life (HRQL) measures when compared with age matched norms.[37,38]

In areas hit hard by the pandemic, ICU staffing shortages may contribute to limited patient mobilization, a preventative measure known to reduce the risk of ICU-acquired weakness.[39] Indeed, the receipt of care in overwhelmed and understaffed hospitals has been associated with adverse outcomes.[25,40] Other risk factors for long-term physical sequelae of critical illness in COVID-19 survivors include frequent use of prone positioning and arterial line placement, which can each increase the risk of neuropathy.[41] Corticosteroids and prolonged used of neuromuscular blocking agents, which are prescribed to treat COVID-19 pneumonia and manage severe acute respiratory distress syndrome, respectively, further increase the risk of CIM when used in combination.[42,43]

Psychological Impairment

The psychological sequelae of PICS are estimated to occur in up to a third of survivors, with PTSD, depression, and anxiety as the predominant conditions.[13,44] While it can be situational for some, others have symptoms that persist for months to years after discharge, disrupting daily functioning and reducing overall quality of life; ICU survivors also have a higher incidence of suicide and self-harm when compared with hospital survivors who never required ICU admission.[45,46] The psychological sequelae extend beyond the patient to those in the family as well, collectively known as PICS-Family (PICS-F).[7] Having a critically ill family member has been shown to have profound effects on relatives, with over two-thirds reporting anxiety or depression when visiting their loved ones, and 30% suffering from anxiety, depression, or PTSD beyond discharge.[47,48] Further, the complex interactions of the various domains of PICS, as outlined above, amplify the burden on patient's families as well as dramatically increase the cost for health care systems.[49,50] Patients with COVID-19 have similarly been found to have high rates of PTSD, anxiety, depression, and insomnia, likely due to both disease-specific and pandemic-related factors including stigmatization, social isolation, and media sensationalism, among others.[51] Existing studies suggest that approximately 30%, 20%, 13%, and 27% of COVID-19 survivors suffer from anxiety, depression, PTSD, and insomnia, respectively.[26]

As PICS has profound effects across mental, cognitive, and physical domains, a first step involves recognizing the comorbidities that predispose to developing it in the first place. To date, there have been many studies evaluating the risk factors associated with PICS, although the mechanisms continue to be poorly understood. While certain risk factors are preexisting and thus nonmodifiable, others are ICU-specific, and thus have the potential to be optimized (**Fig. 2**).[13,52–54] For example, delirium, which is associated with increased mortality, ICU length of stay, and long-term cognitive impairment, may represent one modifiable risk factor.[12,55–57] As such, multicomponent ICU-level strategies, such as the "ABCDEF bundle," have been used with success.[12,56] This systematic method of pain assessment, both spontaneous awakening and breathing trials, choosing safe and effective medication regimens for managing pain and agitation, delirium monitoring, exercise/early mobility, and family engagement, has been shown to reduce the amount of sedative use, duration of

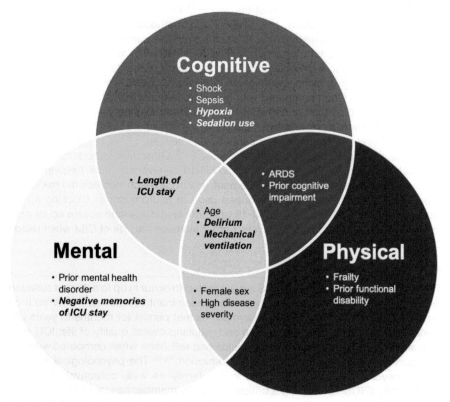

Fig. 2. Risk factors associated with PICS. Each circle represents the PICS domain associated with each risk factor. Those in *italics* represent potentially modifiable risk factors; others are preexisting.

delirium, and ICU length of stay.[58–60] With the COVID-19 pandemic bringing a growing number of patients to the ICU, it is becoming increasingly imperative to identify additional modifiable risk factors for PICS so that new preventative interventions can be developed in the future.

Health Care Utilization and Disability

While symptoms of PICS may improve over time, survivors of critical illness still face a number of long-term challenges, including increased mortality, rehospitalization, reduced quality of life, and financial loss. A study of US Medicare beneficiaries comparing ICU survivors to age, sex, and race-matched controls from the general population found that ICU survivors have increased mortality at 3 years (39.5% vs 14.9%)[61]; similar findings were seen in Dutch[62] and Scottish[63] cohorts. Long-term mortality in mechanically ventilated ICU survivors is markedly increased, with rates of 41% to 58% reported in multicenter cohorts.[61,64,65] Similarly, health care utilization, including hospital readmission, increases after critical illness. In an observational study comparing health care utilization among ICU survivors before and after critical illness, ICU survivors in the year following critical illness were found to have an increase in outpatient visits, emergency department visits, and hospitalizations of 8%, 33%, and 60%, respectively, when compared with the prior year.[66] Expectedly, postdischarge health care costs are also greater than costs in the year before critical illness. Less predictably, health care costs can remain increased from baseline for up to 5 years following discharge.[63]

Functional status and HRQL also suffer after critical illness.[67–74] At least partial disability in activities of daily living is seen in one-fifth of previously independent individuals 1 year after discharge.[69] Frailty, which is associated with new-onset disability,[75] is also common among survivors of critical illness. In a recent multicenter study, transition to a state of increased frailty occurred in 40% of ICU survivors at 1 year, including 23% of patients who were not frail at baseline.[76] Likewise, HRQL is worse in ICU survivors compared with population norms. However, it remains unclear to what degree post-ICU HRQL is a reflection of premorbid quality of life. HRQL has also been found to improve over time, particularly during the first year following ICU discharge.[68,71–73]

Patients with COVID-19 similarly suffer from increased health care utilization and risk of death, with estimates suggesting a 1 in 5 risk of readmission and a 1 in 10 risk of death among hospitalized COVID-19 patients in the first 60 days after discharge.[77] Beyond readmission and death, survivors also have decreased HRQL, increased outpatient health care visits, and increased pharmacotherapy utilization of opioid pain medications, antidepressants, anxiolytics, and more.[78,79]

Social and Financial Considerations

The COVID-19 pandemic has brought increased attention to the role of socioeconomic status in critical illness. Indeed, lower socioeconomic position and social vulnerability are associated with increased risk of critical illness and death from COVID-19 infection.[80,81] However, an inverse relationship between socioeconomic position and health outcomes in ICU survivors has previously been established, with lower socioeconomic position associated with increased risk of long-term mortality and reduced HRQL.[82,83]

Just as socioeconomic status affects outcomes in the critically ill, critical illness itself has an impact on subsequent social and economic outcomes. Job loss and delayed return to work are common after critical illness, likely a result of post-ICU impairments. Of patients who were previously employed, only 56% to 60% return to work 1 year after critical illness, and one-third remain jobless after 5 years.[84,85] While the long-term work implications in critically ill COVID-19 survivors are still being investigated, preliminary evidence suggests similar findings, with less than half of patients surviving COVID-19 critical illness returning to work at 3 to 4 months after discharge.[79] Consequently, loss of income is common, reported in 71% of ICU survivors in the year following critical illness,[86] as are other elements of financial toxicity, such as loss of health care coverage, depletion of savings, and medical bills.[86–88] Family structure and roles may be also altered, as one-quarter of ICU survivors report needing a caregiver 1 year after critical illness. The vast majority of care is provided by family members, half of whom report a resultant negative impact on employment.[89,90]

EVALUATION OF POSTACUTE SEQUELAE OF SARS-CoV-2 INFECTION IN SURVIVORS OF CRITICAL ILLNESS

While limited evidence exists to inform the optimal evaluation of PASC, significant experience in the post-ICU arena can help guide these efforts.[91] Indeed, to evaluate for PICS and the constellation of downstream effects outlined above, post-ICU clinics have been developed.[92] Guidelines from the United Kingdom recommend that all adults who have stayed in an ICU for more than 4 days be followed after discharge, though implementation barriers have hampered widespread adoption of this policy in the UK and elsewhere.[93] As many patients transfer first to facilities such as skilled nursing facilities or acute rehabilitation units before discharging to home, coordinating the ideal timing of the first post-ICU visit can be challenging. Consensus guidelines recommend an assessment 2 to 4 weeks after hospital discharge.[94]

Experience from centers specializing in post-ICU care suggests that a discharge navigator can be particularly useful in identifying and recruiting eligible patients,[95,96] and may be associated with decreased readmission rates and decreased loss to follow-up.[96] The navigator role may be filled by one of many different providers, including nurse practitioners, social workers, respiratory therapists, or case managers. In this role, the provider can connect with patients while still hospitalized, schedule and share information about the post-ICU clinic visit, and serve as a point of contact for the patients and their families as they navigate the transition out of the hospital. In settings where access to post-ICU follow-up may be more limited, navigators may choose to screen for risk factors to identify patients at particularly high risk for PICS and prioritize these patients for follow-up.

To address all of the components of PICS, post-ICU clinics are typically composed of a multidisciplinary team. Providers have debated which medical specialty is best equipped to lead these clinics (ie, intensivists vs rehabilitation specialists), yet this debate seems to only further highlight the importance of the interdisciplinary approach.[97,98] We believe it is important to incorporate an ICU provider in the clinic, as studies suggest that this can facilitate longitudinal care delivery for patients, circle back to improve processes for future patients in the ICU, and reduce ICU staff burnout.[92,99,100] In addition to an intensivist, a number of other clinicians typically comprise the multidisciplinary team, including a specialist to assess for physical debility (eg, a physical therapist, physiatrist, and/or respiratory therapist), psychological sequelae (eg, a psychologist and/or social worker), and cognitive impairment (eg, an occupational therapist, speech/language pathologist, or neurocognitive specialist). Additional team members may include a pharmacist, nutritionist, chaplain, case manager, or palliative care specialist.

During the clinic visit, standardized tools should be adopted to systemically evaluate PICS and track progression over time (**Fig. 3**). Although further research into the optimal assessment tools are needed, guidelines have been developed based on expert opinion.[94,101] Current guidelines recommend using the Hospital Anxiety

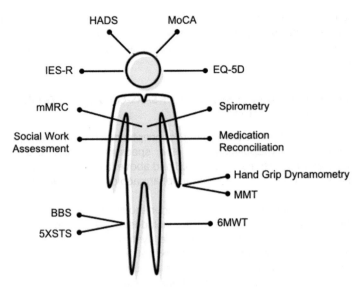

Fig. 3. Outpatient evaluation of PASC in survivors of critical illness. HADS, Hospital Anxiety and Depression Scale; MoCA, Montreal Cognitive Assessment; IESR, Impact of Event Scale-Revised; EQ-5D, EuroQol-5D; mMRC, Modified Medical Research Council; BBS, Borg Balance Scale; 5XSTS, Five Times Sit-to-Stand; MMT, Manual Muscle Testing; 6MWT, Six-Minute Walk Test

and Depression Scale (HADS) to assess for anxiety and depression, as well as either the Impact of Events Scale-Revised (IES-R) or the shorter IES-6 to evaluate for post-traumatic stress disorder.[94,101] While expert consensus has not been reached regarding the optimal cognitive screening tool, the Montreal Cognitive Assessment (MOCA) or MOCA-Blind may be used to screen for cognitive impairment.[94] To evaluate for physical and pulmonary function, the Society of Critical Care Medicine suggests using the 6-minute walk test[94]; our center also uses bedside spirometry and the Modified Medical Research Council dyspnea scale as further assessments of pulmonary function. Some experts also suggest further evaluation of ICU-acquired weakness, including CIM and CIN, through the use of manual muscle testing and handgrip dynamometry; our center also uses the Borg Balance Scale (BBS) and Five Times Sit to Stand (5XSTS) instruments for further assessment of physical disability.[101] Finally, the EuroQol-5D (EQ-5D) questionnaire can be used to evaluate both HRQL and pain.[101]

In addition to using these screening assessments, a complete medication reconciliation should be performed to reduce the risk of polypharmacy. Our center's practice also includes evaluation for new or persistent symptoms, appropriate referrals to further assist with ongoing physical and medical recovery, and screening for health care maintenance gaps such as immunizations. To help educate the patient and family, we summarize the patient's ICU course, counsel on expected ICU recovery and supports available, and answer any questions. We also include family members in this process, as the adverse psychological effects that an ICU stay can have on family members, or PICS-Family, have become increasingly appreciated.[7] Finally, we ask for feedback to help with ongoing quality improvement efforts within the ICU.

While these appointments have traditionally been performed in-person, the expanding role of telemedicine amidst the COVID-19 pandemic has opened up possibilities for expanding the reach of post-ICU clinics.[102] This can be particularly useful in the post-ICU population, where limited patient mobility, large geographic distances, financial strain, and reduced access to transportation services can make in-person visits challenging.[103]

MANAGEMENT OF POSTACUTE SEQUELAE OF SARS-CoV-2 INFECTION IN SURVIVORS OF CRITICAL ILLNESS

As PICS and PASC remain relatively novel concepts, much of the management rests on expert opinion or extrapolation from other specialties. Similar to the multidisciplinary approach to assessment that is outlined above, a cross-disciplinary approach incorporating both pharmacologic and nonpharmacological domains will often need to be used.

In treating cognitive dysfunction, the provider should first evaluate for and manage any potentially reversible etiologies. This includes psychiatric conditions such as depression that can manifest with cognitive dysfunction, polypharmacy that may occur due to inadvertently-continued ICU medications on discharge (eg, atypical antipsychotics), sleep disorders, and metabolic or nutritional disturbances. Once these have been addressed, other treatment options such as cognitive therapy and exercise can be considered. Cognitive rehabilitation therapy aims to improve thought processes and behavior through multimodal strategies such as memory training exercises and/or the incorporation of organizational devices such as phone reminders.[104] This has been evaluated in a limited number of studies on ICU survivors and may lead to improvements in cognitive functioning, and particularly executive function, though further studies are needed.[105] For appropriate patients, exercise therapy has been shown to improve cognitive function in patients with mild cognitive impairment, and may similarly be of benefit to patients with PICS-associated cognitive impairment.[106]

We typically refer patients with ongoing physical limitations to physical therapy and/or occupational therapy for ongoing recovery, with the acknowledgment that there are limited studies for rehabilitation in CIM and CIN at present.[107] In addition, randomized trials of rehabilitation-based programs for ICU survivors have not yet shown benefit for HRQL metrics.[108–110] Nevertheless, given its potential to improve functional capacity, we continue to recommend physical and occupational therapy in this patient population. Rehabilitation specialists may also assist with recommendations regarding mobility aides and environmental adjustments. For COVID-19 survivors specifically, providers should avoid prolonging corticosteroid courses in the outpatient setting unless an alternative condition such as organizing pneumonia exists.[111] In addition, given parallels between myalgic encephalomyelitis/chronic fatigue syndrome and the fatigue that many recovering patients with COVID-19 describe, patients should be counseled on the importance of graded exercise increase to decrease the risk of setbacks and postexertional malaise.[112]

Patients with pulmonary limitations due to post-ARDS fibrosis are managed with both supportive and preventative care. The prevalence of post-ARDS fibrosis in patients with and without COVID-19 remains unclear, but can be evaluated with serial pulmonary function testing and imaging.[113] Thus far, evidence suggests that the majority of these patients experience improvement in both physiologic testing and radiographic changes over time.[67,114,115] In this population, providers can thus assist with oxygen weaning, radiographic and pulmonary function test follow-up, and pulmonary rehabilitation referrals when indicated. Pulmonary rehabilitation, which involves supervised graded aerobic exercise training, strength training, and education on topics such as breathing techniques, inhaler use, and red flag symptoms, has been shown to improve pulmonary function and HRQL in ARDS survivors.[116] We also ensure that vaccinations against *Streptococcus pneumoniae*, influenza, and COVID-19 are up to date. In spite of these measures, a minority of patients might not improve and may ultimately need to be referred to a center specializing in interstitial lung disease.

Patients with persistent psychiatric impairments after ICU survival benefit from referral to a mental health professional for appropriate management. Treatment frequently involves a combination of pharmacotherapy and psychotherapy. Patients with depression can be treated with either an antidepressant or psychotherapy alone, as each has shown efficacy in randomized trials, though data also suggest that combination therapy may be more efficacious than either treatment individually.[117–119] For anxiety, cognitive behavioral therapy remains the most studied, and thus first-line, psychotherapeutic option, though mindfulness-based therapies are gaining increasing attention and may be more feasible for patients to initiate themselves during the initial recovery period.[120] Pharmacotherapy for generalized anxiety disorder may also be considered for patients who meet diagnostic criteria. First-line treatment of posttraumatic stress disorder involves trauma-focused therapies such as cognitive behavioral therapy and exposure-based therapy, with medications reserved for individuals with a strong preference toward this.[121] Some post-ICU centers also offer peer support groups through either in-person or virtual platforms, which have been shown to have a myriad of beneficial effects for patients.[122,123] An additional challenge we have found during the COVID-19 pandemic is that after discharge, recovered patients are frequently hesitant to leave their homes due to fear of contracting the virus again, inadvertently restricting their opportunities for mobilization, which can exacerbate deconditioning and functional limitations, and also lead to worsened quality of life. In these situations, providers should evaluate for anxiety, agoraphobia, and PTSD and refer for treatment when applicable. They can also reinforce masking and social distancing precautions, and assess for appropriate COVID-19 vaccination timing. We have also found that a minority of patients can become consumed with media reports and social medial rabbit holes on long COVID-19, which often focus on outlier patients and can thus paint an overly negative picture of COVID-19 recovery. Similar stressors have been described in survivors of the SARS pandemic.[124] Providers can assist by counseling patients on an expected recovery trajectory, normalizing their experience, and validating their progress.[125]

BEYOND COVID-19: THE ROLE OF POST-ICU CLINICS IN QUALITY IMPROVEMENT AND RESEARCH

In response to the COVID-19 pandemic, multidisciplinary post-ICU clinics have been newly created by centers worldwide.[40] While these clinics currently serve a crucial role in meeting the needs of patients recovering from COVID-19, they also provide a number of opportunities for improving care for all critically ill patients. On a center level, previously undetected issues can be identified during outpatient follow-up and serve as targets for ICU quality improvement. From the standpoint of clinician education, witnessing a patient's recovery process may result in greater reflective practice in the ICU, influencing clinical decision-making and improving accuracy in predicting outcomes.[126]

Post-ICU clinics also provide a much-needed avenue for conducting long-term outcomes research, which has been methodologically challenging in critical care. Loss to follow-up is a common limitation in long-term ICU outcomes studies, likely resulting in the exclusion of some of the most severely ill patients, who may have physical or

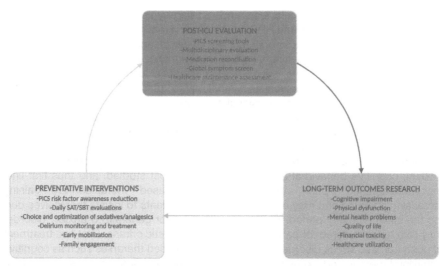

Fig. 4. Role of PICS clinics in improving ICU care. Multidisciplinary evaluation in post-ICU clinics can provide a basis for long-term research, which in turn can inform future preventative interventions in the ICU. PICS, Post-Intensive Care Syndrome; SAT, Spontaneous Awakening Trial; SBT, Spontaneous Breathing Trial.

cognitive deficits leading to study withdrawal.[127] Such patients may potentially be more likely to present for clinical care than for research follow-up. As more patients survive a critical illness, improving care in the ICU will increasingly need to focus on preventing morbidity, and creating additional opportunities for postdischarge assessment is invaluable. The proliferation of post-ICU clinics during the COVID-19 pandemic may ultimately help improve care for all critically ill patients (**Fig. 4**).

SUMMARY

Amidst a growing appreciation of the wide-ranging and long-term public health effects of COVID-19, PICS represents a useful contextual framework for diagnosing and treating PASC in critically ill survivors of COVID-19. While these conditions are not one and the same, there is substantial overlap, and providers can draw on existing knowledge of PICS when treating COVID-19 survivors. Further research into the prevention, diagnosis, and treatment of both PICS and PASC are needed as we move into the new frontier of COVID-19 survivorship.

CLINICS CARE POINTS

- Patients recovering from critical illness after COVID-19 infection are at increased risk of cognitive impairment, ICU-acquired weakness, and psychiatric illness including anxiety, depression, PTSD, and insomnia.
- Multidisciplinary management approaches, including non-pharmacologic options such as cognitive rehabilitation therapy, psychotherapy, and peer support groups, represent cornerstones of treatment in postintensive care syndrome.
- Further research into the optimal treatment of PASC in critically ill patients is needed.

CONFLICT OF INTEREST

All authors report no relevant conflicts of interest.

REFERENCES

1. Center for systems science and Engineering at Johns Hopkins University COVID-19 Dashboard. Available at: https://coronavirus.jhu.edu/map.html. Accessed September 15 2021.
2. Tan E, Song J, Deane AM, et al. Global impact of Coronavirus disease 2019 infection requiring admission to the ICU: a systematic review and meta-analysis. Chest 2021;159:524–36.
3. Domecq JP, Lal A, Sheldrick CR, et al. Outcomes of patients with Coronavirus disease 2019 Receiving organ support therapies: the international viral infection and respiratory illness Universal study Registry. Crit Care Med 2021;49:437–48.
4. Carfì A, Bernabei R, Landi F. Persistent symptoms in patients after acute COVID-19. Jama 2020;324:603–5.
5. Carvalho-Schneider C, Laurent E, Lemaignen A, et al. Follow-up of adults with noncritical COVID-19 two months after symptom onset. Clin Microbiol Infect 2021;27:258–63.
6. Chopra V, Flanders SA, O'Malley M, et al. Sixty-day outcomes among patients hospitalized with COVID-19. Ann Intern Med 2021;576–8.
7. Needham DM, Davidson J, Cohen H, et al. Improving long-term outcomes after discharge from intensive care unit: report from a stakeholders' conference. Crit Care Med 2012;40:502–9.
8. Marra A, Pandharipande PP, Girard TD, et al. Co-occurrence of post-intensive care syndrome Problems among 406 survivors of critical illness. Crit Care Med 2018;46:1393–401.
9. Zimmerman JE, Kramer AA, Knaus WA. Changes in hospital mortality for United States intensive care unit admissions from 1988 to 2012. Crit Care 2013;17:R81.
10. Martin GS, Mannino DM, Eaton S, et al. The epidemiology of sepsis in the United States from 1979 through 2000. N Engl J Med 2003;348:1546–54.
11. Herridge MS, Moss M, Hough CL, et al. Recovery and outcomes after the acute respiratory distress syndrome (ARDS) in patients and their family caregivers. Intensive Care Med 2016;42:725–38.
12. Jackson JC, Pandharipande PP, Girard TD, et al. Depression, post-traumatic stress disorder, and functional disability in survivors of critical illness in the BRAIN-ICU study: a longitudinal cohort study. Lancet Respir Med 2014;2: 369–79.
13. Desai SV, Law TJ, Needham DM. Long-term complications of critical care. Crit Care Med 2011;39:371–9.
14. Bruck E, Schandl A, Bottai M, et al. The impact of sepsis, delirium, and psychological distress on self-rated cognitive function in ICU survivors-a prospective cohort study. J Intensive Care 2018;6:2.
15. Mikkelsen ME, Shull WH, Biester RC, et al. Cognitive, mood and quality of life impairments in a select population of ARDS survivors. Respirology 2009;14: 76–82.
16. Sukantarat K, Greer S, Brett S, et al. Physical and psychological sequelae of critical illness. Br J Health Psychol 2007;12:65–74.
17. Bienvenu OJ, Colantuoni E, Mendez-Tellez PA, et al. Cooccurrence of and remission from general anxiety, depression, and posttraumatic stress disorder

symptoms after acute lung injury: a 2-year longitudinal study. Crit Care Med 2015;43:642–53.

18. Marra A, Pandharipande PP, Girard TD, et al. Co-occurrence of post-intensive care syndrome Problems among 406 survivors of critical illness. Crit Care Med 2018;46:1393–401.

19. Pandharipande PP, Girard TD, Ely EW. Long-term cognitive impairment after critical illness. N Engl J Med 2014;370:185–6.

20. Iwashyna TJ, Ely EW, Smith DM, et al. Long-term cognitive impairment and functional disability among survivors of severe sepsis. JAMA 2010;304:1787–94.

21. Sukantarat KT, Burgess PW, Williamson RC, et al. Prolonged cognitive dysfunction in survivors of critical illness. Anaesthesia 2005;60:847–53.

22. Hopkins RO, Weaver LK, Pope D, et al. Neuropsychological sequelae and impaired health status in survivors of severe acute respiratory distress syndrome. Am J Respir Crit Care Med 1999;160:50–6.

23. Rothenhausler HB, Ehrentraut S, Stoll C, et al. The relationship between cognitive performance and employment and health status in long-term survivors of the acute respiratory distress syndrome: results of an exploratory study. Gen Hosp Psychiatry 2001;23:90–6.

24. Rodriguez-Morales AJ, Cardona-Ospina JA, Gutierrez-Ocampo E, et al. Clinical, laboratory and imaging features of COVID-19: a systematic review and meta-analysis. Trav Med Infect Dis 2020;34:101623.

25. Pun BT, Badenes R, Heras La Calle G, et al. Prevalence and risk factors for delirium in critically ill patients with COVID-19 (COVID-D): a multicentre cohort study. Lancet Respir Med 2021;9:239–50.

26. Groff D, Sun A, Ssentongo AE, et al. Short-term and long-term rates of Postacute sequelae of SARS-CoV-2 infection: a systematic review. JAMA Netw Open 2021; 4:e2128568.

27. Harvey MA, Davidson JE. Postintensive care syndrome: Right care, Right Now...and later. Crit Care Med 2016;44:381–5.

28. Griffiths J, Hatch RA, Bishop J, et al. An exploration of social and economic outcome and associated health-related quality of life after critical illness in general intensive care unit survivors: a 12-month follow-up study. Crit Care 2013;17: R100.

29. Ohtake PJ, Lee AC, Scott JC, et al. Physical impairments associated with post-intensive care syndrome: systematic review based on the World health Organization's international Classification of functioning, disability and health framework. Phys Ther 2018;98:631–45.

30. Le Maguet P, Roquilly A, Lasocki S, et al. Prevalence and impact of frailty on mortality in elderly ICU patients: a prospective, multicenter, observational study. Intensive Care Med 2014;40:674–82.

31. Latronico N, Bolton CF. Critical illness polyneuropathy and myopathy: a major cause of muscle weakness and paralysis. Lancet Neurol 2011;10:931–41.

32. Stanojcic M, Finnerty CC, Jeschke MG. Anabolic and anticatabolic agents in critical care. Curr Opin Crit Care 2016;22:325–31.

33. Fan E, Dowdy DW, Colantuoni E, et al. Physical complications in acute lung injury survivors: a two-year longitudinal prospective study. Crit Care Med 2014;42:849–59.

34. Stevens RD, Marshall SA, Cornblath DR, et al. A framework for diagnosing and classifying intensive care unit-acquired weakness. Crit Care Med 2009;37: S299–308.

35. Dinglas VD, Aronson Friedman L, Colantuoni E, et al. Muscle weakness and 5-year survival in acute respiratory distress syndrome survivors. Crit Care Med 2017;45:446–53.
36. Fan E, Cheek F, Chlan L, et al. An official American Thoracic Society Clinical Practice guideline: the diagnosis of intensive care unit-acquired weakness in adults. Am J Respir Crit Care Med 2014;190:1437–46.
37. Bagshaw SM, Stelfox HT, Johnson JA, et al. Long-term association between frailty and health-related quality of life among survivors of critical illness: a prospective multicenter cohort study. Crit Care Med 2015;43:973–82.
38. Baldwin MR, Reid MC, Westlake AA, et al. The feasibility of measuring frailty to predict disability and mortality in older medical intensive care unit survivors. J Crit Care 2014;29:401–8.
39. Schweickert WD, Pohlman MC, Pohlman AS, et al. Early physical and occupational therapy in mechanically ventilated, critically ill patients: a randomised controlled trial. Lancet 2009;373:1874–82.
40. Churpek MM, Gupta S, Spicer AB, et al. Hospital-level Variation in death for critically ill patients with COVID-19. Am J Respir Crit Care Med 2021;204:403–11.
41. Hosey MM, Needham DM. Survivorship after COVID-19 ICU stay. Nat Rev Dis Primers 2020;6:60.
42. Sterne JAC, Murthy S, Diaz JV, et al. Association between Administration of systemic corticosteroids and mortality among critically ill patients with COVID-19: a meta-analysis. Jama 2020;324:1330–41.
43. Moss M, Huang DT, Brower RG, et al. Early neuromuscular blockade in the acute respiratory distress syndrome. N Engl J Med 2019;380:1997–2008.
44. Hatch R, Young D, Barber V, et al. Anxiety, depression and post traumatic stress disorder after critical illness: a UK-wide prospective cohort study. Crit Care 2018;22:310.
45. Myhren H, Ekeberg O, Toien K, et al. Posttraumatic stress, anxiety and depression symptoms in patients during the first year post intensive care unit discharge. Crit Care 2010;14:R14.
46. Fernando SM, Qureshi D, Sood MM, et al. Suicide and self-harm in adult survivors of critical illness: population based cohort study. BMJ 2021;373:n973.
47. Zante B, Camenisch SA, Schefold JC. Interventions in post-intensive care syndrome-family: a systematic literature review. Crit Care Med 2020;48:e835–40.
48. Gries CJ, Engelberg RA, Kross EK, et al. Predictors of symptoms of posttraumatic stress and depression in family members after patient death in the ICU. Chest 2010;137:280–7.
49. Needham DM, Feldman DR, Kho ME. The functional costs of ICU survivorship. Collaborating to improve post-ICU disability. Am J Respir Crit Care Med 2011;183:962–4.
50. Dowdy DW, Eid MP, Dennison CR, et al. Quality of life after acute respiratory distress syndrome: a meta-analysis. Intensive Care Med 2006;32:1115–24.
51. Mazza MG, De Lorenzo R, Conte C, et al. Anxiety and depression in COVID-19 survivors: role of inflammatory and clinical predictors. Brain Behav Immun 2020;89:594–600.
52. Bienvenu OJ, Colantuoni E, Mendez-Tellez PA, et al. Depressive symptoms and impaired physical function after acute lung injury: a 2-year longitudinal study. Am J Respir Crit Care Med 2012;185:517–24.

53. Davydow DS, Gifford JM, Desai SV, et al. Posttraumatic stress disorder in general intensive care unit survivors: a systematic review. Gen Hosp Psychiatry 2008;30:421–34.
54. Mikkelsen ME, Christie JD, Lanken PN, et al. The adult respiratory distress syndrome cognitive outcomes study: long-term neuropsychological function in survivors of acute lung injury. Am J Respir Crit Care Med 2012;185:1307–15.
55. Ely EW, Gautam S, Margolin R, et al. The impact of delirium in the intensive care unit on hospital length of stay. Intensive Care Med 2001;27:1892–900.
56. Duggan MC, Wang L, Wilson JE, et al. The relationship between executive dysfunction, depression, and mental health-related quality of life in survivors of critical illness: results from the BRAIN-ICU investigation. J Crit Care 2017; 37:72–9.
57. Ely EW, Shintani A, Truman B, et al. Delirium as a predictor of mortality in mechanically ventilated patients in the intensive care unit. JAMA 2004;291: 1753–62.
58. Vasilevskis EE, Ely EW, Speroff T, et al. Reducing iatrogenic risks: ICU-acquired delirium and weakness–crossing the quality chasm. Chest 2010;138:1224–33.
59. Balas MC, Vasilevskis EE, Olsen KM, et al. Effectiveness and safety of the awakening and breathing coordination, delirium monitoring/management, and early exercise/mobility bundle. Crit Care Med 2014;42:1024–36.
60. Hsieh SJ, Otusanya O, Gershengorn HB, et al. Staged implementation of awakening and breathing, coordination, delirium monitoring and management, and early mobilization bundle improves patient outcomes and reduces hospital costs. Crit Care Med 2019;47:885–93.
61. Wunsch H, Guerra C, Barnato AE, et al. Three-year outcomes for Medicare beneficiaries who survive intensive care. JAMA 2010;303:849–56.
62. Brinkman S, de Jonge E, Abu-Hanna A, et al. Mortality after hospital discharge in ICU patients. Crit Care Med 2013;41:1229–36.
63. Lone NI, Gillies MA, Haddow C, et al. Five-year mortality and hospital costs associated with surviving intensive care. Am J Respir Crit Care Med 2016; 194:198–208.
64. Wang CY, Calfee CS, Paul DW, et al. One-year mortality and predictors of death among hospital survivors of acute respiratory distress syndrome. Intensive Care Med 2014;40:388–96.
65. Fernando SM, Qureshi D, Tanuseputro P, et al. Mortality and costs following extracorporeal membrane oxygenation in critically ill adults: a population-based cohort study. Intensive Care Med 2019;45:1580–9.
66. Hirshberg EL, Wilson EL, Stanfield V, et al. Impact of critical illness on Resource utilization: a Comparison of Use in the Year before and after ICU admission. Crit Care Med 2019;47:1497–504.
67. Herridge MS, Cheung AM, Tansey CM, et al. One-year outcomes in survivors of the acute respiratory distress syndrome. New Engl J Med 2003;348:683–93.
68. Cuthbertson BH, Roughton S, Jenkinson D, et al. Quality of life in the five years after intensive care: a cohort study. Crit Care 2010;14:R6.
69. Jackson JC, Pandharipande PP, Girard TD, et al. Depression, post-traumatic stress disorder, and functional disability in survivors of critical illness in the BRAIN-ICU study: a longitudinal cohort study. Lancet Respir Med 2014;2: 369–79.
70. Pfoh ER, Wozniak AW, Colantuoni E, et al. Physical declines occurring after hospital discharge in ARDS survivors: a 5-year longitudinal study. Intensive Care Med 2016;42:1557–66.

71. Gerth AMJ, Hatch RA, Young JD, et al. Changes in health-related quality of life after discharge from an intensive care unit: a systematic review. Anaesthesia 2019;74:100–8.
72. Hofhuis JGM, Schrijvers AJP, Schermer T, et al. Health-related quality of life in ICU survivors—10 years later. Scientific Rep 2021;11.
73. Oeyen SG, Vandijck DM, Benoit DD, et al. Quality of life after intensive care: a systematic review of the literature. Crit Care Med 2010;38:2386–400.
74. Herridge MS, Tansey CM, Matté A, et al. Functional disability 5 Years after acute respiratory distress syndrome. New Engl J Med 2011;364:1293–304.
75. Vermeiren S, Vella-Azzopardi R, Beckwee D, et al. Frailty and the prediction of negative health outcomes: a meta-analysis. J Am Med Dir Assoc 2016;17:1163 e1–e17.
76. Brummel NE, Girard TD, Pandharipande PP, et al. Prevalence and course of frailty in survivors of critical illness. Crit Care Med 2020;48:1419–26.
77. Donnelly JP, Wang XQ, Iwashyna TJ, et al. Readmission and death after initial hospital discharge among patients with COVID-19 in a large Multihospital system. Jama 2021;325:304–6.
78. Al-Aly Z, Xie Y, Bowe B. High-dimensional characterization of post-acute sequelae of COVID-19. Nature 2021;594:259–64.
79. Garrigues E, Janvier P, Kherabi Y, et al. Post-discharge persistent symptoms and health-related quality of life after hospitalization for COVID-19. J Infect 2020;81:e4–6.
80. Riou J, Panczak R, Althaus CL, et al. Socioeconomic position and the COVID-19 care cascade from testing to mortality in Switzerland: a population-based analysis. Lancet Public Health 2021;6:e683–91.
81. Karmakar M, Lantz PM, Tipirneni R. Association of social and Demographic factors with COVID-19 incidence and death rates in the US. JAMA Netw Open 2021;4:e2036462.
82. Jones JRA, Berney S, Connolly B, et al. Socioeconomic position and health outcomes following critical illness. Crit Care Med 2019;47:e512–21.
83. Bastian K, Hollinger A, Mebazaa A, et al. Association of social deprivation with 1-year outcome of ICU survivors: results from the FROG-ICU study. Intensive Care Med 2018;44:2025–37.
84. Mcpeake J, Mikkelsen ME, Quasim T, et al. Return to employment after critical illness and its association with Psychosocial outcomes. A systematic review and meta-analysis. Ann Am Thorac Soc 2019;16:1304–11.
85. Kamdar BB, Suri R, Suchyta MR, et al. Return to work after critical illness: a systematic review and meta-analysis. Thorax 2020;75:17–27.
86. Kamdar BB, Huang M, Dinglas VD, et al. Joblessness and Lost Earnings after acute respiratory distress syndrome in a 1-year National multicenter study. Am J Respir Crit Care Med 2017;196:1012–20.
87. Hauschildt KE, Seigworth C, Kamphuis LA, et al. Financial toxicity after acute respiratory distress syndrome: a National Qualitative cohort study. Crit Care Med 2020;48:1103–10.
88. Iwashyna TJ, Kamphuis LA, Gundel SJ, et al. Continuing Cardiopulmonary symptoms, disability, and financial toxicity 1 Month after hospitalization for third-Wave COVID-19: early results from a US Nationwide cohort. J Hosp Med 2021;16.
89. Griffiths J, Hatch RA, Bishop J, et al. An exploration of social and economic outcome and associated health-related quality of life after critical illness in

general intensive care unit survivors: a 12-month follow-up study. Crit Care 2013;17:R100.

90. Johnson CC, Suchyta MR, Darowski ES, et al. Psychological sequelae in family caregivers of critically Ill intensive care Unit patients. A systematic review. Ann Am Thorac Soc 2019;16:894–909.

91. Parker AM, Brigham E, Connolly B, et al. Addressing the post-acute sequelae of SARS-CoV-2 infection: a multidisciplinary model of care. Lancet Respir Med 2021;9(11):1328–41.

92. Sevin CM, Jackson JC. Post-ICU clinics should Be staffed by ICU clinicians. Crit Care Med 2019;47:268–72.

93. Connolly B, Douiri A, Steier J, et al. A UK survey of rehabilitation following critical illness: implementation of NICE Clinical Guidance 83 (CG83) following hospital discharge. BMJ Open 2014;4:e004963.

94. Mikkelsen ME, Still M, Anderson BJ, et al. Society of critical care Medicine's international consensus conference on prediction and Identification of long-term impairments after critical illness. Crit Care Med 2020;48:1670–9.

95. Eaton TL, McPeake J, Rogan J, et al. Caring for survivors of critical illness: current practices and the role of the nurse in intensive care Unit Aftercare. Am J Crit Care 2019;28:481–5.

96. Bloom SL, Stollings JL, Kirkpatrick O, et al. Randomized clinical trial of an ICU recovery Pilot program for survivors of critical illness. Crit Care Med 2019;47: 1337–45.

97. Meyer J, Brett SJ, Waldmann C. Should ICU clinicians follow patients after ICU discharge? Yes. Intensive Care Med United States 2018;44:1539–41.

98. Vijayaraghavan BKT, Willaert X, Cuthbertson BH. Should ICU clinicians follow patients after ICU discharge? No. Intensive Care Med United States:1542-1544.

99. Haines KJ, Sevin CM, Hibbert E, et al. Key mechanisms by which post-ICU activities can improve in-ICU care: results of the international THRIVE collaboratives. Intensive Care Med 2019;45:939–47.

100. Jarvie L, Robinson C, MacTavish P, et al. Understanding the patient journey: a mechanism to reduce staff burnout? Br J Nurs 2019;28:396–7.

101. Needham DM, Sepulveda KA, Dinglas VD, et al. Core outcome measures for clinical research in acute respiratory failure survivors. An international modified Delphi consensus study. Am J Respir Crit Care Med 2017;196:1122–30.

102. Santhosh L, Block B, Kim SY, et al. Rapid Design and implementation of post-COVID-19 clinics. Chest 2021;160:671–7.

103. Jalilian L, Cannesson M, Kamdar N. Post-ICU recovery clinics in the Era of Digital health and Telehealth. Crit Care Med 2019;e796–7.

104. Cicerone KD, Goldin Y, Ganci K, et al. Evidence-based cognitive rehabilitation: systematic review of the literature from 2009 through 2014. Arch Phys Med Rehabil 2019;100:1515–33.

105. Muradov O, Petrovskaya O, Papathanassoglou E. Effectiveness of cognitive interventions on cognitive outcomes of adult intensive care unit survivors: a scoping review. Aust Crit Care 2021;34:473–85.

106. Petersen RC, Lopez O, Armstrong MJ, et al. Practice guideline update summary: mild cognitive impairment: report of the guideline Development, Dissemination, and implementation Subcommittee of the American Academy of Neurology. Neurology 2018;90:126–35.

107. Mehrholz J, Pohl M, Kugler J, et al. Physical rehabilitation for critical illness myopathy and neuropathy: an abridged version of Cochrane Systematic Review. Eur J Phys Rehabil Med 2015;51:655–61.

108. Cuthbertson BH, Rattray J, Campbell MK, et al. The PRaCTICaL study of nurse led, intensive care follow-up programmes for improving long term outcomes from critical illness: a pragmatic randomised controlled trial. Bmj 2009;339: b3723.

109. Walsh TS, Salisbury LG, Merriweather JL, et al. Increased hospital-based physical rehabilitation and information Provision after intensive care Unit discharge: the RECOVER randomized clinical trial. JAMA Intern Med 2015; 175:901–10.

110. McDowell K, O'Neill B, Blackwood B, et al. Effectiveness of an exercise programme on physical function in patients discharged from hospital following critical illness: a randomised controlled trial (the REVIVE trial). Thorax 2017;72: 594–5.

111. Myall KJ, Mukherjee B, Castanheira AM, et al. Persistent post-COVID-19 interstitial lung disease. An observational study of corticosteroid treatment. Ann Am Thorac Soc 2021;18:799–806.

112. Nath A. Long-haul COVID. Neurology 2020;559–60.

113. George PM, Barratt SL, Condliffe R, et al. Respiratory follow-up of patients with COVID-19 pneumonia. Thorax 2020;75:1009–16.

114. Han X, Fan Y, Alwalid O, et al. Six-month follow-up chest CT findings after severe COVID-19 pneumonia. Radiology 2021;299. E177-e86.

115. van den Borst B, Peters JB, Brink M, et al. Comprehensive health assessment 3 Months after recovery from acute Coronavirus disease 2019 (COVID-19). Clin Infect Dis 2021;73:e1089–98.

116. Hsieh MJ, Lee WC, Cho HY, et al. Recovery of pulmonary functions, exercise capacity, and quality of life after pulmonary rehabilitation in survivors of ARDS due to severe influenza A (H1N1) pneumonitis. Influenza Other Respir Viruses 2018; 12:643–8.

117. Kupfer DJ, Frank E, Phillips ML. Major depressive disorder: new clinical, neurobiological, and treatment perspectives. Lancet 2012;379:1045–55.

118. Cuijpers P, Dekker J, Hollon SD, et al. Adding psychotherapy to pharmacotherapy in the treatment of depressive disorders in adults: a meta-analysis. J Clin Psychiatry 2009;70:1219–29.

119. Cuijpers P, van Straten A, Warmerdam L, et al. Psychotherapy versus the combination of psychotherapy and pharmacotherapy in the treatment of depression: a meta-analysis. Depress Anxiety 2009;26:279–88.

120. Hoge EA, Bui E, Marques L, et al. Randomized controlled trial of mindfulness meditation for generalized anxiety disorder: effects on anxiety and stress reactivity. J Clin Psychiatry 2013;74:786–92.

121. Summary of the clinical practice guideline for the treatment of posttraumatic stress disorder (PTSD) in adults. Am Psychol 2019;74:596–607.

122. McPeake J, Iwashyna TJ, Boehm LM, et al. Benefits of peer support for intensive care Unit survivors: Sharing experiences, care Debriefing, and Altruism. Am J Crit Care 2021;30:145–9.

123. Lassen-Greene CL, Nordness M, Kiehl A, et al. Peer support group for intensive care Unit survivors: Perceptions on supportive recovery in the Era of social distancing. Ann Am Thorac Soc 2021;18:177–82.

124. Tansey CM, Louie M, Loeb M, et al. One-year outcomes and health care utilization in survivors of severe acute respiratory syndrome. Arch Intern Med 2007; 167:1312–20.

125. McPeake J, Boehm LM, Hibbert E, et al. Key components of ICU recovery programs: what Did patients report provided benefit? Crit Care Explorations 2020; 2:e0088.
126. Haines KJ, Sevin CM, Hibbert E, et al. Key mechanisms by which post-ICU activities can improve in-ICU care: results of the international THRIVE collaboratives. Intensive Care Med 2019;45:939–47.
127. Wilcox ME, Ely EW. Challenges in conducting long-term outcomes studies in critical care. Curr Opin Crit Care 2019;25:473–88.

COVID-19 and Acute Kidney Injury

James Hilton, MBBS, MRCP[a,b], Naomi Boyer, BSc, MBBS[a,b], Mitra K. Nadim, MD, FASN[c], Lui G. Forni, BSc, PhD, MBBS, MRCPI, AFICM, JFCMI[a,b,d,*], John A. Kellum, MD, MCCM[e]

KEYWORDS

- Acute kidney injury • Renal replacement therapy • Blood purification techniques
- COVID-19 • Cytokines

KEY POINTS

- AKI is common in patients with COVID-19.
- Increasing age, diabetes, hypertension and CKD are the major risk factors for developing covid-19 associated AKI.
- No specific therapies are available for treatment of AKI associated with COVID-19 and therefore practitioners should follow accepted local management guidelines.
- The use of blood purification techniques should be adopted with caution although preliminary data shows promise.
- The consequences of COVID-19 associated AKI in the longer term are as yet unknown

INTRODUCTION

In December 2019, a novel severe acute respiratory syndrome coronavirus 2 (SARS-CoV-2) was discovered in Wuhan, China, the rapid spread of which culminated in a global pandemic and critical pressure on health care resources.[1,2] The presentation of COVID-19 varies considerably from asymptomatic individuals and those presenting with mild respiratory symptoms to the more severe spectrum of disease requiring hospitalization. In more severe cases, the development of multi-organ failure may ensue. Overall, mortality from COVID-19 infection is approximately 1% population-wide but may reach 50% or more in those requiring intensive care.[3,4]

[a] Department of Critical Care, Royal Surrey Hospital, Egerton Road, Guildford, Surrey GU2 7XX, UK; [b] SPACeR Group (Surrey Peri-Operative, Anaesthesia & Critical Care Collaborative Research Group), Royal Surrey Hospital, Egerton Road, Guildford, Surrey GU2 7XX, UK; [c] Division of Nephrology and Hypertension, Department of Medicine, Keck School of Medicine, University of Southern California, 1520 San Pablo Street, Suite 4300, Los Angeles, CA 90033, USA; [d] Department of Clinical & Experimental Medicine, Faculty of Health Sciences, University of Surrey, Stag Hill, Guildford GU2 7XH, UK; [e] Center for Critical Care Nephrology, University of Pittsburgh, 3347 Forbes Avenue #220, Pittsburgh, PA 15213, USA
* Corresponding author. Department of Critical Care, Royal Surrey Hospital, Egerton Road, Guildford, Surrey GU2 7XX, UK.
E-mail address: luiforni@nhs.net

Crit Care Clin 38 (2022) 473–489
https://doi.org/10.1016/j.ccc.2022.01.002
0749-0704/22/© 2022 Elsevier Inc. All rights reserved.
criticalcare.theclinics.com

EPIDEMIOLOGY OF COVID-19-ASSOCIATED ACUTE KIDNEY INJURY

Initial reports suggested that acute kidney injury (AKI) as defined by the Kidney Disease Improving Global Outcomes (KDIGO) criteria was uncommon following acute COVID-19 infection.[5,6] However, subsequent data from the US and Europe did not support this finding particularly in the critically ill whereby AKI rates in excess of 40% were reported.[7,8] The incidence of C19-AKI continues to demonstrate regional variability among patients hospitalized for COVID-19. For example, a recent international meta-analysis including 49,048 patients found 28.6% of hospitalized individuals with COVID-19 were diagnosed with AKI in Europe and the USA, compared with only 5.5% of inpatients in China.[9] Similar results have been shown by others,[10] with data from the UK demonstrating C19-AKI rates in intensive care patients of greater than 45% in the period February to July 2020.[11] This disparity, may, in part, be explained by the difference in thresholds dictating hospital admission, for example, in China admission of any suspected COVID-19 infection was mandatory, whereas this was not the case in Europe and the USA.[9]

What is clear is that the development of AKI is a poor prognostic factor for individuals with COVID-19 infection with a risk ratio (RR) of 4.6 for mortality when compared with patients with COVID-19 but without AKI.[9] Cheng and colleagues were able to demonstrate that age over 65, male sex and severe COVID-19 infection were independent risk factors for in-hospital mortality. After adjusting for these, they found a significant increase in mortality with worsening AKI stage, dipstick proteinuria above 1+, and the presence of hematuria.[12]

RISK FACTORS FOR COVID-19-ASSOCIATED ACUTE KIDNEY INJURY

Boxes 1 and **2** outline the main risk factors for the development of AKI in patients with COVID-19 infection. Unsurprisingly, there is considerable overlap with factors known to contribute to the development of AKI in patients without COVID-19 infection.[13] A recent retrospective study from a New York City health system demonstrated a higher incidence of AKI among patients with COVID-19 infection compared with a historical cohort (56.9% vs 25.1%).[14] Factors independently associated with the development of stage 2 or 3 C19-AKI included older age, black race, male sex, diabetes mellitus, nursing home resident, and initial respiratory rate. The median time to development of AKI was 6.5 days in one study in a cohort suffering from severe COVID-19 pneumonitis.[15] Given this delay, predicting those at risk of C19-AKI may influence management and several studies have identified potential candidates for developing C19-AKI including higher levels of α_1-microglobulin excretion.[16]

Box 1
Risk factors for the development of C19-AKI

- Patient factors
  - Obesity[15]
  - Increasing age[15,122,123]
  - Renal transplant recipient[10]
  - Chronic kidney disease[124]

- Disease factors
  - Invasive mechanical ventilation[15,124]
  - Severe COVID-19[122,123]
  - Nephrotoxic drugs exposure[123]
  - Vasopressor requirement[124]

Box 2
Causes of renal impairment in COVID-19 infection

- Hypotension/hypovolemia
- Vascular
  - Macrovascular thrombosis
  - Microthrombi
  - Endothelialitis
  - Thrombotic microangiopathies (atypical hemolytic uremic syndrome, thrombotic thrombocytopenic purpura)
- Acute tubular necrosis
- Viral infection of renal parenchyma
- Collapsing glomerulopathy
- Glomerulonephritis
- Drug-induced acute interstitial nephritis
- Drug-induced acute tubular necrosis

PATHOPHYSIOLOGY

Given that AKI, rather than being a distinct phenotype, is often multifactorial in nature, C19-AKI may also be due to a variety of concomitant factors with a number of potential pathophysiological processes implicated. These include direct kidney injury as well as indirect mechanisms leading to C19-AKI (**Fig. 1**).[17,18]

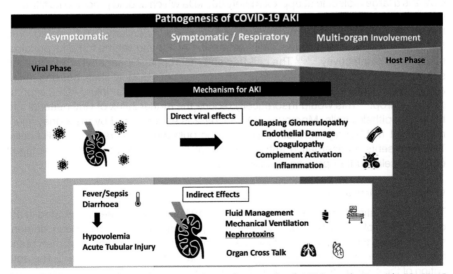

Fig. 1. Pathogenesis of COVID-19 AKI. The pathogenesis of AKI in patients with COVID-19 (COVID-19 AKI) is likely multifactorial, involving both the direct effects of the SARS-CoV-2 virus on the kidney and the indirect mechanisms resulting from systemic consequences of viral infection or effects of the virus on distant organs including the lung, in addition to mechanisms relating to the management of COVID-19. (*From* Acute Disease Quality Initiative 25, www.ADQI.org, CC BY 2.0 (https://creativecommons.org/licenses/by/2.0/).)

Tubular and Glomerular Damage

Acute tubular injury is the most frequent finding on autopsy studies reported in C19-AKI although the findings are often mild despite significant serum creatinine elevation with often evidence of preexisting comorbidities such as hypertensive nephrosclerosis associated with kidney disease.[19,20] In keeping with these findings, proteinuria when demonstrated in C19-AKI has a low molecular weight, pointing to a tubular rather than glomerular injury pattern.[21] In a multicentre study from France including 47 patients who underwent kidney biopsy in those who had severe AKI, the histopathological pattern was almost exclusively tubular injury, whereas none in their comparator group outside the ICU had evidence of acute tubular injury. Interestingly, in those outside the ICU with proteinuria and/or AKI glomerular collapsing glomerulosclerosis characterized by the segmental collapse of the glomerular tuft, parietal cell hypertrophy, or obliteration of the capillary loop or podocyte, was observed. This phenotype has also been described elsewhere predominantly in individuals with high-risk APOL1 genotypes.[22] The APOL1 gene encodes apolipoprotein-1 (apol1), part of high-density lipoprotein complex and genetic variants are common in the peoples of western Africa and carriers of APOL1 variants are at higher risk of chronic kidney disease (CKD) including a 17 times higher risk of developing focal segmental glomerulosclerosis.[23,24]

Viral Tropism in the Kidney

Evidence for direct renal tropism by COVID-19 is controversial. Although a few studies have been able to demonstrate evidence of the presence of viral particles in renal tissue many have not.[25–27] Furthermore, the timing of renal biopsies and autopsy studies are often days to weeks after the onset of the associated AKI, putatively beyond the infectious period of SARS-CoV-2. However, the trimeric spike protein of SARS-CoV-2 is a large molecule at approximately 600 kDa which should preclude its filtration in the healthy glomerulus suggesting the infection of the renal tubular cells, the urothelium or filtration occurring through damaged glomeruli.[28] Similarly to the related virus SARS-CoV, SARS-CoV-2 enters cells expressing ACE2 and seems to be its principal mechanism of infectivity.[29,30] The cell-free and macrophage-phagocytosed virus can spread to other organs and infect ACE2-expressing cells at local sites, causing multiorgan injury.[31] Interestingly, in murine models of ischemic tubular injury ACE2 expression may drop.[32] This would theoretically reduce the further influx of viral material into the renal epithelial cells. Moreover, SARS-CoV-2 is endocytosed by the kidney injury molecule-1 (KIM-1) glycoprotein expressed on pulmonary and renal epithelial cells. This represents an alternative entry mechanism for the virus into already damaged epithelial cells, further prolonging infectivity.[33]

Complement Activation

The immune/inflammatory response to COVID-19 infection has been implicated in the development of C19-AKI. For example, complement activation has been demonstrated within the kidney with evidence of complement deposition and membrane attack complex in nephron vessels and the tubular basement membrane.[34] The activation of the complement cascade has previously been shown to lead to chronic renal inflammation and subsequent tubulointerstitial fibrosis.[35] This has led to studies administering the complement C5a inhibitor eculizumab in patients with COVID-19.[36] Although preliminary results show promise, these are proof of concept studies with insufficient numbers to demonstrate any significant effects on C19-AKI or the need for RRT.

Cytokine Activation

The inflammatory response to COVID-19 infection has been described as a "cytokine storm" contributing to organ dysfunction. Although poorly defined, cytokine storm syndrome (macrophage activation syndrome) is a life-threatening inflammatory response involving high levels of circulating cytokines and immune cell hyperactivation triggered by multiple mechanisms including sepsis. The proinflammatory cytokines interleukin (IL)-1, IL-6, and tumor necrosis factor-alpha (TNFα) are 3 of the most important cytokines of the innate immune system and are implicated in the development of a cytokine storm. Although in COVID-19 elevated levels of monocytes and macrophages have been demonstrated, particularly in the lungs, and are thought to account for the high levels of IL-1, IL-6, and TNFα observed in some individuals other data suggest that levels of circulating cytokines are often lower in patients with COVID-19 than in patients with acute respiratory distress syndrome (ARDS) due to causes other than COVID-19.[37–39] Nevertheless, monoclonal antibodies against IL-6 have been trialed in patients with the RECOVERY trial demonstrating that the anti-IL-6 monoclonal antibody tocilizumab had a positive effect in moderate COVID-19 pneumonitis, contradicting the results of a smaller multicentre Italian study which found no benefit.[40,41] However, in the critically ill, the data are more contentious. The REMAP-CAP trial demonstrated a reduction in the duration of cardiorespiratory support in an intensive care population when administering tocilizumab or sarilumab, another anti-IL-6 monoclonal antibody.[42] The excess cytokine production resulting in ARDS maybe associated with disease severity in COVID-19; however, its role in the contribution toward kidney damage is vague. IL-6 has been implicated in the development of AKI given that elevated IL-6 levels may induce renal endothelium cells to secrete other proinflammatory cytokines and chemokines contributing to microvascular dysfunction.[43] Moreover, in patients with a greater than 100-fold increase in IL-6 levels increased rates of AKI have been observed although this is not a consistent finding.[44,45]

COVID-19-Associated Coagulopathy

The extrapulmonary clinical manifestations of COVID-19-infection are likely to be related to associate widespread vascular pathology given prominent pulmonary as well as systemic endotheliitis represents a distinguishable and distinct feature of COVID-19 infection.[46] The prothrombotic nature of COVID-19-associated sepsis has been well described.[47] Platelet-rich thrombi have been observed in the microvasculature of the heart, brain, kidney, and liver and renal infarction secondary to arterial thrombi have also been described.[48,49] Although prophylactic anticoagulation with low-molecular-weight subcutaneous heparin or enoxaparin (a low-molecular-weight heparin) was shown to provide a mortality benefit in inpatients with COVID-19 from the US Veterans database this finding was confirmed only in moderate COVID-19 pneumonitis, failing to show benefit in the critical care population.[50,51] Furthermore, no effect on AKI rates was observed. Thrombotic microangiopathy characterized by thrombocytopenia and microthrombi which may lead to ischemic tissue injury has been observed both in the pulmonary vasculature and kidneys of patients with severe COVID-19.[52–54] In addition, significant alterations of the von Willebrand factor (VWF)-ADAMTS13 axis in patients with COVID-19 have been observed with an elevated VWF:Ag to ADAMTS13 activity ratio being strongly associated with disease severity. Such an imbalance enhances the hypercoagulable state of patients with COVID-19 and their risk of microthrombosis.[55]

Indirect Kidney Injury

Indirect mechanisms include damage from the therapeutic interventions to manage critical illness as well as the systemic effects of COVID-19 infection (see **Fig. 1**).

Insensible losses leading to hypovolemia and kidney injury, through an increased work of breathing, pyrexia, and gastrointestinal manifestations of infection may be significant in individuals with COVID-19. Moreover, hemodynamic instability and fluid restrictive strategies in patients with ARDS may further exacerbate kidney injury. The relationship between the underlying pulmonary pathology and the kidney may also exacerbate C19-AKI. The consequence of respiratory failure and subsequent hypoxemia on the kidney are well documented with increased renovascular resistance, exacerbated by hypercapnia, leading to a reduction in glomerular filtration rate (GFR).[56] Furthermore, increases in pulmonary artery and intrathoracic pressure may lead to right ventricular dysfunction and renal venous congestion, effects exacerbated by the use of mechanical ventilation and the application of positive end-expiratory pressure (PEEP).[57,58] This effect may be exaggerated in severe COVID-19, whereby high PEEP levels and high peak and plateau pressures are often required to achieve adequate oxygenation in the context of COVID-19 ARDS.[59] Administration of nephrotoxic medications, such as antibiotics, may also contribute to the development of AKI in patients already at high risk.

ASSESSMENT AND INVESTIGATION OF ACUTE KIDNEY INJURY

Initial assessment of any patient with COVID-19 infection should include a full medical history focusing on those comorbidities and patient factors identified as being associated with higher risk for AKI development.[13,46,60] Clinical examination should include the evaluation of volume status and whereby appropriate, hemodynamic assessment. AKI in COVID-19 is defined and classified by the KDIGO criteria-based serum creatinine and urine output changes.[5] Urinalysis is mandatory as it may help to differentiate various causes of AKI and give an indication of potential glomerular involvement, even whereby alterations in kidney function as defined by KDIGO criteria are absent. This has been observed in one study whereby urinalysis was positive for proteinuria in 65.8% and hematuria in 41.7%, while only 4.7% of the patients met KDIGO criteria for AKI.[61]

Biomarkers of Acute Kidney Injury

Novel biomarkers of AKI in the evaluation of C19-AKI have been evaluated in several studies. Neutrophil gelatinase-associated lipocalin (NGAL) is produced in the distal nephron and its synthesis is upregulated in response to kidney injury and may predict the need for RRT requirement and in-hospital mortality.[62,63] A small observational trial of 17 patients with COVID-19-positive admitted to a Japanese ICU showed that elevated urinary NGAL on admission to the ICU was associated with the development of AKI during their stay.[64] Of note, patients with elevated urinary NGAL had a longer duration of mechanical ventilation and ICU length of stay which may reflect the effect of AKI; however, increased NGAL levels have also been observed in ventilator-associated lung injury.[65] The type-1 transmembrane glycoprotein KIM-1 is expressed in proximal tubular epithelial cells and has been shown to be associated with AKI development.[66] A recent study has shown that KIM-1 was significantly elevated in patients with COVID-19 with, compared with those without AKI ($P = .005$) and was significantly elevated in the patients with COVID-19 that had to be transferred to the ICU.[67] The use of other biomarkers such as tissue inhibitor of metaloproteinases-2 (TIMP-2) and insulin-like growth factor binding protein-7 (IGFBP-7) has also been proposed in assessing patients with COVID-19 and a recent study demonstrated that the use of this biomarker combination may identify patients with AKI and infection early.[68,69] Also, increased requirement for RRT in individuals with C19-AKI and high levels of [TIMP-2]x[IGFBP-7], has been observed. While a further study in a cohort of 352 patients found admission soluble urokinase plasminogen activator receptor (suPAR) levels to be predictive of in-hospital AKI and the requirement for RRT.[16,70]

MANAGEMENT OF C19-ACUTE KIDNEY INJURY

As the syndrome of C19-AKI has multiple etiologies, no generalized single management plan can be proposed for use in all cases and there is no evidence that the treatment of C-19 AKI should be managed differently to other causes of AKI in hospitalized patients.[13] Patients admitted with COVID-19 are often intravascularly deplete and fluid resuscitation until euvolemic with vasopressor support whereby required, should be administered according to usual best practice and individualized whereby possible. This is in keeping with recent evidence showing that targeted resuscitation through dynamic hemodynamic assessment reduces the risk of both AKI and respiratory failure.[71] Fluid choice for initial resuscitation should be crystalloid, preferably balanced in those who are critically ill. It has been shown that a composite outcome of death, new RRT, or persistent kidney dysfunction among critically ill patients was reduced with the administration of balanced crystalloids over 0.9% saline. Similar findings in noncritically ill patients were also generated.[72,73] Although subsequent meta-analysis failed to demonstrate a definite benefit for balanced crystalloids over 0.9% saline, other indications, such as hypochloremia or hypernatremia may guide the clinician toward using balanced solutions.[74] Although recent data from a randomized trial on over 11,000 patients in Brazil did not demonstrate a difference in mortality between saline and balanced solutions these data are not directly transferable to severely ill patients with COVID-19 with AKI.[75] These data were from patients with lower acuity (median APACHE II score 12 and SOFA 4) and 40% of the patients were not hypotensive. Median volumes of trial fluid administered were low (mean < 1 L/d) and 68% of all patients received fluid before randomization with significant crossover. Furthermore, following randomization, approximately 30% of the total fluid received by day 3 was nonstudy crystalloid. General management should follow the KDIGO guidelines and include glucose monitoring and control, relevant given the potential association between diabetes, insulin resistance, and COVID-19 infection.[76] Preferably pharmacy lead medication review should be undertaken and pharmacokinetics and drug clearance should be considered as a dose adjustment may be required in AKI for both COVID-19 specific acute therapies as well as other medications. General guidance for nutritional assessment and support in critically ill patients with AKI should be followed especially as COVID-19 infection which is associated with an inflammatory hypercatabolic state, reduced oral intake, and immobilization predisposing to malnutrition and muscle wasting.[77] Where mechanical ventilation is needed lung-protective low tidal volume ventilation strategies as per general ARDS management should be followed.[78–80] Prone ventilation has been reported as beneficial in patients with COVID-19 pneumonitis, and at present no evidence suggests that any effect on intraabdominal pressure and renal blood flow impact on the risk of AKI.[81–83]

COVID-19-SPECIFIC THERAPIES

Several therapeutic agents have emerged as potentially beneficial in COVID-19 infection. Remdesivir, an inhibitor of the viral RNA-dependent RNA polymerase was studied in the Adaptive COVID-19 Treatment Trial (ACTT-1) and demonstrated that compared with placebo, remdesivir shortened the time to recovery although no significant mortality benefit was seen.[84] Of note, however, patients with AKI or CKD were excluded and as such, the clinical effect of remdesivir in C19-AKI remains largely unknown. The RECOVERY trial examined the use of the glucocorticoid dexamethasone at a dose of 6 mg/d for up to 10 days. The use of dexamethasone reduced the mortality of hospitalized patients receiving invasive mechanical ventilation or oxygen therapy at the time of randomization with further evidence supporting this approach from meta-analysis of systemic cortico-steroids in COVID-19.[85,86] The RECOVERY trial also demonstrated a reduced need for RRT in patients not requiring RRT at the time of randomization, with a risk ratio of 0.61 (95% CI 0.48–0.76). More recently a small pilot study from France has also shown a reduction in AKI in COVID-19 infection.[87]

As outlined, there may be significant systemic inflammation complicating COVID-19 infection. This has led to the use of immunomodulatory therapies such as Tocilizumab, an anti-IL-6 receptor monoclonal antibody. The use of Tocilizumab improved survival in critically ill patients receiving organ support in intensive care with an observed reduction in the need for RRT, while the RECOVERY trial demonstrated a reduced 28-day mortal-ity, probability of discharge at 28 days and reduced progression to the composite outcome of mechanical ventilation and death in those not already ventilated in hospital-ized patients with hypoxia and systemic inflammation (defined as CRP $\geq$ 75 mg/L).[40,42] Although other therapies have been considered for COVID-19 at the time of writing there is insufficient evidence of clinical efficacy in the management ofC19-AKI.

RENAL REPLACEMENT THERAPY

The indications for RRT in C19-AKI do not differ from AKI complicating other conditions and should consider both patient and disease factors. However, resource limitations in the setting of the pandemic may require further consideration of potential for benefit at the individual patient level.[13] Vascular access should be through the internal jugular and femoral sites with ultrasound directed placement as this increases success rate and re-duces complications.[5,13,88,89] Internal jugular access may be associated with lower infection rates compared with femoral in patients with elevated body mass index, but left internal jugular access is associated with higher rates of vascular access dysfunc-tion.[90,91] Internal jugular access may also be preferable in patients whereby prone venti-lation is anticipated.[13] In the absence of an emergent indication, multiple trials have failed to demonstrate any impact on mortality using either early/accelerated versus delayed initiation of RRT, and indeed, premature start may be associated with adverse outcomes.[92,93] However, it must be remembered that the ELAIN trial and more recently, the AKIKI2 trial found that an overly delayed strategy may be associated with harm (ref-erences) This implies that the exact timing of initiation of RRT in COVID-19 should be on a patient by patient basis considering the full clinical context, not just the degree of kid-ney dysfunction as measured by conventional means.[94,95] Use of maximal medical management, whereby safe, including loop diuretics, potassium binders, and sodium bicarbonate should be considered before committing to RRT, especially whereby re-sources may be limited in surge situations. Continuous RRT, prolonged intermittent renal replacement therapy (PIRRT), and intermittent hemodialysis may all be considered depending on local familiarity and resources given there is no evidence for superior out-comes with any one modality of RRT over another. However, continuous RRT may allow more fluid removal and tends to cause less hemodynamic instability, which may be a consideration in critically ill patients with COVID-19.[96] During peak admissions associ-ated with the COVID-19 pandemic, the demand for ICU care and RRT was stretched, and shortages of RRT devices, disposables, and dialysis fluid were described.[97] Ap-proaches to mitigate this included moderating RRT intensity to conserve fluids, running accelerated high clearance RRT or PIRRT to allow machine sharing, in-house prepara-tion of dialysis fluid, and early transition to IHD.[98–100] Peritoneal dialysis (PD) is rarely used in critical care due to concerns regarding unpredictable fluid balance, variable dialysis adequacy, potential peritoneal infection, and compromised ventilation due to diaphragmatic restriction. Also from a practical standpoint, there may be substantial challenges involved in delivering PD to patients who are ventilated in the prone position and intra-abdominal pressure may be increased. Despite these reservations during surge conditions PD was successfully implemented under certain conditions.[101–103]

Anticoagulation is recommended for RRT unless contra-indicated especially given the proinflammatory and prothrombotic nature of COVID-19 infection. This is especially relevant given that reduced RRT circuit life has been widely reported which has implications on the dose delivered as well as increasing the consumption of consumables and potential exposure of staff to infection risk.[13,104,105] Regional citrate anticoagulation has been shown to be superior to systemic heparin for anticoagulation with RRT and although some centers have reported reduced effectiveness of citrate in patients with COVID-19 others have suggested superiority over heparin.[106,107] Choice of anticoagulation regime is likely to be center dependent, but it is important that if issues with filter lifespan are identified a stepwise approach to optimizing anticoagulation is taken, with the consideration of a shift in modality to IHD, PIRRT, or acute peritoneal dialysis if possible if issues persist.

EXTRACORPOREAL BLOOD PURIFICATION

There has been considerable interest in the use of extracorporeal blood purification (EBP) therapies to modify or remove circulating inflammatory mediators with the aim of mitigating organ damage, including AKI.[108] Given the inflammatory profile associated with COVID-19 this provides the rationale for such a treatment, but, as discussed earlier, the degree of cytokine production is generally not as pronounced in COVID-19 infection as in other causes of ARDS or bacterial sepsis which may confound this approach. Despite these reservations, several extracorporeal blood purification filters received emergency use authorization from the US FDA for the treatment of severe COVID-19 pneumonia in patients with respiratory failure not specifically for AKI. To-date, several single-center case series have been produced with variable results. In a time-series analysis of 44 consecutive COVID-19 cases treated with the AN69ST (oXiris) cytokine adsorbing hemodiafilter a decrease in acute phase proteins was demonstrated with a reduction in IL-6 levels and an observed mortality of 36.3% across the cohort.[109] In a further study on 5 patients using the AN69ST filter a reduction in cytokines levels and improvement of hemodynamic status was also observed and similarly in 37 patients in a further single-center study a reduction in expected mortality was also seen (8.3% compared with the expected rate as calculated by APACHE IV).[110,111] Several studies have reported benefits on the use of the hemadsorption filter Cytosorb whereby improvements in catecholamine use as well as decreases in inflammatory markers were seen.[112] A multi-centre study enrolled 61 patients with COVID-19 treated with the Seraph 100 microbind affinity sorbent hemoperfusion filter which contains polyethylene beads coated with immobilized heparin and allows for broad-spectrum pathogen removal.[113] An overall mortality of 37.3% was observed compared with 67.4% in historical controls ($P = .003$). In addition, multivariable logistic regression analysis yielded an odds ratio of 0.27 (95% confidence interval 0.09–0.79, $P = .016$) in favor of the treatment. However, there are important caveats principally that this was a retrospective analysis with differing local criteria for initiating extracorporeal blood purification therapy and hence the potential for significant selection bias.[114] However, not all EBP interventions have demonstrated such positive findings as a recent randomized controlled pilot study examined cytokine adsorption during the first 72 h after the initiation of venovenous ECMO in severe

COVID-19 demonstrates. Of the 34 patients assessed for eligibility, 17 (50%) were treated with cytokine adsorption but cytokine adsorption did not result in reduced interleukin-6 concentrations after 72 h, compared with the control group. One patient in each group died before 72 h. Survival after 30 days was 3 (18%) of 17 with cytokine adsorption and 13 (76%) of 17 without cytokine adsorption ($P = 0.0016$) These findings were in contrast with the hypothesis of a treatment benefit for patients in the cytokine adsorption group although the study was not powered to detect a mortality benefit, the results are of interest.[115,116] These variable results show that although control of inflammation in the critically ill through immunomodulation may hold promise, more data from large, multicentre trials with robust yet pragmatic endpoints are required.

LONG-TERM OUTCOMES

Early observational data suggest that approximately 50% of patients who have had AKI associated with COVID-19 infection had not recovered to baseline by the time of hospital discharge.[61,117] Similarly, emerging data suggest that C19-AKI may be associated with an increased decline in GFR postdischarge than patients who had AKI from other causes.[118] Data from New York showed that in survivors from AKI who required RRT, 30.6% remained dialysis dependent on discharge with a history of CKD being the only independent risk factor for this association (adjusted OR, 9.3 [95% CI, 2.3–37.8]).[119] In another US-based cohort study from 67 hospitals, 1 in 5 patients developed AKI-RRT, 63% of whom died during hospitalization. Among those who survived to discharge, 1 in 3 remained dialysis dependent at discharge, and 1 in 6 remained dialysis dependent 60 days after ICU admission.[120] Similar results were observed in a German study whereby 67% of patients who had required RRT were dialysis free at hospital discharge and encouragingly at a mean follow-up of 151 days over 90% were dialysis independent.[121]

SUMMARY

Despite early reports, AKI complicating COVID-19 infection is common in hospitalized patients. The development of AKI increases the risk of mortality significantly and therefore, efforts should be made to minimize the occurrence of AKI and limit the progression to more severe stages. Treatment should follow accepted practice guidelines for the general management of AKI given the heterogeneous nature of the potential causes of AKI in this group. To-date, no specific therapies have demonstrated a benefit for patients with C19-AKI. Extracorporeal blood therapies show promise but should be adopted with caution and preferably within a clinical trial. Long-term outcomes from C19-AKI may not be as poor as initially suggested although data are still accumulating.

CLINICS CARE POINTS

- COVID-19 associated AKI resembles AKI due to other causes and therefore these should be excluded where possible.
- Although no specific therapies are available for the treatment of AKI associated with COVID-19 practitioners should follow accepted management guidelines for the treatment of AKI.
- Where possible follow up of patients who have sustained severe AKI should occur to minimise longer term sequelae such as CKD.

DISCLOSURE

The authors have nothing to disclose.

REFERENCES

1. Zhu N, Zhang D, Wang W, et al. A novel coronavirus from patients with pneumonia in China, 2019. N Engl J Med 2020;382(8):727–33.
2. Tangcharoensathien V, Bassett MT, Meng Q, et al. Are overwhelmed health systems an inevitable consequence of COVID-19? Experiences from China, Thailand, and New York State. BMJ 2021;372:n83.
3. Wang C, Wang Z, Wang G, et al. COVID-19 in early 2021: current status and looking forward. Signal Transduct Target Ther 2021;6(1):114.
4. Wang D, Hu B, Hu C, et al. Clinical characteristics of 138 hospitalized patients with 2019 novel coronavirus–infected pneumonia in Wuhan, China. JAMA 2020; 323(11):1061–9.
5. Acute Kidney Injury Work G. Kidney disease: improving global outcomes (KDIGO). Kidney Int Suppl 2012;2:1–138.
6. Wang L, Li X, Chen H, et al. Coronavirus disease 19 infection does not result in acute kidney injury: an analysis of 116 hospitalized patients from Wuhan, China. Am J Nephrol 2020;51(5):343–8.
7. Hirsch JS, Ng JH, Ross DW, et al. Acute kidney injury in patients hospitalized with COVID-19. Kidney Int 2020;98(1):209–18.
8. Richardson S, Hirsch JS, Narasimhan M, et al. Presenting characteristics, comorbidities, and outcomes among 5700 patients hospitalized with COVID-19 in the New York city area. JAMA 2020;323(20):2052.
9. Fu EL, Janse RJ, de Jong Y, et al. Acute kidney injury and kidney replacement therapy in COVID-19: a systematic review and meta-analysis. Clin Kidney J 2020;13(4):550–63.
10. Yang X, Tian S, Guo H. Acute kidney injury and renal replacement therapy in COVID-19 patients: a systematic review and meta-analysis. Int Immunopharmacol 2021;90:107159.
11. Doidge JC, Gould DW, Ferrando-Vivas P, et al. Trends in intensive care for patients with COVID-19 in England, Wales, and Northern Ireland. Am J Respir Crit Care Med 2021;203(5):565–74.
12. Cheng Y, Luo R, Wang K, et al. Kidney disease is associated with in-hospital death of patients with COVID-19. Kidney Int 2020;97(5):829–38.
13. Nadim MK, Forni LG, Mehta RL, et al. COVID-19-associated acute kidney injury: consensus report of the 25th Acute Disease Quality Initiative (ADQI) Workgroup. Nat Rev Nephrol 2020;16(12):747–64.
14. Fisher M, Neugarten J, Bellin E, et al. AKI in hospitalized patients with and without COVID-19: a comparison study. J Am Soc Nephrol 2020;31(9):2145–57.
15. Casas-Aparicio GA, Leon-Rodriguez I, Alvarado-de la Barrera C, et al. Acute kidney injury in patients with severe COVID-19 in Mexico. PLoS One 2021; 16(2):e0246595.
16. Husain-Syed F, Wilhelm J, Kassoumeh S, et al. Acute kidney injury and urinary biomarkers in hospitalized patients with coronavirus disease-2019. Nephrol Dial Transplant 2020;35(7):1271–4.
17. Sharma P, Ng JH, Bijol V, et al. Pathology of COVID-19-associated acute kidney injury. Clin Kidney J 2021;14(Suppl 1):i30–9.
18. Legrand M, Bell S, Forni L, et al. Pathophysiology of COVID-19-associated acute kidney injury. Nat Rev Nephrol 2021;17(11):751–64.

19. Santoriello D, Khairallah P, Bomback AS, et al. Postmortem kidney pathology findings in patients with COVID-19. J Am Soc Nephrol 2020;31(9):2158–67.

20. Sharma P, Uppal NN, Wanchoo R, et al. COVID-19-Associated kidney injury: a case series of kidney biopsy findings. J Am Soc Nephrol 2020;31(9):1948–58.

21. Ferlicot S, Jamme M, Gaillard F, et al. The spectrum of kidney biopsies in hospitalized patients with COVID-19, acute kidney injury, and/or proteinuria. Nephrol Dial Transplant 2021. https://doi.org/10.1093/ndt/gfab042.

22. Shetty AA, Tawhari I, Safar-Boueri L, et al. COVID-19-associated glomerular disease. J Am Soc Nephrol 2021;32(1):33–40.

23. Kopp JB, Nelson GW, Sampath K, et al. APOL1 genetic variants in focal segmental glomerulosclerosis and HIV-associated nephropathy. J Am Soc Nephrol 2011;22(11):2129–37.

24. Foster MC, Coresh J, Fornage M, et al. APOL1 variants associate with increased risk of CKD among African Americans. J Am Soc Nephrol 2013;24(9):1484–91.

25. Hassler L, Reyes F, Sparks M, et al. Evidence for and against direct kidney infection by SARS-CoV-2 in Patients with COVID-19. Clin J Am Soc Nephrol 2021;16(11):1755–65.

26. Puelles VG, Lutgehetmann M, Lindenmeyer MT, et al. Multiorgan and renal tropism of SARS-CoV-2. N Engl J Med 2020;383(6):590–2.

27. Westhoff TH, Seibert FS, Bauer F, et al. Allograft infiltration and meningoencephalitis by SARS-CoV-2 in a pancreas-kidney transplant recipient. Am J Transplant 2020;20(11):3216–20.

28. Yao H, Song Y, Chen Y, et al. Molecular architecture of the SARS-CoV-2 virus. Cell 2020;183(3):730–8.e3.

29. Zhou P, Yang XL, Wang XG, et al. A pneumonia outbreak associated with a new coronavirus of probable bat origin. Nature 2020;579(7798):270–3.

30. Walls AC, Park YJ, Tortorici MA, et al. Structure, function, and antigenicity of the SARS-CoV-2 spike glycoprotein. Cell 2020;183(6):1735.

31. Ni W, Yang X, Yang D, et al. Role of angiotensin-converting enzyme 2 (ACE2) in COVID-19. Crit Care 2020;24(1):422.

32. Nath KA, Grande JP, Garovic VD, et al. Expression of ACE2 in the intact and acutely injured kidney. Kidney360 2021;2:1095–106.

33. Ichimura T, Mori Y, Aschauer P, et al. KIM-1/TIM-1 is a receptor for SARS-CoV-2 in lung and kidney. medRxiv 2020. https://doi.org/10.1101/2020.09.16.20190694.

34. Pfister F, Vonbrunn E, Ries T, et al. Complement activation in kidneys of patients with COVID-19. Front Immunol 2020;11:594849.

35. Choudhry N, Li K, Zhang T, et al. The complement factor 5a receptor 1 has a pathogenic role in chronic inflammation and renal fibrosis in a murine model of chronic pyelonephritis. Kidney Int 2016;90(3):540–54.

36. Annane D, Heming N, Grimaldi-Bensouda L, et al. Eculizumab as an emergency treatment for adult patients with severe COVID-19 in the intensive care unit: a proof-of-concept study. EClinicalMedicine 2020;28:100590.

37. Sinha P, Matthay MA, Calfee CS. Is a "cytokine storm" relevant to COVID-19? JAMA Intern Med 2020;180(9):1152.

38. Ragab D, Salah Eldin H, Taeimah M, et al. The COVID-19 cytokine storm; what we know so far. Front Immunol 2020;11:1446.

39. Soy M, Keser G, Atagunduz P, et al. Cytokine storm in COVID-19: pathogenesis and overview of anti-inflammatory agents used in treatment. Clin Rheumatol 2020;39(7):2085–94.

40. Abani O, Abbas A, Abbas F, et al. Tocilizumab in patients admitted to hospital with COVID-19 (RECOVERY): a randomised, controlled, open-label, platform trial. Lancet 2021;397(10285):1637–45.

41. Salvarani C, Dolci G, Massari M, et al. Effect of tocilizumab vs standard care on clinical worsening in patients hospitalized with COVID-19 pneumonia: a randomized clinical trial. JAMA Intern Med 2021;181(1):24–31.

42. The REMAP-CAP investigatorsInterleukin-6 receptor antagonists in critically ill patients with covid-19. New England Journal of Medicine 2021;384(16):1491–502.

43. Desai TR, Leeper NJ, Hynes KL, et al. Interleukin-6 causes endothelial barrier dysfunction via the protein kinase C pathway. J Surg Res 2002;104(2):118–23.

44. Li XQ, Liu H, Meng Y, et al. Critical roles of cytokine storm and secondary bacterial infection in acute kidney injury development in COVID-19: a multi-center retrospective cohort study. J Med Virol 2021;93(12):6641–52.

45. Fajgenbaum DC, June CH. Cytokine storm. N Engl J Med 2020;383(23):2255–73.

46. Cottam D, Nadim MK, Forni LG. Management of acute kidney injury associated with COVID-19: what have we learned? Curr Opin Nephrol Hypertens 2021;30(6):563–70.

47. Klok FA, Kruip M, van der Meer NJM, et al. Incidence of thrombotic complications in critically ill ICU patients with COVID-19. Thromb Res 2020;191:145–7.

48. Rapkiewicz AV, Mai X, Carsons SE, et al. Megakaryocytes and platelet-fibrin thrombi characterize multi-organ thrombosis at autopsy in COVID-19: a case series. EClinicalMedicine 2020;24:100434.

49. Post A, den Deurwaarder ESG, Bakker SJL, et al. Kidney infarction in patients with COVID-19. Am J Kidney Dis 2020;76(3):431–5.

50. Rentsch CT, Beckman JA, Tomlinson L, et al. Early initiation of prophylactic anticoagulation for prevention of coronavirus disease 2019 mortality in patients admitted to hospital in the United States: cohort study. BMJ 2021;372:n311.

51. Investigators R-C, Investigators AC-a, Investigators A, et al. Therapeutic anticoagulation with heparin in critically ill patients with COVID-19. N Engl J Med 2021;385(9):777–89.

52. Ackermann M, Verleden SE, Kuehnel M, et al. Pulmonary vascular endothelialitis, thrombosis, and angiogenesis in COVID-19. N Engl J Med 2020;383(2):120–8.

53. Akilesh S, Nast CC, Yamashita M, et al. Multicenter clinicopathologic correlation of kidney biopsies performed in COVID-19 patients presenting with acute kidney injury or proteinuria. Am J Kidney Dis 2021;77(1):82–93.e81.

54. Bascunana A, Mijaylova A, Vega A, et al. Thrombotic microangiopathy in a kidney transplant patient with COVID-19. Kidney Med 2021;3(1):124–7.

55. Mancini I, Baronciani L, Artoni A, et al. The ADAMTS13-von Willebrand factor axis in COVID-19 patients. J Thromb Haemost 2021;19(2):513–21.

56. Sharkey RA, Mulloy EM, O'Neill SJ. Acute effects of hypoxaemia, hyperoxaemia and hypercapnia on renal blood flow in normal and renal transplant subjects. Eur Respir J 1998;12(3):653–7.

57. Koyner JL, Murray PT. Mechanical ventilation and the kidney. Blood Purif 2010;29(1):52–68.

58. Joannidis M, Forni LG, Klein SJ, et al. Lung–kidney interactions in critically ill patients: consensus report of the Acute Disease Quality Initiative (ADQI) 21 Workgroup. Intensive Care Med 2020;46(4):654–72.

59. Swenson KE, Swenson ER. Pathophysiology of acute respiratory distress syndrome and COVID-19 lung injury. Crit Care Clin 2021;37(4):749–76.

60. Alvarez-Belon L, Sarnowski A, Forni LG. COVID-19 infection and the kidney. Br J Hosp Med (Lond) 2020;81(10):1–8.

61. Pei G, Zhang Z, Peng J, et al. Renal involvement and early prognosis in patients with COVID-19 pneumonia. J Am Soc Nephrol 2020;31(6):1157–65.

62. Haase M, Bellomo R, Devarajan P, et al. Accuracy of neutrophil gelatinase-associated lipocalin (NGAL) in diagnosis and prognosis in acute kidney injury: a systematic review and meta-analysis. Am J Kidney Dis 2009;54(6):1012–24.

63. Albert C, Zapf A, Haase M, et al. Neutrophil gelatinase-associated lipocalin measured on clinical laboratory platforms for the prediction of acute kidney injury and the associated need for dialysis therapy: a systematic review and meta-analysis. Am J Kidney Dis 2020;76(6):826–41.e1.

64. Komaru Y, Doi K, Nangaku M. Urinary neutrophil gelatinase-associated lipocalin in critically ill patients with coronavirus disease 2019. Crit Care Explor 2020;2(8): e0181.

65. Xiao R, Chen R. Neutrophil gelatinaseassociated lipocalin as a potential novel biomarker for ventilatorassociated lung injury. Mol Med Rep 2017;15(6): 3535–40.

66. Han WK, Bailly V, Abichandani R, et al. Kidney Injury Molecule-1 (KIM-1): a novel biomarker for human renal proximal tubule injury. Kidney Int 2002;62(1):237–44.

67. Vogel MJ, Mustroph J, Staudner ST, et al. Kidney injury molecule-1: potential biomarker of acute kidney injury and disease severity in patients with COVID-19. J Nephrol 2021;34(4):1007–18.

68. Fanelli V, Fiorentino M, Cantaluppi V, et al. Acute kidney injury in SARS-CoV-2 infected patients. Crit Care 2020;24(1):155.

69. Kellum JA, Artigas A, Gunnerson KJ, et al. Use of biomarkers to identify acute kidney injury to help detect sepsis in patients with infection. Crit Care Med 2021;49(4):e360–8.

70. Azam TU, Shadid HR, Blakely P, et al. Soluble urokinase receptor (SuPAR) in COVID-19-related AKI. J Am Soc Nephrol 2020;31(11):2725–35.

71. Douglas IS, Alapat PM, Corl KA, et al. Fluid response evaluation in sepsis hypotension and shock: a randomized clinical trial. Chest 2020;158(4):1431–45.

72. Self WH, Semler MW, Wanderer JP, et al. Balanced crystalloids versus saline in noncritically ill adults. N Engl J Med 2018;378(9):819–28.

73. Semler MW, Self WH, Wanderer JP, et al. Balanced crystalloids versus saline in critically ill adults. N Engl J Med 2018;378(9):829–39.

74. Antequera Martín AM, Barea Mendoza JA, Muriel A, et al. Buffered solutions versus 0.9% saline for resuscitation in critically ill adults and children. Cochrane Database Syst Rev 2019;7:CD012247.

75. Zampieri FG, Machado FR, Biondi RS, et al. Effect of intravenous fluid treatment with a balanced solution vs 0.9% saline solution on mortality in critically ill patients: the BaSICS randomized clinical trial. JAMA 2021;326(9):1–12.

76. Santos A, Magro DO, Evangelista-Poderoso R, et al. Diabetes, obesity, and insulin resistance in COVID-19: molecular interrelationship and therapeutic implications. Diabetology Metab Syndr 2021;13(1):23.

77. Thibault R, Seguin P, Tamion F, et al. Nutrition of the COVID-19 patient in the intensive care unit (ICU): a practical guidance. Crit Care 2020;24(1):447.

78. Acute Respiratory Distress Syndrome N, Brower RG, Matthay MA, et al. Ventilation with lower tidal volumes as compared with traditional tidal volumes for acute

lung injury and the acute respiratory distress syndrome. N Engl J Med 2000; 342(18):1301–8.

79. Briel M, Meade M, Mercat A, et al. Higher vs lower positive end-expiratory pressure in patients with acute lung injury and acute respiratory distress syndrome: systematic review and meta-analysis. JAMA 2010;303(9):865–73.

80. Griffiths M, Meade S, Summers C, et al. RAND appropriateness panel to determine the applicability of UK guidelines on the management of acute respiratory distress syndrome (ARDS) and other strategies in the context of the COVID-19 pandemic. Thorax 2021. https://doi.org/10.1136/thoraxjnl-2021-216904.

81. Shelhamer MC, Wesson PD, Solari IL, et al. Prone positioning in moderate to severe acute respiratory distress syndrome due to COVID-19: a cohort study and analysis of physiology. J Intensive Care Med 2021;36(2):241–52.

82. Weiss TT, Cerda F, Scott JB, et al. Prone positioning for patients intubated for severe acute respiratory distress syndrome (ARDS) secondary to COVID-19: a retrospective observational cohort study. Br J Anaesth 2021;126(1):48–55.

83. Hering R, Wrigge H, Vorwerk R, et al. The effects of prone positioning on intra-abdominal pressure and cardiovascular and renal function in patients with acute lung injury. Anesth Analg 2001;92(5):1226–31.

84. Beigel JH, Tomashek KM, Dodd LE, et al. Remdesivir for the treatment of covid-19 — final report. New England Journal of Medicine 2020;383(19):1813–26.

85. Group TRC. Dexamethasone in hospitalized patients with COVID-19. N Engl J Med 2020.

86. Group WHOREAfC-TW, Sterne JAC, Murthy S, et al. Association between administration of systemic corticosteroids and mortality among critically ill patients with COVID-19: a meta-analysis. JAMA 2020;324(13):1330–41.

87. Orieux A, Khan P, Prevel R, et al. Impact of dexamethasone use to prevent from severe COVID-19-induced acute kidney injury. Crit Care 2021;25(1):249.

88. Brass P, Hellmich M, Kolodziej L, et al. Ultrasound guidance versus anatomical landmarks for internal jugular vein catheterization. Cochrane Database Syst Rev 2015;1:CD006962.

89. Brass P, Hellmich M, Kolodziej L, et al. Ultrasound guidance versus anatomical landmarks for subclavian or femoral vein catheterization. Cochrane Database Syst Rev 2015;2015(1):CD011447.

90. Parienti J-J, Mégarbane B, Fischer M-O, et al. Catheter dysfunction and dialysis performance according to vascular access among 736 critically ill adults requiring renal replacement therapy: a randomized controlled study. Crit Care Med 2010;38(4):1118–25.

91. Parienti J-J, Thirion M, Mégarbane B, et al. Femoral vs jugular venous catheterization and risk of nosocomial events in adults requiring acute renal replacement therapy: a randomized controlled trial. JAMA 2008;299(20):2413.

92. Gaudry S, Hajage D, Benichou N, et al. Delayed versus early initiation of renal replacement therapy for severe acute kidney injury: a systematic review and individual patient data meta-analysis of randomised clinical trials. Lancet 2020; 395(10235):1506–15.

93. STARRT-AKI Investigators; Canadian Critical Care Trials Group; Australian and New Zealand Intensive Care Society Clinical Trials Group; United Kingdom Critical Care Research Group; Canadian Nephrology Trials Network; Irish Critical Care Trials Group, Bagshaw SM, Wald R, Adhikari NKJ, et al. Timing of initiation of renal-replacement therapy in acute kidney injury. N Engl J Med 2020;383(3): 240–51.

94. Gaudry S, Hajage D, Martin-Lefevre L, et al. Comparison of two delayed strategies for renal replacement therapy initiation for severe acute kidney injury (AKIKI 2): a multicentre, open-label, randomised, controlled trial. Lancet 2021; 397(10281):1293–300.

95. Zarbock A, Kellum JA, Schmidt C, et al. Effect of early vs delayed initiation of renal replacement therapy on mortality in critically ill patients with acute kidney injury: the ELAIN randomized clinical trial. JAMA 2016;315(20):2190–9.

96. Khwaja A. KDIGO clinical practice guidelines for acute kidney injury. Nephron Clin Pract 2012;120(4):c179–84.

97. Chua H-R, MacLaren G, Choong LH-L, et al. Ensuring sustainability of continuous kidney replacement therapy in the face of extraordinary demand: lessons from the COVID-19 pandemic. Am J Kidney Dis 2020;76(3):392–400.

98. Burgner A, Ikizler TA, Dwyer JP. COVID-19 and the inpatient dialysis unit: managing resources during contingency planning pre-crisis. Clin J Am Soc Nephrol 2020;15(5):720–2.

99. Adapa S, Aeddula NR, Konala VM, et al. COVID-19 and renal failure: challenges in the delivery of renal replacement therapy. J Clin Med Res 2020;12(5):276–85.

100. Lumlertgul N, Tunstell P, Watts C, et al. In-house production of dialysis solutions to overcome challenges during the coronavirus disease 2019 pandemic. Kidney Int Rep 2021;6(1):200–6.

101. Shamy OE, Patel N, Abdelbaset MH, et al. Acute start peritoneal dialysis during the COVID-19 pandemic: outcomes and experiences. J Am Soc Nephrol 2020; 31(8):1680–2.

102. Srivatana V, Aggarwal V, Finkelstein FO, et al. Peritoneal dialysis for acute kidney injury treatment in the United States: Brought to You by the COVID-19 Pandemic. Kidney360 2020;1(5):410–5.

103. Bowes E, Joslin J, Braide-Azikiwe DCB, et al. Acute peritoneal dialysis with percutaneous catheter insertion for COVID-19–associated acute kidney injury in intensive care: experience from a UK Tertiary Center. Kidney Int Rep 2021; 6(2):265–71.

104. Wen Y, LeDoux JR, Mohamed M, et al. Dialysis filter life, anticoagulation, and inflammation in COVID-19 and acute kidney injury. Kidney360. 2020;1(12): 1426–31.

105. Shankaranarayanan D, Muthukumar T, Barbar T, et al. Anticoagulation Strategies and Filter Life in COVID-19 patients receiving continuous renal replacement therapy: a single-center experience. Clin J Am Soc Nephrol 2021;16(1):124–6.

106. Zarbock A, Küllmar M, Kindgen-Milles D, et al. Effect of regional citrate anticoagulation vs systemic heparin anticoagulation during continuous kidney replacement therapy on dialysis filter life span and mortality among critically ill patients with acute kidney injury: a randomized clinical trial. JAMA 2020; 324(16):1629–39.

107. Arnold F, Westermann L, Rieg S, et al. Comparison of different anticoagulation strategies for renal replacement therapy in critically ill patients with COVID-19: a cohort study. BMC Nephrol 2020;21(1):486.

108. Ronco C, Reis T. Kidney involvement in COVID-19 and rationale for extracorporeal therapies. Nat Rev Nephrol 2020;16(6):308–10.

109. Rosalia RA, Ugurov P, Neziri D, et al. Extracorporeal Blood Purification in moderate and severe COVID-19 patients: a prospective cohort study. medRxiv 2020. 2020.2010.2010.20210096.

110. Zhang H, Zhu G, Yan L, et al. The absorbing filter Oxiris in severe coronavirus disease 2019 patients: a case series. Artif Organs 2020;44(12):1296–302.

111. Villa G, Romagnoli S, De Rosa S, et al. Blood purification therapy with a hemo-diafilter featuring enhanced adsorptive properties for cytokine removal in patients presenting COVID-19: a pilot study. Crit Care 2020;24(1):605.

112. Nassiri AA, Hakemi MS, Miri MM, et al. Blood purification with CytoSorb in critically ill COVID-19 patients: a case series of 26 patients. Artif Organs 2021; 45(11):1338–47.

113. Seffer MT, Cottam D, Forni LG, et al. Heparin 2.0: a new approach to the infection crisis. Blood Purif 2021;50(1):28–34.

114. Chitty SA, Mobbs S, Rifkin BS, et al. A multicenter evaluation of blood purification with seraph 100 microbind affinity blood filter for the treatment of severe COVID-19: a preliminary report. medRxiv 2021. 2021.2004.2020.21255810.

115. Rieder M, Duerschmied D, Zahn T, et al. Cytokine adsorption in severe acute respiratory failure requiring veno-venous extracorporeal membrane oxygenation. ASAIO J 2021;67(3):332–8.

116. Supady A, Weber E, Rieder M, et al. Cytokine adsorption in patients with severe COVID-19 pneumonia requiring extracorporeal membrane oxygenation (CY-COV): a single centre, open-label, randomised, controlled trial. Lancet Respir Med 2021;9(7):755–62.

117. Bowe B, Cai M, Xie Y, et al. Acute kidney injury in a national cohort of hospitalized US veterans with COVID-19. Clin J Am Soc Nephrol 2020;16(1):14–25.

118. Nugent J, Aklilu A, Yamamoto Y, et al. Assessment of acute kidney injury and longitudinal kidney function after hospital discharge among patients with and without COVID-19. JAMA Netw Open 2021;4(3):e211095.

119. Ng JH, Hirsch JS, Hazzan A, et al. Outcomes among patients hospitalized with COVID-19 and acute kidney injury. Am J Kidney Dis 2021;77(2):204–15.e201.

120. Gupta S, Coca SG, Chan L, et al. AKI treated with renal replacement therapy in critically ill patients with COVID-19. J Am Soc Nephrol 2021;32(1):161.

121. Stockmann H, Hardenberg JB, Aigner A, et al. High rates of long-term renal recovery in survivors of coronavirus disease 2019-associated acute kidney injury requiring kidney replacement therapy. Kidney Int 2021;99(4):1021–2.

122. Lin L, Wang X, Ren J, et al. Risk factors and prognosis for COVID-19-induced acute kidney injury: a meta-analysis. BMJ Open 2020;10(11):e042573.

123. See YP, Young BE, Ang LW, et al. Risk factors for development of acute kidney injury in COVID-19 patients: a retrospective observational cohort study. Nephron 2021;145(3):256–64.

124. Geri G, Darmon M, Zafrani L, et al. Acute kidney injury in SARS-CoV2-related pneumonia ICU patients: a retrospective multicenter study. Ann Intensive Care 2021;11(1):86.

Role of Acute Thrombosis in Coronavirus Disease 2019

Derek V. Gibbs, MD[a], Satya S. Shreenivas, MD, MBA[b],
Kristin M. Hudock, MD, MSTR[c,d],*

KEYWORDS

- COVID • Thrombosis • Coronary thrombus • Anticoagulation • NETs • D-dimer

KEY POINTS

- Patients infected with the SARS CoV-2 virus are at increased risk of thrombosis and coagulopathy.
- Patients with cardiovascular disease are predisposed to COVID-19 infection, and once infected, they are at elevated risk for cardiovascular complications.
- Most patients with COVID-19 who experienced strokes developed ischemic stroke.
- D-dimer is very commonly elevated during acute SARS-CoV-2 infection, particularly in hospitalized patients, rendering D-dimer alone of limited use in the assessment of VTE.
- Moderately ill patients with COVID-19 have a significant benefit from therapeutic-dose heparin compared with usual care-dose heparin in organ-free support days.

INTRODUCTION

Severe acute respiratory syndrome coronavirus 2 (SARS-CoV-2) rapidly spread across the world in late 2019 and early 2020 causing mild to severe multisystem disease. In addition to respiratory symptoms, coronavirus disease 2019 (COVID-19) causes coagulopathy, particularly in critically ill patients.[1–3] Thrombosis is crucial in infection to protect the host by limiting dissemination of viral and other pathogens, but when uncontrolled can cause tissue damage.[4,5] The pathogenesis of SARS-CoV-2 is exacerbated by microthrombi and macrothrombi that compromise circulation and threaten organ function.[6] In addition to limiting blood flow, the positive feedback loop of the immune response perpetuating clots further exacerbates inflammation and contributes to disease burden in COVID-19. Herein, the latest

The authors have nothing to disclose.
[a] Division of General Internal Medicine, Department of Medicine, University of Cincinnati School of Medicine, 231 Albert Sabin Way, MSB 6065, Cincinnati, OH 45267, USA; [b] Division of Cardiology, The Christ Hospital, 2139 Auburn Avenue, Cincinnati, OH 45219, USA; [c] Division of Pulmonary, Critical Care & Sleep Medicine, Department of Medicine, University of Cincinnati School of Medicine, 231 Albert Sabin Way, MSB 6053, Cincinnati, OH 45267, USA; [d] Division of Pulmonary Biology, Cincinnati Children's Hospital Medical Center, 3333 Burnet Avenue, Cincinnati, OH 45229, USA
* Corresponding author. 231 Albert Sabin Way, MSB 6053, Cincinnati, OH 45267.
E-mail address: Kristin.Hudock@uc.edu

Crit Care Clin 38 (2022) 491–504
https://doi.org/10.1016/j.ccc.2022.03.003
0749-0704/22/© 2022 Elsevier Inc. All rights reserved.
criticalcare.theclinics.com

Abbreviations	
NETs	neutrophil extracellular traps
MPO	myeloperoxidase
NE	neutrophil elastase
IL	interleukin
COVID-19	coronavirus disease 2019
SARS-CoV-2	severe acute respiratory syndrome coronavirus 2
CVA	cerebrovascular accident
VTE	venous thromboembolism
DVT	deep vein thrombosis

epidemiology, biologic mechanisms, organ-specific considerations, and therapeutic trials regarding thrombosis in COVID-19 are reviewed.

PATHOGENESIS OF CORONAVIRUS DISEASE 2019-INDUCED THROMBOSIS

The mechanisms by which SARS-CoV-2 infection promotes coagulopathy include host- and virus-related factors. Neutrophil extracellular traps (NETs) are weblike structures composed of DNA, histones, and immunomodulatory proteins that trap and kill microorganisms.[7,8] NETs have been implicated in thrombus formation via multiple mechanisms.[9–12] The SARS-CoV-2 virus and plasma from patients with COVID-19 can induce neutrophils to form NETs ex vivo.[13,14] NETs—detected by the presence of MPO-DNA and/or NE-DNA complexes—are increased in the blood of hospitalized patients with COVID-19 compared with healthy controls.[13,15,16] NET concentrations correlate with severity of SARS-CoV-2 disease.[14,16] Histologic analysis of autopsy tissue from patients who died of COVID-19 showed NETs within vascular thrombi, although whether NETs initiate clots or NET formation is activated by platelets at the site of preformed clots remains unclear.[15,17] The authors have demonstrated that NETs can cause human airway epithelia to increase secretion of interleukin IL-1 cytokines, another potential mechanism by which NETs could contribute to COVID-19 pathogenesis.[18] Drugs that affect NETs in COVID are currently being trialed. Endothelial, complement, and platelet activation also contribute to coagulopathy in COVID-19, the details of which are described in recent excellent reviews.[19,20]

EPIDEMIOLOGY OF VASCULAR THROMBI IN CORONAVIRUS DISEASE 2019

Patients infected with the SARS-CoV-2 virus are at increased risk of thrombosis and coagulopathy for reasons previously described, with coagulopathy itself predicting worse prognosis. In an early study of 184 Dutch patients in the intensive care unit (ICU), 27% of patients were found to have a venous thromboembolism (VTE)—most commonly due to pulmonary embolism (PE)—whereas 3.7% had an arterial thrombus. This study was evaluating symptomatic thrombotic events and did not include a universal screen; however, it demonstrated an overall thrombosis rate of 31%, which was higher than seen in other studies.[21] A study that included lower-extremity Dopplers on admission for 26 patients with COVID-19 in 2 French ICUs found an overall VTE rate of 69%. Moreover, high rates of PE and deep vein thrombosis (DVT) were observed on subsequent imaging, even in those treated with therapeutic anticoagulation.[22] Another small study using routine lower extremity Dopplers in a French ICU found DVTs in 22 (65%) patients on admission and 27 (79%) after 48 hours.[23] Of note, all 3 of these studies were limited to 1 to 2 centers and were performed early in the pandemic when treatment and anticoagulation protocols varied significantly across institutions.

A large cohort study evaluated the incidence of VTE in greater than 3000 patients in the United States within 2 weeks of ICU admission. Only 3 of the 67 sites did routine screening with imaging, for most patients radiographic evaluation was at the discretion of the treating team. The VTE incidence was found to be 6.3% in greater than 3000 patients.[24] This incidence is significantly lower than the initial studies of VTE in COVID-19; however, this US study did not include a universal screening protocol and excluded patients with confirmed or suspected DVT at the time of study enrollment.[24] Given the lack of a universal screening protocol, it is possible that many patients have thrombi that go undetected because they are asymptomatic or the contribution of microthrombi and macrothrombi were underrecognized. Furthermore, it is possible that if these studies were repeated now, rates of VTE may be further altered by our evolved standard-of-care treatments, for example, dexamethasone, for COVID-19.[71] Moreover, we agree with the National Institutes of Health (NIH) guidelines that recommend imaging for thrombi as part of the assessment of patients with COVID-19 with significant clinical deteriorations, if not contraindicated.[25]

CVA IN CORONAVIRUS DISEASE 2019

There have been varying reports on the risk of stroke in COVID-19 with rates ranging from 0.5% to 6%.[72,73] Initial reports from China suggested that the overall rate of strokes and vascular interventions for the general population was decreased during COVID-19.[74] However, this may have been due to external factors including reduced health care utilization and decreased use of vascular imaging during initial phases of the pandemic. A cross-sectional study using data from a New York health care system discharge and billing database of 24,808 patients (566 of whom were COVID-19 positive) showed an odds ratio (OR) of 0.25 of developing stroke compared with age- and comorbidity-matched COVID-19-negative patients.[26] More recent large meta-analyses suggest an incidence closer to 1.3% to 1.5%. When looking at the patients with COVID-19 who developed cerebrovascular events, they were approximately 4.5 to 6 years younger than their noninfected counterparts in the general population.[27,28] These patients often had the same cardiovascular risk factors such as coronary artery disease, hypertension, and diabetes. One important risk factor for development of stroke is COVID-19 disease severity.[28,29] In one meta-analysis, patients with severe COVID-19 had an incidence of 3.37%, whereas patients without severe disease had an incidence of 0.6%.[30] It is difficult to know the true incidence of stroke in COVID-19, in part due to critically ill patients—who are at the highest risk of stroke—often being intubated. We suspect that incidence of CVA in critically ill patients is underestimated because (1) patients are too sick to be transported for brain imaging, (2) neurologic examinations are limited in patients on sedation used for mechanical ventilation/proning leading to an underappreciation of potential deficits, and (3) patients die before imaging can occur or a meaningful neurologic examination can be completed.

Most patients with COVID-19 with strokes developed ischemic stroke (around 87%). In addition, 44.7% of strokes were cryptogenic and 21.9% were cardioembolic. The absence of atherosclerotic disease as a significant cause of stroke in this population is one possible explanation for the earlier age of onset. Compared with patients without COVID-19 infection, large vessel occlusion was seen around two and a half times more often.[28]

CORONARY THROMBOSIS IN CORONAVIRUS DISEASE 2019

Patients with cardiovascular disease are predisposed to COVID-19 infection, and once infected, they are at elevated risk for cardiovascular complications.[31] A significant source of COVID-19-related cardiac risk comes from myocardial injury related to coronary thrombosis. Case series from New York and Wuhan in early 2020 showed patients presenting with ST elevation on electrocardiogram and elevated cardiac biomarkers of injury (troponin).[32,33] Troponin elevation as a sign of myocardial injury is an important marker of adverse prognosis in patients with COVID-19; patients with abnormally elevated troponin levels in the setting of COVID-19 are more likely to be admitted to the ICU and are more likely to die.[34] Case series have reported the incidence of acute myocardial injury (defined as both elevated levels of biomarkers and electrocardiographic abnormalities) in patients with COVID-19 ranging from 12% to 19.7%.[35,36] However, other than small case series, the true incidence of myocardial injury with COVID-19 is unclear because these series are mostly in hospitalized patients and we know that patients with comorbidities of coronary artery disease such as hypertension and diabetes are also more likely to be hospitalized with COVID-19. In addition, several case series only examined patients who had undergone coronary angiograms to define the incidence of coronary thrombosis. In many parts of the world, the COVID-19 pandemic changed practice patterns due to health care rationing such that patients who might have routinely undergone invasive cardiac testing were instead managed conservatively. For example, in Wuhan, one hospital system's published algorithm for patients with COVID-19 presenting with ST-elevation myocardial infarction articulated a delay in management of coronary thrombosis in patients with severe pneumonia and in those with less severe pulmonary disease, a fibrinolytic first strategy was recommended.[37]

PATHOPHYSIOLOGY OF CARDIAC THROMBUS IN COVID-19

The burden of coronary thrombosis varies widely, ranging from nonobstructive thrombus to large thrombi burden in multiple vessels.[38] Patients with COVID-19 with myocardial infarction can have coronary thrombus in epicardial vessels that can be associated with coronary stenosis or plaque rupture, similar to patients without COVID-19. However, there are also numerous reports of patients with COVID-19 with epicardial thrombus without any evidence of coronary artery atherosclerotic plaque or stenosis and cases in which no epicardial vessel thrombus was seen during coronary angiogram.[39] In these cases, it is likely that microemboli or thrombosis in vessels that are not visible to the naked eye on coronary angiogram could still be causing significant myocardial injury. In a case series of postmortem examinations of 40 hearts from patients who died of COVID-19, 35% had evidence of myocardial necrosis.[40] Of these cases, only 2 (14.2%) had evidence of epicardial coronary artery thrombi, whereas the rest had evidence of microthrombi in myocardial capillaries, arterioles, and small muscular arteries.[40]

Timing of coronary thrombosis during a COVID-19 infection also needs further elucidation, but there is some evidence that this is an early phenomenon. In one case series from Lombardy, Italy, 85% of patients diagnosed with coronary thrombosis by coronary angiogram presented with chest pain and ST-segment elevations before diagnosis of COVID-19 and the remainder were diagnosed with ST-segment elevation myocardial infarction during the hospitalization.[41] Owing to the heterogeneous patient population (including many patients who are at high risk for coronary events due to many cardiac comorbidities), it is important to have myocardial ischemia as a differential diagnosis for new patients presenting with COVID-19 and for patients with COVID-19 who clinically decompensate during a hospitalization.

There are several potential mechanisms for why COVID-19 may cause coronary thrombosis. There are many similarities between the potential causes of coronary thrombosis and the postulated causative role of COVID-19 in thrombosis in other vascular distributions. Specifically, there are 4 proposed hypotheses, which are not mutually exclusive, to explain the large role that cardiovascular system plays in morbidity and mortality in COVID-19. (1) Cardiac tissue is a substrate for SARS-CoV-2 binding. (2) The role of SARS-CoV-2-induced endothelial dysfunction causes acute thrombosis. (3) Proinflammatory immune responses to the virus cause acute thrombosis. (4) COVID-19 preferentially affects people with cardiovascular risk factors.

The SARS-CoV-2 virus has an affinity for the angiotensin-converting enzyme (ACE) receptor, which is highly concentrated in myocardial tissue, and this could explain the role of COVID-19 in causing coronary thrombosis, myocarditis, and arrhythmias. The ACE receptor is also found on vascular endothelium, and endothelial dysfunction could result in the inciting injury that is further propagated by the proinflammatory state of acute infection associated with severe COVID-19 infection. The proinflammatory cascade is known to interfere with the coagulation to form a prothrombotic milieu that can then proceed to acute myocardial infarction, as has been shown in other types of acute infection including other types of pneumonia.[42,43] Finally, all of this is occurring in a patient group with multiple coronary artery disease risk factors including preexisting coronary artery disease, older age, hypertension, and diabetes.[44] The combination of high affinity for myocardial tissue for SARS-CoV-2 binding, endothelial dysfunction, proinflammatory state, and the at-risk patient cohort contributes to the risk for coronary thrombosis in patients with COVID-19.

TREATMENT OF CORONARY THROMBUS IN CORONAVIRUS DISEASE 2019

In cases of suspected coronary thrombosis with ST-segment elevation myocardial infarction the recommendation of the American College of Cardiology is to proceed with primary percutaneous coronary intervention (PCI) unless there are limitations in local resources that might result in delayed care.[45] In situations that may result in delay to primary PCI, a fibrinolytic first strategy could be considered. This is similar to recommendations for the care of ST-segment elevation myocardial infarctions in the general population where geography, weather, or other systemic delays in care sometimes prevent a primary PCI strategy and fibrinolytics are still used. In cases of non-ST elevation myocardial infarction or in cases in which an ST elevation diagnosis is not clear, efforts should be made to differentiate between demand ischemia from occlusive coronary thrombosis. Tools that could help with such differentiation include trending biomarkers, serial electrocardiograms, and point-of-care echocardiography. If the patient is clinically stable and symptom free—depending on the local resources needed for the care of other patients—a deferred strategy can be considered with medical treatment with antiplatelet and antithrombotic agents. Of note, patients with COVID-19 frequently present with thrombocytopenia with one study showing 36% of patients diagnosed with COVID-19 presenting with a platelet count of less than 150,000/μL.[46] The risk/benefit for antiplatelet and antithrombotic therapy in these patients needs to be individualized, and careful monitoring for both bleeding and thrombotic complications is essential. Finally, in cases in which a patient undergoes a coronary angiogram and no occlusive epicardial disease is found, consideration should then turn toward other causes of elevated troponin levels including myocarditis, stress-induced cardiomyopathy (Takotsubo), and microvascular coronary ischemia.

CURRENT EVIDENCE FOR PREVENTION OF MICROTHROMBI AND MACROTHROMBI IN CORONAVIRUS DISEASE 2019

There has been a substantial amount of research on whether anticoagulation or antiplatelet therapy changes outcomes and rates of thrombosis in patients with COVID-19. Earlier studies primarily focused on an end point of thrombosis and mortality; however, when most of those were negative or showed no benefit to anticoagulation, later studies began to focus on risk stratification with severity of illness, location of treatment (ICU vs floor), and laboratory evaluation. In addition, as described herein, the presence of PE or stroke significantly increases mortality. Because of this, there was significant interest in prevention of thrombosis with multicenter clinical trials testing full-dose versus prophylactic-dose anticoagulation as well as different antithrombotic agents.

Although most trials focused on anticoagulation on the inpatient side, there are several studies in progress to assess the use of prophylactic dose anticoagulation as an outpatient during SARS-CoV-2 infection. PREVENT-HD trial assessed the safety and efficacy of Xarelto 10 mg daily on an outpatient basis for 35 days.[47] Two trials, the OVID trial and the early thromboprophylaxis in covid-19 (ETHIC) trial, are comparing 40 mg subcutaneous lovenox daily versus placebo.[48,75] The accelerating covid-19 therapeutic interventions and vaccines (ACTIV-4b trial studied apixaban (2.5 or 5 mg twice daily) versus 81mg of aspirin daily versus placebo. This trial was stopped early at an interim evaluation due to lack of thrombotic events in all arms of the study.[49] At present, there are insufficient data to support routine use of prophylactic anticoagulation on an outpatient basis.

XARELTO

The anticoagulation coronavirus (ACTION) trial was one of the early trials, and it compared treatment-dose Xarelto (20 mg or 15mg daily) in stable patients and lovenox at 1 mg/kg twice a day or IV unfractionated heparin in unstable patients with prophylactic dosing anticoagulation in hospitalized patients followed by Xarelto, all totaling 30 days.[50] Clinically unstable patients had severe COVID-19, a life-threatening comorbidity and required mechanical ventilation or the ICU. It should be noted that in this trial, only 39 of the 615 patients were deemed clinically unstable. There was no difference in the primary outcome of mortality (11.3% in therapeutic arm, 7.6% in prophylactic), but there was a trend toward higher mortality in the treatment arm. There were nonsignificant trends toward lower VTE rate (3.5% in treatment arm, 5.9% in prophylactic arm). The only clinical end point to reach significance was ISTH-defined bleeding, which occurred in 8.3% of patients in the treatment group compared with 2.3% of the patients receiving prophylactic doses of anticoagulation.[50]

APIXABAN

A trial of prophylactic apixaban versus subcutaneous low-molecular-weight heparin (LMWH) demonstrated a significant decrease in mortality with prophylactic-dose apixaban or prophylactic-dose enoxaparin when compared with no anticoagulation at all. The investigators also saw a decrease in mortality in the therapeutic-dose anticoagulation arms; however, there was no significant difference between therapeutic and prophylactic. A subgroup analysis revealed that patients with COVID-19 with a normal D-dimer level less than 1.0 did not benefit from anticoagulation, whereas patients with very high levels of D-dimers (>10) did.[51]

ASPIRIN

The randomized evaluation of covid-19 therapy (RECOVERY) trial was a large multi-center trial in the United Kingdom looking at treatment of patients with COVID-19 admitted in a hospital with moderate-dose 150 mg aspirin daily to see if the anti-inflammatory effects had any significant decrease in hospitalization stay, progression to ventilator support, or mortality. In total, 14,892 patients were randomized. There was no difference in 28-day mortality or progression to invasive mechanical ventilation between those who did and did not receive aspirin. There was a small but significant increase in discharge from hospital alive at 28 days (OR 1.06) and shorter duration of hospital stay in patients in the aspirin arm. For every 1000 patients treated with aspirin, there were 6 major bleeding episodes and 6 fewer thromboembolic events. Overall, aspirin did not show evidence of improving mortality or reducing progression of disease.[52] Trials of additional antiplatelet agents are currently ongoing in patients with moderate and severe COVID-19, for example, NCT04505774.

HEPARIN AND LOW-MOLECULAR-WEIGHT HEPARINS

Most data regarding anticoagulation tested heparin, the historical agent of choice in VTE prophylaxis. There are multiple factors that make heparin more attractive than some other agents, such as avoiding drug interactions with tocilizumab that are seen with Xarelto or apixaban and the potential to reduce inflammation. Three multicenter, international, platform trials assessed the use of heparin: randomized, embedded multifactorial adaptive platform trial for community acquired pneumona (REMAP-CAP), ACTIV-4A, and antithrombotic therapy to ameliorate complications of covid-19 (ATTACC).[53,54] All these studies included a group of patients with critical COVID-19-related illness (severe) and a group of patients with moderate COVID-19. The definition of critically ill varied slightly between these trials. REMAP-CAP included patients admitted to the ICU, and ACTIV-4A enrolled severe patients on greater than 20L NC O2, regardless of their physical location (taking into accounting that many hospitals were having to expand ICU care beyond the ICU). In an effort to maximize enrollment and rapidly answer urgent clinical questions, these groups combined their data and analyzed the results together.[53,54]

The enrollment of critically ill patients was stopped early in December 2020 when no significant difference was seen in the primary outcome of organ support-free days for those who received therapeutic-dose heparin versus usual care dosing (prophylactic- or intermediate-dose subcutaneous (SQ) heparin). Sixty-two percent of 534 patients in the therapeutic heparin arm compared with 64.5% of the 564 patients in the usual care arm survived to hospital discharge. There were fewer thrombotic events noted with full-dose anticoagulation (7.2% vs 11.1%), and rates of major bleeding episodes (3.8% vs 2.3%) were similar between groups. It is important to note that the standard-of-care/prophylactic-dose anticoagulation arm used an intermediate-dose strategy in 51% of the patients.[54]

In contrast to the critically ill group, the moderately ill patients with COVID-19 had a significant benefit from therapeutic-dose heparin compared with usual care-dose heparin. After enrolling 2219 across the 3 platforms of hospitalized patients, there was a 98.6% probability of increasing organ support-free days with an OR of 1.27. When stratifying by patients with high and low levels of D-dimers the results were unchanged. Major bleeding did occur slightly more frequently in the therapeutic-dose group at 1.9% versus 0.9% prophylaxis group, although this did not reach statistical significance. Many of the secondary outcomes in this trial were promising. The rate of major thrombotic event (8.0% vs 9.9%; OR, 0.72; 95% confidence interval [CI], 0.53–0.90) were lower, and the rate of survival without organ support at 28 days (79.3% vs 75.4%; OR, 1.3; 95% CI, 1.05–1.61) was higher in the treatment-dose group. Patients on full-dose heparin had an 80.2% of survival to hospital discharge, compared with 76.4% in the usual care group, which did not reach statistical significance. As occurred in the severe group, there were moderate patients in the standard-of-care arm treated with an intermediate dose of heparin or LMWH; however, it was only about a quarter of patients. In addition, 20% of patients in the experimental group received lower than full therapeutic dose of heparin in the first 2 days after randomization.[53]

RAPID was a randomized controlled trial evaluating treatment of hospitalized non-ICU patients with either treatment dose or prophylactic dose anticoagulation.[55] This study enrolled 465 patients and at interim analysis was found to be underpowered to reach their primary end point, which was a composite of ICU admission, noninvasive or invasive ventilation, or mortality at 28 days. There was, however, a significant decrease in the individual secondary outcomes of all-cause mortality (1.8% vs 7.6%) and an increase in mean ventilator-free days. There was no significant difference in need for ICU admission, venous or arterial thromboembolism, or international society on thrombosis and haemostasis (ISTH)-defined major bleeding. In addition, unlike the results of the pooled multiplatform trials, only 1.7% of the prophylactic-dose patients received an "intermediate" dose for standard of care (SOC) and 2.6% of the treatment-dose-arm patients received a reduced "therapeutic" dose.[55]

In addition to therapeutic- versus prophylactic-dose anticoagulation, a trial designed specifically to test the intermediate-dose strategy was proposed to minimize bleeding risk in severely ill patients. The INSPIRATION trial enrolled 562 patients in an ICU setting randomized to prophylactic-dose enoxaparin 40 mg daily (with adjustments for renal function) versus an intermediate-dose regimen of 1 mg/kg daily. In this study, there was no significant difference in the rate of venous or arterial thrombosis, organ support on extracorporeal membrane oxygenation, or mortality at 30 days.[56]

Utilization of D-Dimer in Coronavirus Disease 2019

Many clinical laboratories have been proposed to prognosticate risk of thrombosis in COVID-19, with D-dimer receiving considerable attention. D-dimer is a degradation product of fibrin formation and, before COVID-19, was used to rule out PE in patients with a low pretest probability.[57] In COVID-19, many studies have demonstrated that elevated D-dimer levels are associated with an increased risk of disease progression and/or mortality.[44,58–60] In one study, only 24% of survivors of COVID-19 were found to have a D-dimer level greater than 1 μg/mL, whereas 81% of nonsurvivors had a D-dimer level greater than 1 μg/mL.[35] A similar study found that 85% of patients with a D-dimer level greater than 3 μg/mL did not survive, suggesting prognostic value to the test.[2]

D-dimer level is very commonly elevated during acute SARS-CoV-2 infection, particularly in hospitalized patients, rendering D-dimer of limited use in the assessment of VTE.[54,61] In a study of people with suspected PEs with COVID-19, 91% of patients without PEs had an elevated D-dimer level (0.05 μg/mL or greater). The same D-dimer cutoff yielded a 100% negative predictive value but only a 14% positive predictive value.[62] Another study evaluating patients with COVID-19 with D-dimer levels greater than 1000 ng/mL found that only 14.7% had asymptomatic DVT.[63] Although higher cutoff values were more likely to be associated with DVT, there is currently no consensus on the D-dimer cutoff that should prompt further imaging.

D-dimer elevations may be due to microthrombotic events and disseminated intravascular coagulation, which are not assessed by imaging modalities. Specifically, at high risk is microthrombosis within the pulmonary vasculature due to regional inflammatory response. Owing to this concern, researchers began looking at whether anticoagulation would affect outcomes in patients with COVID-19 with elevated D-dimer levels. Notably, treatment effects stratified by D-dimer yielded inconsistent results. One study of ~450 patients, which found no overall difference in 28-day mortality with anticoagulation in hospitalized patients with COVID-19, demonstrated a significant reduction in mortality in patients with sepsis-induced coagulopathy (SIC) score greater than 4 or a D-dimer level greater than 6 times upper limit of normal.[64] A subsequent study in which there was a prespecified analysis of patients stratified by D-dimer, reported no significant differences in treatment effect in critically ill patients with high versus low D-dimer levels.[54] In noncritically ill patients with COVID-19, the probability of superiority for therapeutic anticoagulation was slightly more in the high D-dimer group (97.3%) compared with the low D-dimer group (92.9%), but regardless of the D-dimer value, therapeutic anticoagulation was superior to prophylactic dosing.[53]

There are several caveats when assessing the use of D-dimer in COVID-19. D-dimer can be measured using numerous assays, protocols vary across clinical laboratories, and the results are reported in many different units, collectively, making comparison across institutions challenging.[65] Before COVID-19, studies using age-adjusted values for D-dimer were better able to exclude PE in patients.[66] Age adjustment of D-dimer was done in few studies described herein, despite older patients being well represented in clinical trials of COVID-19.[62] D-dimer elevations can persist in 25% of people for at least 4 months after acute SARS-CoV-2 infection.[62,67] In addition, many factors can elevate a D-dimer level including age, liver disease, malignancy, pregnancy, and sepsis, rendering interpretation in patients with COVID-19 with other conditions less straightforward.[65]

In summary, an elevated D-dimer level is common in COVID-19, particularly in critically ill patients. If a patient with COVID-19 has a low D-dimer level, VTE is unlikely. Multiple studies demonstrate that the higher the D-dimer level, the greater the likelihood of VTE and poor clinical outcomes, but there is no consensus across studies regarding the cutoff value for D-dimer level to prompt imaging for VTE in COVID-19. Further study is needed before an isolated elevation in a D-dimer is sufficient to justify empiric full-dose anticoagulation or trigger evaluations for PE or DVTs in the setting of SARS-CoV-2 infection.

SUMMARY OF CURRENT GUIDELINES

The American Society of Hematology (ASH) suggests the use of prophylactic- over intermediate-dose (recommendation 1A) and prophylactic- over therapeutic-dose anticoagulation (recommendation 1B) in critically ill patients with COVID-19. These suggestions apply to patients who should be admitted to an ICU due to "an immediate life-threatening condition" and do not have suspected or confirmed VTE. ASH suggests the use of therapeutic-dose over prophylactic-dose anticoagulation (recommendation 1B) in patients with acute illness due to COVID-19. This recommendation applies to patients who are not critically ill, do not have suspected or confirmed VTE, or do not have another condition requiring treatment-dose anticoagulation.[68]

The NIH recommends therapeutic heparin dosing for hospitalized patients on low-flow oxygen with elevated D-dimer levels who are not in the ICU and without known contraindications (CIIa); it recommends prophylactic heparin dosing in patients in the ICU with COVID-19 (AI). For patients transferred from the floor to the ICU the NIH recommends switching from therapeutic- to prophylactic-dose heparin (BIII). The NIH does not recommend prophylactic anticoagulation or antiplatelet therapy in outpatients with COVID-19 (AIIa). The aforementioned recommendations apply to patients with COVID-19 without confirmed or suspected VTE. The NIH reports insufficient evidence to recommend routine screening for VTE in all patients with COVID-19, irrespective of their coagulation values; however, in hospitalized patients with sudden clinical deteriorations they recommend assessment for VTE (AIII). The NIH recommends patients on chronic anticoagulation or antiplatelet treatments at home continue those during their acute COVID-19 illness (AIII).[25]

MANAGEMENT SUMMARY

Given the aforementioned reduction in organ support-free days shown in ACTIV-4A, the authors recommend use of full-dose intravenous heparin to treat moderately ill patients (those on < 20 L NC O_2) admitted to the hospital with COVID-19;. This effect may reflect the impact of heparin beyond ATIII inhibition including degradation of NETs and mitigation of the SARS-CoV-2 spike protein binding, but further mechanistic studies are needed.[15,69,70]

SUMMARY

Patients with COVID-19 are prone to venous, cerebrovascular, and coronary thrombi, particularly those with severe disease. The pathogenesis is multifactorial involving proinflammatory cascades and development of coagulopathy, but further investigations are needed to elucidate the mechanisms by which host-viral interactions promote thrombus formation. Elevated D-dimer levels are common in patients with COVID-19 and cannot be used in isolation to predict VTE in people with SARS-CoV-2. If given early in hospital admission, therapeutic-dose heparin improves clinical outcomes in patients with moderate COVID-19. To date antithrombotics have not improved outcomes in patients with severe COVID-19, possibly because significant tissue damage has already occurred. Finally, prompt recognition of extrapulmonary thrombi—particularly in the brain and heart—may be beneficial, but additional studies are needed and interventional response times may be limited by local resources.

CLINICS CARE POINTS

- The pathogenesis of SARS-CoV-2 is exacerbated by microthrombi and macrothrombi that compromise circulation and threaten organ function.
- Imaging for thrombi should be included as part of the assessment of patients with COVID-19 with significant sudden clinical deteriorations.
- To date, severely ill patients with COVID-19 do not significantly benefit from full-dose antithrombotic therapy.

ACKNOWLEGDGMENTS

Funding sources are : NIH NHLBI 1K08HL124191, CFF K Boost HUDOCK20, NIH NHLBI K08HL124191-04S1

REFERENCES

1. Iba T, Levy JH, Levi M, et al. Coagulopathy in COVID-19. J Thromb Haemost 2020;18(9):2103–9.
2. Tang N, Li D, Wang X, et al. Abnormal coagulation parameters are associated with poor prognosis in patients with novel coronavirus pneumonia. J Thromb Haemost 2020;18(4):844–7.
3. Polimeni A, Leo I, Spaccarotella C, et al. Differences in coagulopathy indices in patients with severe versus non-severe COVID-19: a meta-analysis of 35 studies and 6427 patients. Sci Rep 2021;11(1):10464–x.
4. Gaertner F, Massberg S. Blood coagulation in immunothrombosis-at the frontline of intravascular immunity. Semin Immunol 2016;28(6):561–9.
5. Gollomp K, Sarkar A, Harikumar S, et al. Fc-modified HIT-like monoclonal antibody as a novel treatment for sepsis. Blood 2020;135(10):743–54.
6. Becker RC. COVID-19 update: covid-19-associated coagulopathy. J Thromb Thrombolysis 2020;50(1):54–67.

7. Brinkmann V, Reichard U, Goosmann C, et al. Neutrophil extracellular traps kill bacteria. Science 2004;303(5663):1532–5.

8. Szturmowicz M, Demkow U. Neutrophil extracellular traps (NETs) in severe SARS-CoV-2 lung disease. Int J Mol Sci 2021;22(16):8854.

9. Fuchs TA, Brill A, Duerschmied D, et al. Extracellular DNA traps promote thrombosis. Proc Natl Acad Sci U S A 2010;107(36):15880–5.

10. Caudrillier A, Kessenbrock K, Gilliss BM, et al. Platelets induce neutrophil extracellular traps in transfusion-related acute lung injury. J Clin Invest 2012;122(7):2661–71.

11. Gollomp K, Kim M, Johnston I, et al. Neutrophil accumulation and NET release contribute to thrombosis in HIT. JCI Insight 2018;3(18):e99445.

12. Kimball AS, Obi AT, Diaz JA, et al. The emerging role of NETs in venous thrombosis and immunothrombosis. Front Immunol 2016;7:236.

13. Veras FP, Pontelli MC, Silva CM, et al. SARS-CoV-2-triggered neutrophil extracellular traps mediate COVID-19 pathology. J Exp Med 2020;217(12):e20201129.

14. Middleton EA, He XY, Denorme F, et al. Neutrophil extracellular traps contribute to immunothrombosis in COVID-19 acute respiratory distress syndrome. Blood 2020;136(10):1169–79.

15. Leppkes M, Knopf J, Naschberger E, et al. Vascular occlusion by neutrophil extracellular traps in COVID-19. EBioMedicine 2020;58:102925.

16. Zuo Y, Yalavarthi S, Shi H, et al. Neutrophil extracellular traps in COVID-19. JCI Insight 2020;5(11):e138999.

17. Radermecker C, Detrembleur N, Guiot J, et al. Neutrophil extracellular traps infiltrate the lung airway, interstitial, and vascular compartments in severe COVID-19. J Exp Med 2020;217(12):e20201012.

18. Hudock KM, Collins MS, Imbrogno M, et al. Neutrophil extracellular traps activate IL-8 and IL-1 expression in human bronchial epithelia. Am J Physiol Lung Cell Mol Physiol 2020;319(1):L137–47.

19. Perico L, Benigni A, Casiraghi F, et al. Immunity, endothelial injury and complement-induced coagulopathy in COVID-19. Nat Rev Nephrol 2021;17(1):46–64. https://www.ncbi.nlm.nih.gov/pubmed/33077917.

20. Loo J, Spittle DA, Newnham M. COVID-19, immunothrombosis and venous thromboembolism: biological mechanisms. Thorax 2021;76(4):412–20. https://doi.org/10.1136/thoraxjnl-2020-216243.

21. Klok FA, Kruip MJHA, van der Meer NJM, et al. Incidence of thrombotic complications in critically ill ICU patients with COVID-19. Thromb Res 2020;191:145–7.

22. Llitjos JF, Leclerc M, Chochois C, et al. High incidence of venous thromboembolic events in anticoagulated severe COVID-19 patients. J Thromb Haemost 2020;18(7):1743–6.

23. Nahum J, Morichau-Beauchant T, Daviaud F, et al. Venous thrombosis among critically ill patients with coronavirus disease 2019 (COVID-19). JAMA Netw Open 2020;3(5):e2010478.

24. Al-Samkari H, Gupta S, Leaf RK, et al. Thrombosis, bleeding, and the observational effect of early therapeutic anticoagulation on survival in critically ill patients with COVID-19. Ann Intern Med 2021;174(5):622–32.

25. NIH COVID-19 treatment guidelines in COVID-19: antithrombotic therapy. Available at: https://www.covid19treatmentguidelines.nih.gov/therapies/antithrombotic-therapy/. Accessed March 1, 2022.

26. Bekelis K, Missios S, Ahmad J, et al. Ischemic stroke occurs less frequently in patients with COVID-19: a multicenter cross-sectional study. Stroke 2020;51(12):3570–6.

27. Qureshi AI, Baskett WI, Huang W, et al. Acute ischemic stroke and COVID-19: an analysis of 27 676 patients. Stroke 2021;52(3):905–12.

28. Nannoni S, de Groot R, Bell S, et al. Stroke in COVID-19: a systematic review and meta-analysis. Int J Stroke 2021;16(2):137–49.

29. Siepmann T, Sedghi A, Simon E, et al. Increased risk of acute stroke among patients with severe COVID-19: a multicenter study and meta-analysis. Eur J Neurol 2021;28(1):238–47.

30. Lu Y, Zhao JJ, Ye MF, et al. The relationship between COVID-19's severity and ischemic stroke: a systematic review and meta-analysis. Neurol Sci 2021;42(7): 2645–51.

31. Li B, Yang J, Zhao F, et al. Prevalence and impact of cardiovascular metabolic diseases on COVID-19 in China. Clin Res Cardiol 2020;109(5):531–8.

32. Bangalore S, Sharma A, Slotwiner A, et al. ST-segment elevation in patients with covid-19 - a case series. N Engl J Med 2020;382(25):2478–80.

33. Huang C, Wang Y, Li X, et al. Clinical features of patients infected with 2019 novel coronavirus in wuhan, China. Lancet 2020;395(10223):497–506.

34. Lippi G, Lavie CJ, Sanchis-Gomar F. Cardiac troponin I in patients with coronavirus disease 2019 (COVID-19): evidence from a meta-analysis. Prog Cardiovasc Dis 2020;63(3):390–1.

35. Zhou F, Yu T, Du R, et al. Clinical course and risk factors for mortality of adult inpatients with COVID-19 in wuhan, China: a retrospective cohort study. Lancet 2020;395(10229):1054–62.

36. Shi S, Qin M, Shen B, et al. Association of cardiac injury with mortality in hospitalized patients with COVID-19 in wuhan, China. JAMA Cardiol 2020;5(7):802–10.

37. Zhang L, Fan Y, Lu Z. Experiences and lesson strategies for cardiology from the COVID-19 outbreak in wuhan, China, by 'on the scene' cardiologists. Eur Heart J 2020;41(19):1788–90.

38. Choudry FA, Hamshere SM, Rathod KS, et al. High thrombus burden in patients with COVID-19 presenting with ST-segment elevation myocardial infarction. J Am Coll Cardiol 2020;76(10):1168–76.

39. Kurdi H, Obaid DR, UlHaq Z, et al. Multiple spontaneous coronary thrombosis causing ST-elevation myocardial infarction in a patient with COVID-19. Br J Hosp Med (Lond) 2020;81(7):1–6.

40. Pellegrini D, Kawakami R, Guagliumi G, et al. Microthrombi as a major cause of cardiac injury in COVID-19: a pathologic study. Circulation 2021;143(10): 1031–42.

41. Stefanini G, Montorfano M, Trabattoni D, et al. ST-elevation myocardial infarction in patients with COVID-19: clinical and angiographic outcomes. Circulation 2020; 141(25):2113–6. Available at: http://ovidsp.ovid.com/ovidweb.cgi?T=JS&NEWS= n&CSC=Y&PAGE=fulltext&D=ovft&AN=00003017-202006230-00013. Accessed 1 February 2022.

42. McGill SN, Ahmed NA, Christou NV. Endothelial cells: role in infection and inflammation. World J Surg 1998;22(2):171–8.

43. Kwong JC, Schwartz KL, Campitelli MA, et al. Acute myocardial infarction after laboratory-confirmed influenza infection. N Engl J Med 2018;378(4):345–53.

44. Wu C, Chen X, Cai Y, et al. Risk factors associated with acute respiratory distress syndrome and death in patients with coronavirus disease 2019 pneumonia in wuhan, China. JAMA Intern Med 2020;180(7):934–43.

45. Mahmud E, Dauerman HL, Welt FGP, et al. Management of acute myocardial infarction during the COVID-19 pandemic: a position statement from the society for cardiovascular angiography and interventions (SCAI), the american college of

cardiology (ACC), and the american college of emergency physicians (ACEP). J Am Coll Cardiol 2020;76(11):1375–84.

46. Guan WJ, Ni ZY, Hu Y, et al. Clinical characteristics of coronavirus disease 2019 in China. N Engl J Med 2020;382(18):1708–20.

47. Capell WH, Barnathan ES, Piazza G, et al. Rationale and design for the study of rivaroxaban to reduce thrombotic events, hospitalization and death in outpatients with COVID-19: the PREVENT-HD study. Am Heart J 2021;235:12–23.

48. Barco S, Bingisser R, Colucci G, et al. Enoxaparin for primary thromboprophylaxis in ambulatory patients with coronavirus disease-2019 (the OVID study): a structured summary of a study protocol for a randomized controlled trial. Trials 2020;21(1):770–4.

49. Connors JM, Brooks MM, Sciurba FC, et al. Effect of antithrombotic therapy on clinical outcomes in outpatients with clinically stable symptomatic COVID-19: the ACTIV-4B randomized clinical trial. JAMA 2021;326(17):1703–12.

50. Lopes RD, de Barros E Silva PGM, Furtado RHM, et al. Therapeutic versus prophylactic anticoagulation for patients admitted to hospital with COVID-19 and elevated D-dimer concentration (ACTION): an open-label, multicentre, randomised, controlled trial. Lancet 2021;397(10291):2253–63.

51. Billett HH, Reyes-Gil M, Szymanski J, et al. Anticoagulation in COVID-19: effect of enoxaparin, heparin, and apixaban on mortality. Thromb Haemost 2020;120(12):1691–9.

52. Abdulakeem A, Acosta A, Ahmad S, et al. Aspirin in patients admitted to hospital with COVID-19 (RECOVERY): a randomised, controlled, open-label, platform trial. Lancet (British edition) 2022;399(10320):143–51. https://doi.org/10.1016/S0140-6736(21)01825-0. doi: 10.1016/S0140-6736(21)01825-0. Available at:.

53. ATTACC Investigators, ACTIV-4a Investigators, REMAP-CAP Investigators, et al. Therapeutic anticoagulation with heparin in noncritically ill patients with covid-19. N Engl J Med 2021;385(9):790–802.

54. REMAP-CAP Investigators, ACTIV-4a Investigators, ATTACC Investigators, et al. Therapeutic anticoagulation with heparin in critically ill patients with covid-19. N Engl J Med 2021;385(9):777–89.

55. Sholzberg M, Tang GH, Rahhal H, et al. Effectiveness of therapeutic heparin versus prophylactic heparin on death, mechanical ventilation, or intensive care unit admission in moderately ill patients with covid-19 admitted to hospital: RAPID randomised clinical trial. BMJ 2021;375:n2400.

56. INSPIRATION Investigators, Sadeghipour P, Talasaz AH, et al. Effect of intermediate-dose vs standard-dose prophylactic anticoagulation on thrombotic events, extracorporeal membrane oxygenation treatment, or mortality among patients with COVID-19 admitted to the intensive care unit: the INSPIRATION randomized clinical trial. JAMA 2021;325(16):1620–30.

57. Douma RA, Gibson NS, Gerdes VEA, et al. Validity and clinical utility of the simplified wells rule for assessing clinical probability for the exclusion of pulmonary embolism. Thromb Haemost 2009;101(1):197–200. Available at: https://www.narcis.nl/publication/RecordID/oai:pure.amc.nl:publications%2F1f997371-8e88-4407-8edb-97c6c6b4df68. Accessed 1 February 2022.

58. Cummings MJ, Baldwin MR, Abrams D, et al. Epidemiology, clinical course, and outcomes of critically ill adults with COVID-19 in New York city: a prospective cohort study. Lancet (British Edition) 2020;395(10239):1763–70.

59. García-Cervera C, Giner-Galvañ V, Wikman-Jorgensen P, et al. Estimation of admission D-dimer cut-off value to predict venous thrombotic events in hospitalized COVID-19 patients: analysis of the SEMI-COVID-19 registry. J Gen Intern

Med 2021;36(11):3478–86. Available at: https://link.springer.com/article/10.1007/s11606-021-07017-8. Accessed 1 February 2022.

60. Varikasuvu SR, Varshney S, Dutt N, et al. D-dimer, disease severity, and deaths (3D-study) in patients with COVID-19: a systematic review and meta-analysis of 100 studies. Scientific Rep 2021;11(1):21888. Available at: https://search.proquest.com/docview/2594889360. Accessed 1 February 2022.

61. Berger J, Kunichoff D, Adhikari S, et al. Prevalence and outcomes of D-dimer elevation in hospitalized patients with COVID-19. Arterioscler Thromb Vasc Biol 2020;40(10):2539–47. Available at: http://ovidsp.ovid.com/ovidweb.cgi?T=JS&NEWS=n&CSC=Y&PAGE=fulltext&D=ovft&AN=00043605-202010000-00019. Accessed 1 February 2022.

62. Logothetis CN, Weppelmann TA, Jordan A, et al. D-dimer testing for the exclusion of pulmonary embolism among hospitalized patients with COVID-19. JAMA Netw Open 2021;4(10):e2128802.

63. Demelo-Rodríguez P, Cervilla-Muñoz E, Ordieres-Ortega L, et al. Incidence of asymptomatic deep vein thrombosis in patients with COVID-19 pneumonia and elevated D-dimer levels. Thromb Res 2020;192:23–6.

64. Tang N, Bai H, Chen X, et al. Anticoagulant treatment is associated with decreased mortality in severe coronavirus disease 2019 patients with coagulopathy. J Thromb Haemost 2020;18(5):1094–9. Available at: https://onlinelibrary.wiley.com/doi/abs/10.1111/jth.14817. Accessed 1 February 2022.

65. Johnson ED, Schell JC, Rodgers GM. The d-dimer assay. Am J Hematol 2019;94(7):833–9. Available at: https://onlinelibrary.wiley.com/doi/abs/10.1002/ajh.25482. Accessed 1 February 2022.

66. Righini M, Van Es J, Den Exter PL, et al. Age-adjusted D-dimer cutoff levels to rule out pulmonary embolism: the ADJUST-PE study. JAMA 2014;311(11):1117–24.

67. Townsend L, Fogarty H, Dyer A, et al. Prolonged elevation of d-dimer levels in convalescent COVID-19 patients is independent of the acute phase response. J Thromb Haemost 2021;19(4):1064–70. Available at: https://onlinelibrary.wiley.com/doi/abs/10.1111/jth.15267. Accessed 1 February 2022.

68. American society of hematology guidelines on anticoagulation in patients with COVID-19. Available at: https://www.hematology.org/education/clinicians/guidelines-and-quality-care/clinical-practice-guidelines/venous-thromboembolism-guidelines/ash-guidelines-on-use-of-anticoagulation-in-patients-with-covid-19. Accessed March 1, 2022.

69. Clausen TM, Sandoval DR, Spliid CB, et al. SARS-CoV-2 infection depends on cellular heparan sulfate and ACE2. Cell 2020;183(4):1043–57.e15.

70. Paiardi G, Richter S, Oreste P, et al. The binding of heparin to spike glycoprotein inhibits SARS-CoV-2 infection by three mechanisms. J Biol Chem 2022;298(2):101507.

71. The RECOVERY Collaborative Group. Dexamethasone in Hospitalized Patients with COVID-19. New England Journal of Medicine 2021;384(8):693–704.

72. Mao Ling. Neurologic Manifestations of Hospitalized Patients with Coronavirus Disease 2019 in Wuhan, China. JAMA Neurology 2020;77(6):683–90.

73. Annie Frank. Prevalence and Outcomes of Acute Ischemic Stroke Among Patients <50 years of Age with Laboratory Confirmed COVID-19 Infection. American Journal of Cardiology 2020;130:169–70.

74. Liu Jie. A sharp decline in bruden of stroke in rural China during COVID-19 pandemic. Frontiers in Neurology 2021;11:596871.

75. https://clinicaltrials.gov/ct2/show/NCT04492254. Accessed March 5, 2022.

COVID-19 Acute Respiratory Distress Syndrome

One Pathogen, Multiple Phenotypes

Susannah Empson, MD[a],*, Angela J. Rogers, MD[b],
Jennifer G. Wilson, MD, MS[c]

KEYWORDS

- ARDS • COVID-19 • Subtypes • Phenotypes

KEY POINTS

- COVID-19 acute respiratory distress syndrome (ARDS) represents a distinct subset of ARDS.
- Significant clinical heterogeneity exists within COVID-19 ARDS despite a single causative agent.
- Several physiologically, clinically, and biologically derived phenotypes of COVID-19 ARDS have been identified.
- Phenotypic stratification in COVID-19 ARDS has value for both prognostic and predictive enrichment.

INTRODUCTION

Severe acute respiratory syndrome coronavirus 2 (SARS CoV-2) is the novel respiratory virus responsible for the COVID-19 pandemic, which in less than 2 years has caused more than 4.5 million deaths worldwide.[1] In its most severe form, COVID-19 causes acute respiratory distress syndrome (ARDS), a syndrome defined by acute onset hypoxemia ($Pao_2:Fio_2 < 300$) with bilateral infiltrates not otherwise explained by volume overload or cardiac failure.[2]

ARDS is a clinically heterogeneous syndrome arising from multiple causes (pneumonia, aspiration, trauma, sepsis, pancreatitis, and so forth) and with a range of clinical severity. Although the landmark ARDS Network trials showed a mortality benefit from lung protective ventilation, subsequent experimental therapies have failed to demonstrate consistent benefit.[3–9] One plausible explanation for the numerous negative trials, despite high-quality preliminary evidence, is the substantial heterogeneity

[a] Department of Anesthesiology, Perioperative, and Pain Medicine, 300 Pasteur Drive, H3580, Stanford, CA 94305, USA; [b] Department of Pulmonary, Allergy & Critical Care Medicine, 300 Pasteur Drive, H3153, Stanford, CA 94305, USA; [c] Department of Emergency Medicine, 900 Welch Road, Suite 350, Stanford, CA 94305, USA
* Corresponding author.
E-mail address: sfempson@stanford.edu

Crit Care Clin 38 (2022) 505–519
https://doi.org/10.1016/j.ccc.2022.02.001
0749-0704/22/© 2022 Elsevier Inc. All rights reserved.

within the ARDS population; this has led to an interest in identifying more homogeneous subgroups or phenotypes within ARDS for both prognostic and predictive enrichment. Prognostic enrichment enables identification of patients at highest risk for poor outcomes, thereby increasing the power to detect a therapeutic benefit with an intervention, should one exist. Predictive enrichment allows for selection of patients most likely to respond to a given therapy, thereby amplifying the effect of a particular treatment of any given sample size. Both strategies are recommended by the Food and Drug Administration and increase the efficacy of clinical trials.[10] Thus far, several physiologically, clinically, and biologically derived subphenotypes have been identified (**Table 1**) with the potential to more efficiently and effectively test and tailor interventions to the unique profile of the patient.[11,12]

In contrast to the general ARDS population, patients with COVID-19 ARDS have a single unifying causative agent and might therefore be expected to show less clinical heterogeneity. Nevertheless, the spectrum of disease severity observed in COVID-19 can range from asymptomatic to fulminant hypoxemic respiratory failure. The reasons for this marked variation in disease severity are incompletely understood but are hypothesized to include both host and pathogen factors.[13,14] Even among the subset of COVID-19 patients who develop COVID-19 ARDS, there is a spectrum of physiology, biomarker expression, and outcomes, and controversy remains as to which patients should be treated with which therapies. Furthermore, we remain unable to predict, nor can we fully explain, why some patients improve and others develop

Table 1
Proposed acute respiratory distress syndrome and COVID-19 acute respiratory distress syndrome phenotypes

Phenotype	ARDS	COVID-19 ARDS
Physiologic	Hypoxemia (Pao_2:Fio_2) Lung water/weight Dead space fraction Ventilatory ratio Driving pressure	Hypoxemia (level of respiratory support) Lung compliance
Clinical	Direct/indirect Early/late (time of onset, duration) Trauma-related/medical Radiographic patterns (focal/diffuse) Extrapulmonary organ involvement (AKI)	Demographic characteristics Medical comorbidities Radiographic characteristics Early/late (time since symptom onset) Worsening/recovering Extrapulmonary organ involvement

Biological	Genomic (genome-wide association)
	Transcriptomic (microRNA analysis)
	Proteomic (biomarkers)
	• Inflammation
	• Endothelial injury
	• Epithelial injury
	• Impaired coagulation
	Metabolomic
	Hyper/hypoinflammatory
		Genomic
		Transcriptomic
		Proteomic
		• Pathogen Factors
		  ○ Viral variant
		  ○ Viral kinetics (viral load at 7–14 d)
		  ○ Viremia
		• Host Factors
		  ○ Serostatus
		  ○ Hypo-/hyperinflammatory
		  ○ Coagulation profile
		Metabolomic

persistent or fatal disease. As with ARDS in general, therefore, there is substantial interest in identifying more homogeneous subgroups of COVID-19 ARDS within the broader population. In order to be clinically meaningful, however, these subgroups must be more than mere descriptions of different clinical presentations and patterns of disease. Phenotypes of COVID-19 ARDS are valuable only if they are[1] feasibly identifiable and[2] improve our ability to prognosticate or predict treatment response.

In this review, the authors summarize the existing literature on clinically meaningful COVID-19 ARDS phenotypes, including the impact of the timeline of disease progression on phenotypic features, how these phenotypes are compared with known ARDS phenotypes, and how this approach may be leveraged to improve both prognostication and precision therapy.

PHYSIOLOGIC PHENOTYPES IN COVID-19 ACUTE RESPIRATORY DISTRESS SYNDROME
Severity of Hypoxemia

Codified within the Berlin consensus definition of ARDS, severity of hypoxemia has been used to stratify patients with ARDS both pre-COVID-19 and post-COVID-19.[2] Pre-COVID-19, many major clinical trials of ARDS used severity of hypoxemia as an enrichment strategy for their study population, enrolling patients with moderate-to-severe hypoxemia ($Pao_2:Fio_2$ <150).[4,5,15] To date, the most important clinical trials of therapies for acute hypoxemic respiratory failure due to COVID-19 have analyzed treatment effect based on level of respiratory support at the time of randomization. Although in theory level of respiratory support should correlate with degree of hypoxemia, because of institutional variation in timing of intubation and use of noninvasive positive pressure ventilation, this is likely an imperfect proxy. Nonetheless, multiple recent trials have shown important differences in treatment effect based on level of respiratory support at time of randomization. Most notably, the RECOVERY trial of dexamethasone showed maximal benefit in patients receiving invasive mechanical ventilation, less benefit in patients receiving supplemental oxygen but not mechanically ventilated, and a trend toward harm in patients on no oxygen therapy[16]; this raises questions about the mechanisms by which some therapies provide benefit to patients with lower severity of illness, whereas others seem to provide greater benefit to those with more severe disease. As discussed earlier, it may be that the degree of hypoxemia is best understood as a proxy for the time course and underlying biology, providing the clinician with important data on which patient is most likely to benefit from which therapy and when.

Lung Compliance

Early in the pandemic, Marini and Gattinoni noted that severity of hypoxemia alone was not sufficient to understand the "stages" of COVID-19 ARDS. They proposed phenotyping patients with COVID-19 ARDS according to lung compliance and advocated for a ventilation strategy that departed from traditional tenets of lung protective ventilation based on compliance phenotype. It was suggested that patients with preserved compliance (termed "L phenotype") be ventilated with lower PEEP and slightly higher tidal volumes, whereas patients with poor lung compliance ("H phenotype") be managed with a traditional lung protective ventilation strategy.[17] It has since been demonstrated, however, that patients with pre-COVID-19 ARDS also had a range of lung compliance early in disease,[18] and therefore current consensus is that a low tidal volume lung protective ventilation approach is appropriate for all patients with COVID-19 ARDS regardless of their compliance profile.[19] Nonetheless, Marini and Gattinoni introduced 2 fundamental concepts with which most experts now agree[1]: not all patients with COVID-19 ARDS have the same phenotype, and[2] an individual's phenotype may change over time.

CLINICAL PHENOTYPES OF COVID-19 ACUTE RESPIRATORY DISTRESS SYNDROME
Baseline Demographics and Comorbidities

Accepted risk factors for severe or fatal COVID-19 include older age, male sex, obesity, cardiovascular disease, diabetes, chronic lung, liver or kidney disease, immunocompromise, and active cancer.[20,21] Nonwhite race is also associated with higher risk of death from COVID-19 in the Unites States and United Kingdom, a disparity that is largely attributable to underlying socioeconomic disadvantage.[22,23] Age and comorbidities have been used as prognostic enrichment criteria for clinical trials in COVID-19, but once COVID-19 ARDS has developed, all patients are at high risk of death from hypoxemic respiratory failure and worsening extrapulmonary organ dysfunction, so these prognostic enrichment factors may be less important in terms of trial design. Beyond providing prognostic value, however, baseline patient phenotypes may help select patients for trials of more targeted therapies such as monoclonal antibodies in immunocompromised patients or SGLT2 inhibitors in diabetic or obese patients.[24] As with all subgroups of patients with COVID-19 ARDS, however, these baseline phenotypes may be more precisely characterized by combining them with other physiologic, clinical, or biological variables, all of which are discussed in other sections of this review.

Radiographic Findings

As with pre-COVID ARDS, radiographic findings associated with COVID-19 have been well described and correlate with disease severity.[25-29] Increasingly, studies have attempted to identify patterns on computed tomography (CT) that might serve as predictors of disease progression and mortality. Ruch and colleagues demonstrated that visual quantification of affected lung parenchyma on hospital admission CT was independently associated with disease severity.[30] In one retrospective study, the volume of affected lung as well as the rate of progression on serial CT scans performed within 5 days of symptom onset predicted progression to severe disease in advance of clinical decompensation.[31]

Pellegrini and colleagues used chest CT to describe the progression of lung injury in a small cohort of critically ill patients with COVID-19 ARDS, observing initially a predominantly subpleural distribution of hypo- and nonaerated sections of lung.[32] However, in those patients exposed to volutrauma, extensive centripetal progression of disease was noted. Similar radiographic findings were observed in those with a positive fluid balance and elevated ferritin and d-dimer levels and were associated with worsening gas exchange and pulmonary mechanics. Results of this study show that worsening radiographic lung injury correlates with multiple known risk factors for poor outcome, including duration of symptoms, volutrauma, positive fluid balance (and associated increase in lung weight), systemic inflammation, and hypercoagulability. Whether this subset of patients with worsening CT findings represents a distinct phenotype of COVID-19 ARDS or the end stage of disease progression remains unclear, and although radiographic phenotyping can prove prognostically useful, it is uncertain whether or how it should guide management.

Time Since Symptom Onset and Trajectory of Disease

The importance of time since symptom onset in terms of selecting COVID-19 therapies has been apparent from the beginning of the pandemic. Many patients will not develop severe illness until a week or more after onset of symptoms. In light of this, several clinical trials have limited enrollment to patients who are within a certain window from symptom onset or planned subgroup analyses based on time since symptom onset (ACTIV-3, RECOVERY).[16,33] The rationale for this is clearly based on the temporal dynamics of peak viral load and antibody/immune response (**Fig. 1** below).[34] Although point-of-care tests for antibody status are in development, until such tests are available, time since symptom onset may serve as a way to categorize patients, with "earlier" patients more likely to benefit from therapies focused on inhibiting viral replication and enhancing viral clearance (such as antiviral therapy and monoclonal antibodies), and "later" patients more likely to benefit from immunomodulating therapies. In support of this idea, the RECOVERY trial of dexamethasone discussed earlier showed no benefit in patients who were less than 7 days from symptom onset.[16] Of course, the exact timing of onset of symptoms, peak of viral load, and antibody production and inflammasome activation varies from patient to patient. Thus, although time since symptom onset may be a pragmatic way to classify patients, direct measurement of antibody serostatus or inflammatory markers (as discussed in detail later) or combination of time course with other clinical or physiologic markers (such as need for oxygen therapy) is likely a more precise approach to phenotyping patients with COVID-19 with worsening hypoxemic respiratory failure.

Another way to phenotype patients is based on the trajectory of their organ dysfunction. Su and colleagues describe 2 distinct phenotypes of organ failure trajectory among intubated patients with COVID-19 ARDS based on serial daily Sequential Organ Failure Assessment scores over the first 7 days postintubation: worsening or recovering.[35] These 2 groups were identified in all strata of illness severity, and baseline demographics, comorbidities, and organ dysfunction did not differ. Patients with the worsening phenotype in the mild and intermediate illness severity strata had worse outcomes than patients with the highest baseline severity of illness who had a recovering phenotype; this suggests that grouping patients with COVID-19 ARDS according to trajectory of extrapulmonary organ dysfunction postintubation is more prognostic than grouping them by baseline risk factors or severity of illness at time of intubation.

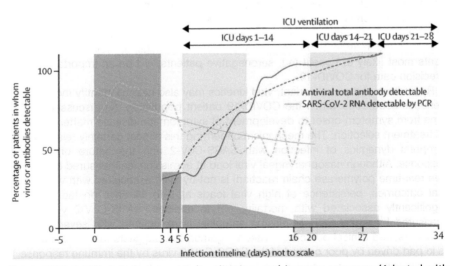

Fig. 1. SARS-CoV-2 clinical course, viral replication, and immune response. (Adapted with permission from https://www.thelancet.com/journals/lanres/article/PIIS2213-2600(20)30230-7/fulltext.)

Further, these findings reinforce the need to investigate the biological pathways driving the progressive extrapulmonary organ dysfunction seen in some but not all patients with COVID-19 ARDS.

Extrapulmonary Organ Dysfunction

Although respiratory failure is the leading cause of death for patients with COVID-19 ARDS, many patients develop multisystem organ dysfunction either before or after the onset of respiratory failure.[36,37] As one would expect, these patients have worse outcomes, and therefore, presence of extrapulmonary organ dysfunction in patients with worsening hypoxemia may be a low-effort, high-yield strategy for prognostic enrichment. Extrapulmonary organ dysfunction attributable to SARS-CoV-2 infection may also provide important clues about the underlying pathophysiology of severe disease in patients with COVID-19 ARDS. Multiple mechanisms by which SARS-CoV-2 causes multiorgan injury have been postulated, including direct viral toxicity, endothelial inflammation and thrombosis, systemic immune response, and dysregulation of the renin-angiotensin-aldosterone system.[38] Focusing future research on the biological profile of this phenotype of patients may therefore help prioritize targets for potential therapeutic intervention.

BIOLOGICAL PHENOTYPES OF COVID-19 ACUTE RESPIRATORY DISTRESS SYNDROME
SARS-CoV-2 Variants and Kinetics

As SARS-CoV-2 mutates over time, different variants of concern have emerged, with the B.1.617.2 (Delta) variant predominant in the United States as of Fall 2021.[39] Different variants may produce different disease manifestations, likely related to variation in angiotensin-converting enzyme 2 receptor binding affinity and degree of immune escape between different strains.[40] Certain therapies proved beneficial during a time when previous variants predominated may work differently in patients infected with a new variant; this has already occurred with combination bamlanivimab and etesevimab monoclonal antibody therapy, which had its emergency use authorization revised based on concern about continued use in areas where resistant variants are prevalent.[41] Thus rather than using a one-size-fits-all approach for COVID-19 therapies, tailoring treatments based on SARS-CoV-2 genomics, as well as targeting patients most likely to benefit (eg, seronegative patients) will be an important part of precision care for COVID-19.

Regardless of the viral variant, viral kinetics may also help us identify more homogeneous subgroups within the COVID-19 patient population. As discussed earlier, time from symptom onset to development of symptomatic disease matters in terms of treatment selection. The mechanism underlying this almost certainly relates to the temporal dynamics of infection with SARS-CoV-2 and the nature of the host response. Although nasopharyngeal viral load at admission (as measured by qualitative real-time polymerase chain reaction) is not by itself associated with worse clinical outcomes, persistence of high viral loads at 7 to 14 days postadmission is significantly associated with mortality.[42,43] In addition, SARS-CoV-2 viremia (as measured by digital PCR in plasma samples) is associated with severe disease and worsened clinical outcomes. Taken together, this suggests that severe disease is in part driven by poor control of the SARS-CoV-2 virus by the immune response.[16] Using viral kinetics and viremia may therefore be a feasible way to identify patients at highest risk for deterioration and most likely to derive benefit from antiviral therapies early in the course of disease.

Host Response: Serostatus

Although monoclonal antibody therapies (largely agents directed at various epitopes on the SARS-CoV-2 spike protein) have demonstrated benefit in high-risk outpatient populations, previous trials of monoclonal antibody therapies in hospitalized patients had failed to show benefit, even when enrollment was limited to patients with less than 12 days of symptoms.[44,45] The more recently released results from the RECOVERY trial of combination casirivimab and imdevimab for hospitalized COVID-19 suggests that the failure of monoclonal antibodies in previous inpatient trials may be explained by the serostatus of the patients enrolled: in this large randomized trial, although there was no benefit of therapy observed in the combined trial population (both seronegative and seropositive at baseline), there was a 20% reduction in mortality rate among patients who were seronegative at baseline.[46] Thus serostatus has already been shown to be a phenotypic feature by which treatment effect of antiviral therapies will differ and is more precise than using time since symptom onset as a surrogate marker. Because rapid turnaround antibody tests may not be available in all settings, time since symptom onset and severe immunocompromise may be important clinical features to consider when antibody testing is not feasible.

Host Response: Overview

The cascade of the immune and inflammatory response to SARS-CoV-2 infection is complex and incompletely understood. However, the proposed pathogenesis of COVID-19 ARDS is characterized by a dysregulated host response, leading to local and systemic inflammatory and thrombotic derangements. More specifically, infection triggers an immune response characterized by both T- and B-cell activation, leading to inflammatory cytokine release, activation of the complement and coagulation cascades, and resulting endothelial injury.[47] Autopsies of deceased patients demonstrate diffuse alveolar damage with leukocyte infiltration, microangiopathy, and thrombosis of the pulmonary capillaries.[48] The terms "endotheliitis" and "thromboinflammation" have been used to describe the pathogenesis of severe disease.[49,50] There has therefore been sustained interest in phenotyping patients according to their cytokine or coagulation profile, each of which is discussed later.

Host Response: Inflammatory Profile

Multiple studies have demonstrated high levels of inflammatory biomarkers in patients with COVID-19, and higher levels correlate with disease severity and clinical outcomes.[26,51–53] These data have therefore sparked an interest in "cytokine storm," as central to the pathogenesis of severe COVID-19.[54] Hypo- and hyperinflammatory phenotypes have been well described in the general ARDS population, and Sinha and colleagues were able to identify similar phenotypes in patients with COVID-19 ARDS.[55–59] As with general ARDS, the hyperinflammatory phenotype was associated with a higher mortality rate but was observed at a much lower prevalence than in the matched non-COVID-19 cohort. Furthermore, although proinflammatory cytokine/cytokine receptor (interleukin-6 [IL-6], soluble tumor necrosis factor receptor) levels were elevated, supporting a state of systemic inflammation, they were similar to or lower than those observed in the matched non–COVID-19-associated ARDS cohort.[60,61] Finally, mortality among both the hypo- and hyperinflammatory COVID-19 cohorts was higher than their matched counterparts. It is therefore hypothesized that COVID-19 ARDS has distinct pathophysiologic features compared with non–COVID-19 ARDS and that severity of disease is incompletely understood and not explained by "cytokine storm."

Nonetheless, multiple clinical trials have now demonstrated benefit to using antiinflammatory therapies in subgroups of patients with COVID-19 ARDS. Dexamethasone is recommended in all patients with COVID-19 who require supplemental oxygen and shows the greatest benefit in patients requiring mechanical ventilation at the time of randomization. In addition, tocilizumab (an anti-IL-6 therapy) and baricitinib (a JAK inhibitor) have now been proved beneficial in patients with markers of systemic inflammation.[62,63] Trials of these therapies used elevated C-reactive protein (CRP) (in the case of tocilizumab) and elevated D-dimer, lactate dehydrogenase, or ferritin (in the case of baricitinib) as enrollment criteria, thereby enriching the trial population for patients at higher risk for poor outcomes and most likely to benefit based on mechanism of these antiinflammatory therapies. Taken together, these studies add to the growing body of evidence that there is a subset of patients with COVID-19 with an inflammatory phenotype amenable to targeted therapy within a distinct time frame of clinical disease progression.

Unfortunately, with the exception of dexamethasone, little evidence exists to guide the use of antiinflammatory therapies in COVID-19 ARDS requiring intubation beyond the choice of initial therapy before or within 24 hours of intubation. The COV-BARRIER study of JAK inhibition excluded patients on mechanical ventilation at time of study entry.[63] The REMAP-CAP trial of anti-IL-6 therapy in the critically ill required randomization within 24 hours of initiating organ support in the intensive care unit, and the RECOVERY trial of anti-IL-6 therapy showed no benefit in patients who were already mechanically ventilated at the time of study entry.[62,64] Thus, an incredibly important question remains of how to manage patients with COVID-19 ARDS who have persistent organ dysfunction or elevated inflammatory markers despite initial treatment with dexamethasone or IL-6/JAK inhibition.

The multisystem inflammatory syndrome in children is a hyperinflammatory syndrome triggered by recent SARS-CoV-2 infection that has recognized diagnostic criteria and guidelines for suggested therapy.[65] There is now a working definition for a multisystem inflammatory syndrome in adults (MIS-A) as well, and glucocorticoids, anakinra (an IL-1 receptor antagonist), and intravenous immunoglobulin have been suggested as therapies for patients with this phenotype.[65–67] Indeed, although several studies have found that inflammatory cytokine levels in patients with COVID-19 ARDS are not markedly different from critically ill patients with sepsis or ARDS from other causes and are lower than those observed in cytokine release syndrome, noncytokine inflammatory biomarkers (D-dimer, CRP, ferritin) are elevated to a greater degree in COVID-19 than in other critical illnesses.[60,68] In addition to identifying patients with COVID-19 ARDS with potential MIS-A, several investigators have suggested that there is a subset of severely ill patients with a "macrophage activation syndrome" phenotype (identified by marked hyperferritinemia or a clinical score known as the H-score) in which IL-1 blockade should be considered.[69–71]

In summary, there are numerous approaches to identifying patients with COVID-19 ARDS who are showing signs of maladaptive inflammation and who may benefit from antiinflammatory therapies. The question of which approach should be used, and how signs of hyperinflammation should be interpreted and treated at different timepoints in the disease course will be a central focus for researchers going forward.[13]

Host Response: Coagulation Profile

As discussed earlier, the interaction between inflammation and hypercoagulability is a notable feature of severe COVID-19, and presence of both micro- and macrovascular thrombosis in patients with severe disease and ARDS has been well documented.[72–75] In addition, serum biomarkers of systemic coagulation have been independently associated with more severe forms of disease and poorer outcomes.[53,76–78] Clinically, coagulopathy most commonly manifests as high rates of venous thromboembolic disease, but microthrombosis of the pulmonary vasculature has also been posited as a mechanism for the increased dead space observed in COVID-19 ARDS.[79] Histopathologically, autopsies of deceased patients with COVID-19 demonstrate widespread platelet-fibrin activation and microthrombi in the alveolar capillaries.[80,81] Although the exact mechanism of coagulopathy is incompletely understood, it is hypothesized that virus-induced endothelial injury leads to inflammation and thrombosis. Furthermore, microthrombosis, coagulopathy, and subsequent endotheliitis have been theorized to play a central role in the development of extrapulmonary complications and multisystem organ failure.[47]

Despite the recognized role of micro- and macrovascular thrombosis in the pathogenesis of COVID-19, a large multiplatform randomized controlled trial of empirical therapeutic anticoagulation in hospitalized patients with COVID-19 yielded different results in critically and noncritically ill cohorts. In the noncritically ill cohort, therapeutic anticoagulation increased the probability of survival to hospital discharge and reduced the need for organ support, regardless of baseline D-dimer (although the effect was slightly greater in those with D-dimer levels >2x ULN).[82] In contrast, no benefit was observed among patients who were critically ill at the time of enrollment, and there was a trend toward harm.[83] One explanation posited for this discrepancy in treatment effect is that by the time patients have progressed to critical illness, the cascade of inflammation, thrombosis, and organ dysfunction has progressed to a degree where anticoagulation can no longer make a meaningful difference on outcomes. In this sense, the choice of anticoagulation dose in COVID-19 may depend not only on selecting patients most likely to benefit based on their coagulation profile but also on identifying the time point at which those patients are most likely to derive that benefit.

Aspirin has also been studied by the RECOVERY platform trial and unfortunately did not reduce 28-day mortality.[84] Studies of P2Y12 inhibitors are ongoing at the time of this review, and other trials of treatments with antithrombotic properties (eg crizanlizumab) are planned. Regardless of the outcomes of these trials, it is clear that endothelial dysfunction and platelet activation are prominent features of severe COVID-19, and future work focuses on identifying subsets of patients with COVID-19 most likely to benefit from antiplatelet and antithrombotic therapies.

Host Response: Genomics and Transcriptomics

The heterogeneity of COVID-19 ARDS has provoked interest in identifying biologically distinct phenotypes, and research has therefore increasingly focused on genomic and transcriptomic signatures with the hope of identifying host factors that predict poor outcomes and pathways for targeted therapies.[85–89] Preliminary work has focused predominantly on the host immune response, inflammatory, and coagulation cascade and has suggested an association between a cluster of genes encoding chemokine receptors and severe disease, as well as upregulation of genes involving inflammation, immunity, coagulation, and interferon signaling.[90–92] Furthermore, several multi-omics studies have identified distinct shifts in immunologic and inflammatory profiles between mild, moderate, and severe disease.[93–95] In addition to identifying targeted pathways for therapeutic intervention, transcriptomics in particular may shed light on the optimal timing of specific interventions. There is, however, significant work to be done to confirm associations between candidate genes, transcriptomic signatures, and clinically meaningful subphenotypes of COVID-19 ARDS. At this point, genomic and transcriptomic phenotyping of COVID-19 ARDS patients remains exploratory and unavailable outside of the research setting.

SUMMARY

Despite a unifying causative agent, the spectrum of disease observed in COVID-19 ARDS is broad, and although research is progressing at a rapid pace, the underlying reasons for this clinical heterogeneity remain incompletely understood. It is becoming increasingly accepted that COVID-19 ARDS is a distinct subset of ARDS with its own subphenotypes that bear some similarities to but also distinct differences from the broader syndrome. As DeMerle and colleagues remind us, however, phenotypic categorization is meaningful only to the extent that it offers plausible, easily identifiable, and reproducible frameworks to prognosticate and tailor treatment.[96] Although many recent and ongoing clinical trials have used combined physiologic, clinical, and biological phenotypes to identify and target patients most likely to benefit from a particular therapy, precision medicine for COVID-19 ARDS is still in its infancy. Years of work have led to identification of biological subphenotypes of sepsis and ARDS, but the clinical importance of these phenotypes has yet to be rigorously established in prospective clinical trials. For the clinician practicing in the midst of a dynamic global pandemic, therefore, keeping current with the outcomes of high-quality clinical trials for COVID-19 ARDS—and adhering to established evidence-based therapies for ARDS in the interim—remains best practice. The clinical relevance of many of the proposed phenotypes discussed in this review require ongoing prospective validation with the ultimate goal of bringing precision therapies for COVID-19 ARDS to the bedside.

CLINICS CARE POINTS

- Patients with COVID-19 ARDS have a similar range of lung compliance as patients with general ARDS, and adherence to classic ARDS strategies, including low tidal volume ventilation, remains the mainstay of care for COVID-19 ARDS.
- Oxygen requirement, markers of systemic inflammation, and timing since symptom onset can help guide treatment.
- Steroids (dexamethasone), anti-IL-6 therapy, and JAK1/2 inhibition have demonstrated therapeutic benefit in subsets of patients hospitalized with COVID-19.
- The clinical applicability of biological phenotypes in COVID-19 ARDS requires ongoing prospective validation.

DISCLOSURE

S. Empson has no conflict of interest to declare. A.J. Rogers is a pulmonary clinical trials advisor for Merck, not relevant to this work. J.G. Wilson has no conflict of interest to declare.

REFERENCES

1. WHO Coronavirus (COVID-19) Dashboard. Available at: https://covid19.who.int. Accessed October 1, 2021.
2. ARDS Definition Task Force, Ranieri VM, Rubenfeld GD, et al. Acute respiratory distress syndrome: the Berlin Definition. JAMA 2012;307(23):2526–33.
3. Ventilation with lower tidal volumes as compared with traditional tidal volumes for acute lung injury and the acute respiratory distress syndrome. N Engl J Med 2000;342(18):1301–8.

4. Papazian L, Forel JM, Gacouin A, et al. Neuromuscular blockers in early acute respiratory distress syndrome. N Engl J Med 2010;363(12):1107–16.

5. Early neuromuscular blockade in the acute respiratory distress syndrome. N Engl J Med 2019;380(21):1997–2008.

6. Rosuvastatin for sepsis-associated acute respiratory distress syndrome. N Engl J Med 2014;370(23):2191–200.

7. McAuley DF, Laffey JG, O'Kane CM, et al. Simvastatin in the acute respiratory distress syndrome. N Engl J Med 2014;371(18):1695–703.

8. Higher versus lower positive end-expiratory pressures in patients with the acute respiratory distress syndrome. N Engl J Med 2004;351(4):327–36.

9. National Heart, Lung, and Blood Institute Acute Respiratory Distress Syndrome (ARDS) Clinical Trials Network, Wiedemann HP, Wheeler AP, et al. Comparison of two fluid-management strategies in acute lung injury. N Engl J Med 2006; 354(24):2564–75.

10. FDA. Enrichment strategies for clinical trials to support approval of human drugs and biological products. Available from https://www-fda-gov.laneproxy.stanford.edu/media/121320/download. Accessed September 15, 2021.

11. Wilson JG, Calfee CS. ARDS subphenotypes: understanding a heterogeneous syndrome. Crit Care Lond Engl 2020;24(1):102.

12. Sinha P, Calfee CS. Phenotypes in acute respiratory distress syndrome: moving towards precision medicine. Curr Opin Crit Care 2019;25(1):12–20.

13. Sinha P, Calfee CS. Immunotherapy in COVID-19: why, who, and when? Lancet Respir Med 2021;9(6):549–51.

14. Gattinoni L, Chiumello D, Caironi P, et al. COVID-19 pneumonia: different respiratory treatments for different phenotypes? Intensive Care Med 2020;46(6): 1099–102.

15. Guérin C, Reignier J, Richard JC, et al. Prone positioning in severe acute respiratory distress syndrome. N Engl J Med 2013;368(23):2159–68.

16. RECOVERY Collaborative Group, Horby P, Lim WS, et al. Dexamethasone in hospitalized patients with Covid-19. N Engl J Med 2021;384(8):693–704.

17. Marini JJ, Gattinoni L. Management of COVID-19 respiratory distress. JAMA 2020;323(22):2329–30.

18. Panwar R, Madotto F, Laffey JG, et al. Compliance phenotypes in early acute respiratory distress syndrome before the COVID-19 Pandemic. Am J Respir Crit Care Med 2020;202(9):1244–52.

19. Botta M, Tsonas AM, Pillay J, et al. Ventilation management and clinical outcomes in invasively ventilated patients with COVID-19 (PRoVENT-COVID): a national, multicentre, observational cohort study. Lancet Respir Med 2021;9(2):139–48.

20. Williamson EJ, Walker AJ, Bhaskaran K, et al. Factors associated with COVID-19-related death using OpenSAFELY. Nature 2020;584(7821):430–6.

21. Harrison SL, Fazio-Eynullayeva E, Lane DA, et al. Comorbidities associated with mortality in 31,461 adults with COVID-19 in the United States: a federated electronic medical record analysis. PLOS Med 2020;17(9):e1003321.

22. Kabarriti R, Brodin NP, Maron MI, et al. Association of race and ethnicity with comorbidities and survival among patients with COVID-19 at an urban medical center in New York. JAMA Netw Open 2020;3(9):e2019795.

23. Muñoz-Price LS, Nattinger AB, Rivera F, et al. Racial disparities in incidence and outcomes among patients with COVID-19. JAMA Netw Open 2020;3(9): e2021892.

24. Kosiborod MN, Esterline R, Furtado RHM, et al. Dapagliflozin in patients with cardiometabolic risk factors hospitalised with COVID-19 (DARE-19): a randomised,

double-blind, placebo-controlled, phase 3 trial. Lancet Diabetes Endocrinol 2021;9(9):586–94.

25. Warren MA, Zhao Z, Koyama T, et al. Severity scoring of lung oedema on the chest radiograph is associated with clinical outcomes in ARDS. Thorax 2018; 73(9):840–6.

26. Huang C, Wang Y, Li X, et al. Clinical features of patients infected with 2019 novel coronavirus in Wuhan, China. Lancet Lond Engl 2020;395(10223):497–506.

27. Shi H, Han X, Jiang N, et al. Radiological findings from 81 patients with COVID-19 pneumonia in Wuhan, China: a descriptive study. Lancet Infect Dis 2020;20(4): 425–34.

28. Chung M, Bernheim A, Mei X, et al. CT imaging features of 2019 novel Corona-virus (2019-nCoV). Radiology 2020;295(1):202–7.

29. Bernheim A, Mei X, Huang M, et al. Chest CT Findings in Coronavirus Disease-19 (COVID-19): Relationship to Duration of Infection. Radiology 2020. https://doi.org/10.1148/radiol.2020200463. 200463.

30. Ruch Y, Kaeuffer C, Ohana M, et al. CT lung lesions as predictors of early death or ICU admission in COVID-19 patients. Clin Microbiol Infect 2020;26(10):1417.e5–8.

31. Li K, Liu X, Yip R, et al. Early prediction of severity in coronavirus disease (COVID-19) using quantitative CT imaging. Clin Imaging 2021;78:223–9.

32. Pellegrini M, Larina A, Mourtos E, et al. A quantitative analysis of extension and distribution of lung injury in COVID-19: a prospective study based on chest computed tomography. Crit Care Lond Engl 2021;25(1):276.

33. University of Minnesota. A multicenter, adaptive, randomized, blinded controlled trial of the safety and efficacy of investigational therapeutics for hospitalized patients with COVID-19. clinicaltrials.gov. 2021. Available at: https://clinicaltrials.gov/ct2/show/NCT04501978. Accessed September 30, 2021.

34. McGrath BA, Brenner MJ, Warrillow SJ, et al. Tracheostomy in the COVID-19 era: global and multidisciplinary guidance. Lancet Respir Med 2020;8(7):717–25.

35. Su C, Xu Z, Hoffman K, et al. Identifying organ dysfunction trajectory-based sub-phenotypes in critically ill patients with COVID-19. Sci Rep 2021;11(1):15872.

36. Elezkurtaj S, Greuel S, Ihlow J, et al. Causes of death and comorbidities in hospitalized patients with COVID-19. Sci Rep 2021;11(1):4263.

37. Gupta S, Hayek SS, Wang W, et al. Factors associated with death in critically ill patients with Coronavirus Disease 2019 in the US. JAMA Intern Med 2020; 180(11):1436–47.

38. Gupta A, Madhavan MV, Sehgal K, et al. Extrapulmonary manifestations of COVID-19. Nat Med 2020;26(7):1017–32.

39. CDC. COVID. Data tracker. Centers for Disease Control and Prevention. 2020. Available at: https://covid.cdc.gov/covid-data-tracker. Accessed September 30, 2021.

40. Khateeb J, Li Y, Zhang H. Emerging SARS-CoV-2 variants of concern and potential intervention approaches. Crit Care 2021;25(1):244.

41. Pica N. Bamlanivimab and Etesevimab Authorized States, Territories, and US Jurisdictions. :2.

42. Argyropoulos KV, Serrano A, Hu J, et al. Association of initial viral load in severe acute respiratory syndrome Coronavirus 2 (SARS-CoV-2) patients with outcome and symptoms. Am J Pathol 2020;190(9):1881–7.

43. Néant N, Lingas G, Le Hingrat Q, et al. Modeling SARS-CoV-2 viral kinetics and association with mortality in hospitalized patients from the French COVID cohort. Proc Natl Acad Sci U S A 2021;118(8). e2017962118.

44. NIH-sponsored ACTIV-3 clinical trial closes enrollment into two Sub-studies. National Institutes of Health (NIH). 2021. Available at: https://www.nih.gov/news-

events/news-releases/nih-sponsored-activ-3-clinical-trial-closes-enrollment-into-two-sub-studies. Accessed September 30, 2021.

45. ACTIV-3/TICO LY-CoV555 Study Group, Lundgren JD, Grund B, et al. A neutralizing monoclonal antibody for hospitalized patients with Covid-19. N Engl J Med 2021;384(10):905–14.

46. Group RC, Horby PW, Mafham M, et al. Casirivimab and Imdevimab in Patients Admitted to Hospital with COVID-19 (RECOVERY): A Randomised, Controlled, Open-Label, Platform Trial.; 2021:2021.06.15.21258542. doi:10.1101/2021.06.15.21258542

47. Osuchowski MF, Winkler MS, Skirecki T, et al. The COVID-19 puzzle: deciphering pathophysiology and phenotypes of a new disease entity. Lancet Respir Med 2021;9(6):622–42.

48. Maiese A, Manetti AC, La Russa R, et al. Autopsy findings in COVID-19-related deaths: a literature review. Forensic Sci Med Pathol 2021;17(2):279–96.

49. Talasaz AH, Sadeghipour P, Kakavand H, et al. Recent randomized trials of antithrombotic therapy for patients with COVID-19: JACC state-of-the-art review. J Am Coll Cardiol 2021;77(15):1903–21.

50. Teuwen LA, Geldhof V, Pasut A, et al. COVID-19: the vasculature unleashed. Nat Rev Immunol 2020;20(7):389–91.

51. Chen G, Wu D, Guo W, et al. Clinical and immunological features of severe and moderate coronavirus disease 2019. J Clin Invest 2020;130(5):2620–9.

52. Ruan Q, Yang K, Wang W, et al. Clinical predictors of mortality due to COVID-19 based on an analysis of data of 150 patients from Wuhan, China. Intensive Care Med 2020;46(5):846–8.

53. Zhou F, Yu T, Du R, et al. Clinical course and risk factors for mortality of adult inpatients with COVID-19 in Wuhan, China: a retrospective cohort study. Lancet Lond Engl 2020;395(10229):1054–62.

54. Mehta P, McAuley DF, Brown M, et al. COVID-19: consider cytokine storm syndromes and immunosuppression. The Lancet 2020;395(10229):1033–4.

55. Calfee CS, Delucchi K, Parsons PE, et al. Subphenotypes in acute respiratory distress syndrome: latent class analysis of data from two randomised controlled trials. Lancet Respir Med 2014;2(8):611–20.

56. Delucchi K, Famous KR, Ware LB, et al. Stability of ARDS subphenotypes over time in two randomised controlled trials. Thorax 2018;73(5):439–45.

57. Famous KR, Delucchi K, Ware LB, et al. Acute respiratory distress syndrome subphenotypes respond differently to randomized fluid management strategy. Am J Respir Crit Care Med 2017;195(3):331–8.

58. Bos LD, Schouten LR, van Vught LA, et al. Identification and validation of distinct biological phenotypes in patients with acute respiratory distress syndrome by cluster analysis. Thorax 2017;72(10):876–83.

59. Sinha P, Calfee CS, Cherian S, et al. Prevalence of phenotypes of acute respiratory distress syndrome in critically ill patients with COVID-19: a prospective observational study. Lancet Respir Med 2020;8(12):1209–18.

60. Wilson JG, Simpson LJ, Ferreira AM, et al. Cytokine profile in plasma of severe COVID-19 does not differ from ARDS and sepsis. JCI Insight 2020;5(17):e140289.

61. Kox M, Waalders NJB, Kooistra EJ, et al. Cytokine levels in critically ill patients with COVID-19 and Other Conditions. JAMA 2020. https://doi.org/10.1001/jama.2020.17052.

62. RECOVERY Collaborative Group. Tocilizumab in patients admitted to hospital with COVID-19 (RECOVERY): a randomised, controlled, open-label, platform trial. Lancet Lond Engl 2021;397(10285):1637–45.

63. Marconi VC, Ramanan AV, Bono S de, et al. Efficacy and safety of baricitinib for the treatment of hospitalised adults with COVID-19 (COV-BARRIER): a randomised, double-blind, parallel-group, placebo-controlled phase 3 trial. Lancet Respir Med 2021;0(0). https://doi.org/10.1016/S2213-2600(21)00331-3.

64. Investigators TRC. Interleukin-6 receptor antagonists in critically ill patients with Covid-19. N Engl J Med 2021. https://doi.org/10.1056/NEJMoa2100433.

65. Henderson LA, Canna SW, Friedman KG, et al. American College of rheumatology clinical guidance for multisystem inflammatory syndrome in children associated with SARS–CoV-2 and hyperinflammation in pediatric COVID-19: Version 1. Arthritis Rheumatol 2020;72(11):1791–805.

66. Multisystem CDC. Inflammatory syndrome (MIS). Centers for Disease Control and Prevention. 2020. Available at: https://www.cdc.gov/mis/mis-a/hcp.html. Accessed September 29, 2021.

67. Ahmad F, Ahmed A, Rajendraprasad SS, et al. Multisystem inflammatory syndrome in adults: a rare sequela of SARS-CoV-2 infection. Int J Infect Dis IJID Off Publ Int Soc Infect Dis 2021;108:209–11.

68. Leisman DE, Ronner L, Pinotti R, et al. Cytokine elevation in severe and critical COVID-19: a rapid systematic review, meta-analysis, and comparison with other inflammatory syndromes. Lancet Respir Med 2020;8(12):1233–44.

69. Cavalli G, De Luca G, Campochiaro C, et al. Interleukin-1 blockade with high-dose anakinra in patients with COVID-19, acute respiratory distress syndrome, and hyperinflammation: a retrospective cohort study. Lancet Rheumatol 2020; 2(6):e325–31.

70. Huet T, Beaussier H, Voisin O, et al. Anakinra for severe forms of COVID-19: a cohort study. Lancet Rheumatol 2020;2(7):e393–400.

71. Dimopoulos G, de Mast Q, Markou N, et al. Favorable anakinra responses in severe Covid-19 patients with Secondary Hemophagocytic Lymphohistiocytosis. Cell Host Microbe 2020;28(1):117–23.e1.

72. Mazzaccaro D, Giannetta M, Fancoli F, et al. COVID and venous thrombosis: systematic review of literature. J Cardiovasc Surg (Torino) 2021. https://doi.org/10.23736/S0021-9509.21.12022-1.

73. Liu Y, Cai J, Wang C, et al. A systematic review and meta-analysis of incidence, prognosis, and laboratory indicators of venous thromboembolism in hospitalized patients with coronavirus disease 2019. J Vasc Surg Venous Lymphat Disord 2021;9(5):1099–111.e6.

74. Kollias A, Kyriakoulis KG, Lagou S, et al. Venous thromboembolism in COVID-19: a systematic review and meta-analysis. Vasc Med Lond Engl 2021;26(4):415–25.

75. Zhang C, Shen L, Le KJ, et al. Incidence of venous thromboembolism in hospitalized coronavirus disease 2019 patients: a systematic review and meta-analysis. Front Cardiovasc Med 2020;7:151.

76. Paliogiannis P, Mangoni AA, Dettori P, et al. D-dimer Concentrations and COVID-19 severity: a systematic review and meta-analysis. Front Public Health 2020; 8:432.

77. Vidali S, Morosetti D, Cossu E, et al. D-dimer as an indicator of prognosis in SARS-CoV-2 infection: a systematic review. ERJ Open Res 2020;6(2): 00260–2020.

78. Al-Samkari H, Karp Leaf RS, Dzik WH, et al. COVID-19 and coagulation: bleeding and thrombotic manifestations of SARS-CoV-2 infection. Blood 2020;136(4): 489–500.
79. Bhatt A, Deshwal H, Luoma K, et al. Respiratory Mechanics and association with inflammation in COVID-19-related ARDS. Respir Care 2021. https://doi.org/10.4187/respcare.09156.
80. Carsana L, Sonzogni A, Nasr A, et al. Pulmonary post-mortem findings in a series of COVID-19 cases from northern Italy: a two-centre descriptive study. Lancet Infect Dis 2020;20(10):1135–40.
81. Fox SE, Akmatbekov A, Harbert JL, et al. Pulmonary and cardiac pathology in African American patients with COVID-19: an autopsy series from New Orleans. Lancet Respir Med 2020;8(7):681–6.
82. Therapeutic anticoagulation with Heparin in noncritically ill patients with Covid-19. N Engl J Med 2021;385(9):790–802.
83. REMAP-CAP Investigators, ACTIV-4a Investigators, ATTACC Investigators, et al. Therapeutic anticoagulation with Heparin in critically ill patients with Covid-19. N Engl J Med 2021;385(9):777–89.
84. Group RC, Horby PW, Pessoa-Amorim G, et al. Aspirin in Patients Admitted to Hospital with COVID-19 (RECOVERY): A Randomised, Controlled, Open-Label, Platform Trial.; 2021:2021.06.08.21258132. doi:10.1101/2021.06.08.21258132
85. Kan M, Shumyatcher M, Himes BE. Using omics approaches to understand pulmonary diseases. Respir Res 2017;18(1):149.
86. Rogers AJ, Contrepois K, Wu M, et al. Profiling of ARDS pulmonary edema fluid identifies a metabolically distinct subset. Am J Physiol Lung Cell Mol Physiol 2017;312(5):L703–9.
87. Zhu Z, Liang L, Zhang R, et al. Whole blood microRNA markers are associated with acute respiratory distress syndrome. Intensive Care Med Exp 2017;5(1):38.
88. Bos LDJ, Scicluna BP, Ong DSY, et al. Understanding heterogeneity in biologic phenotypes of acute respiratory distress syndrome by leukocyte expression profiles. Am J Respir Crit Care Med 2019;200(1):42–50.
89. Morrell ED, Radella F, Manicone AM, et al. Peripheral and alveolar cell transcriptional programs are distinct in acute respiratory distress syndrome. Am J Respir Crit Care Med 2018;197(4):528–32.
90. Pathak GA, Singh K, Miller-Fleming TW, et al. Integrative genomic analyses identify susceptibility genes underlying COVID-19 hospitalization. Nat Commun 2021; 12(1):4569.
91. Sarma A, Christenson S, Mick E, et al. COVID-19 ARDS is characterized by a dysregulated host response that differs from cytokine storm and is modified by dexamethasone. Res Sq 2021. https://doi.org/10.21203/rs.3.rs-141578/v1. rs.3.rs-141578.
92. Bost P, Giladi A, Liu Y, et al. Host-viral infection Maps reveal signatures of severe COVID-19 patients. Cell 2020;181(7):1475–88.e12.
93. Su Y, Chen D, Yuan D, et al. Multi-omics resolves a sharp disease-state shift between mild and moderate COVID-19. Cell 2020;183(6):1479–95.e20.
94. Wilk AJ, Lee MJ, Wei B, et al. Multi-omic profiling reveals widespread dysregulation of innate immunity and hematopoiesis in COVID-19. J Exp Med 2021;218(8): e20210582.
95. Overmyer KA, Shishkova E, Miller IJ, et al. Large-scale multi-omic analysis of COVID-19 severity. Cell Syst 2021;12(1):23–40.e7.
96. DeMerle K, Angus DC, Seymour CW. Precision medicine for COVID-19: phenotype Anarchy or promise realized? JAMA 2021;325(20):2041–2.

COVID-19 in the Critically Ill Pregnant Patient

Matthew Levitus, MD[a],*, Scott A. Shainker, DO, MS[b], Mai Colvin, MD[a]

KEYWORDS

- COVID-19 • Pregnancy • Critically ill • ARDS • ECMO • Fetal monitoring

KEY POINTS

- Critically ill pregnant patients with coronavirus disease 2019 (COVID-19) are at increased risk for adverse outcomes.
- Management should focus on the early identification of life-threatening symptoms and initiation of a multi-modal therapy to treat the spectrum of severe disease ranging from hypoxia requiring noninvasive oxygen delivery to acute respiratory distress syndrome requiring extracorporeal membrane oxygenation.
- Fetal monitoring in the ICU is critical to ensure adequate placental perfusion and fetal acid/base status.
- The timing of delivery must be balanced by the potential benefit toward maternal status with the risk of prematurity.

INTRODUCTION

Information related to coronavirus disease 2019 (COVID-19) caused by severe acute respiratory syndrome coronavirus 2 (SARS-CoV-2) in pregnant patients is limited and continues to emerge. Even less is known about critically ill pregnant patient requiring advanced respiratory support or those that progress to the development of acute respiratory distress syndrome (ARDS). Pregnant patients are more likely to have severe COVID-19 illnesses compared with nonpregnant patients. A large study from the Centers of Disease Control and Prevention (CDC) which reviewed reports of more than 1.3 million women of reproductive age with a laboratory-confirmed SARS-CoV-2 infection showed that among women with COVID-19, pregnant patients were at significantly increased risk for intensive care unit (ICU) admission, mechanical ventilation, receipt of extracorporeal membrane oxygenation (ECMO), and death.[1] Furthermore, they are at greater risk for adverse pregnancy-related outcomes, driven by an increased risk of iatrogenic prematurity.[2–4] Factors such as age above 25 years,

---

[a] Division of Critical Care Medicine, Montefiore Medical Center, Albert Einstein College of Medicine, 111 East 210th Street, Bronx, NY 10467, USA; [b] Department of Obstetrics and Gynecology, Beth Israel Deaconess Medical Center, Harvard Medical School, 330 Brookline Avenue, Boston MA 02215, USA
* Corresponding author.
E-mail address: mlevitus@montefiore.org

Crit Care Clin 38 (2022) 521–534
https://doi.org/10.1016/j.ccc.2022.01.003
0749-0704/22/© 2022 Elsevier Inc. All rights reserved.
criticalcare.theclinics.com

obesity, chronic hypertension, chronic lung disease, gestational diabetes, and pre-eclampsia further increase risks of serious complications.[1,5–7]

The physiologic changes in pregnancy necessitate special considerations when attempting to optimize management. Pregnancy results in hyperemia of the upper airway, increased oxygen consumption, reduction in chest wall compliance, and decreased functional residual capacity, all of which can exacerbate respiratory distress.[8–10] Moreover, pregnancy is a hypercoagulable state, leads to modifications of the immune system, and produces a state of increased cardiac output.[9] Standard COVID-19 management is also affected by the presence of the fetus, as maternal hypoxemia and hypercapnia can be harmful. The utility of treatments and interventions must, therefore, be weighed against their safety and risks to the developing fetus.

Given their increased risk of severe COVID-19, unique physiology, and fetal considerations, the clinician requires a detailed understanding of the management of critically ill pregnant patients. This article will provide a detailed review of the management and care for critically ill pregnant patient with severe COVID-19 pneumonia.

Indications for Intensive Care Unit Admission in Pregnancy

If pregnant women are suspected or proven to be infected with COVID-19, especially in the presence of high-risk factors, prompt clinical evaluation, early identification of severe symptoms, and appropriate triage are necessary to improve their outcomes. The International Society of Infectious Disease in Obstetrics and Gynecology (ISIDOG) guidelines suggest that ICU admission should be considered for the following patients:

(A) "Pregnant patients with severe disease: respiratory rate $\geq$ 30/min, resting oxygen saturation SaO2 < 94%, arterial blood oxygen partial pressure (Pao$_2$)/oxygen concentration (Fio$_2$) (P/F) $\leq$ 300 mm Hg."
(B) "Pregnant patients with oxygen requirement and comorbidities."
(C) "Pregnant patients with critical disease: shock with organ failure, respiratory failure requiring mechanical ventilation or refractory hypoxemia requiring ECMO."[11]

In severe/critical cases or in cases whereby specialized treatment is required, pregnant patients should be referred to a tertiary center immediately.

MANAGEMENT

Overall, there are limited data regarding the management of critically ill pregnant patient with COVID-19 as many studies excluded pregnant patients or had limited participants. After the identification of critical illness, care should focus on specific treatments for the range of the disease caused by COVID-19 including those with acute respiratory failure to those who develop severe ARDS. Furthermore, there should be a focus on the monitoring of the fetus and discussion of treatment decisions regarding a viable versus nonviable fetus (**Fig. 1**).

Steroids

It is well established that antenatal glucocorticoids in patients at high risk of preterm delivery within 7 days improves neonatal outcomes.[12] Treatment typically consists of either two 12 mg doses of betamethasone given intramuscularly (IM) 24 hours apart or four 6 mg doses of dexamethasone administered IM every 12 hours.[12,13] Prolonged use or multiple courses of steroids that readily cross the placenta is controversial as prior studies have shown potential adverse fetal effects such as unfavorable

Practical Approach Algorithm for the Critically Ill Pregnant Covid-19 Patient[a]

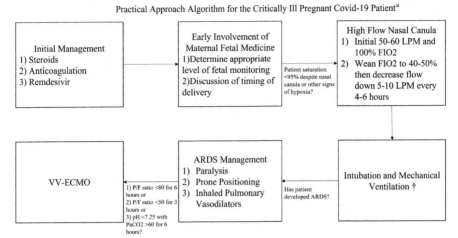

Fig. 1. Practical approach algorithm for the critically ill pregnant COVID-19 patient. [a] All management decisions should be individualized. [b] Similar strategy to nonpregnant patients but with goal SPO2 > 95% with PaO2 > 70 mmHg, avoidance of severe respiratory alkalosis or acidosis, and a plateau pressure greater than 30 mmHg may also be appropriate.

neurologic outcomes, small head circumferences, fetal growth restriction, and increased risk of neonatal hypoglycemia.[12,14,15]

The RECOVERY trial showed that oral or intravenous (IV) dexamethasone at a dose of 6 mg once daily for up to 10 days reduces mortality associated with COVID-19 among patients who required supplemental oxygen or mechanical ventilation compared with those who received standard of care.[16] Pregnant patients were not excluded from the trial, but the trial included only 6 pregnant patients and the protocol was modified to treatment with oral prednisolone 40 mg daily or IV hydrocortisone 80 mg twice daily.

Evidence on the choice and duration of corticosteroid treatment among pregnant patients with COVID-19 is limited and a definitive consensus is lacking. (**Table 1**) Based on the RECOVERY trial results, for patients that do not yet meet criteria for fetal lung maturity the Royal College of Obstetricians and Gynecologists (RCOG) suggests pregnant women who require supplemental oxygen or mechanical ventilators receive oral prednisolone 40 mg once daily or IV hydrocortisone 80 mg twice daily for 10 days or up to discharge.[17] However, Saad and colleagues recommend a total of 32 mg of methylprednisolone orally or IV (which is equivalent to 6 mg dexamethasone) once a day or in divided doses.[15] This is suggested due to the potential harm from additional dexamethasone exposure to the fetus.[15] In contrast, the Society of Maternal–Fetal Medicine (SMFM) recommends the use of dexamethasone in a similar manner to that studied in the RECOVERY trial.[18] The above recommendations are modified for patients that meet criteria for steroids for fetal lung maturity by treatment with dexamethasone 6 mg IM every 12 hours for 4 doses followed by each society's recommended regimen to complete a total of 10 days.

Anticoagulation Strategies

Pregnancy is a hypercoagulable state and pregnant patients have up to a fivefold increased risk of thromboembolism compared with nonpregnant patients.[19,20] Studies have suggested there may be a confounding increased risk of coagulopathy

Table 1
Steroid regimens recommended for the critically ill pregnant Covid-19 patient

Source	If Not Indicated for Fetal Lung Maturity	If Indicated for Fetal Lung Maturity
Royal College of Obstricians and Gynaccologists[17]	Oral prednisolone 40 mg once a day or intravenous hydrocortisone 80 mg twice a day for 10 d or up to discharge, whichever is sooner	Intramuscular dexamethasone 6 mg every 12 h for 4 doses than oral prednisolone 40 mg once a day or intravenous hydrocortisone 80 mg twice a day to complete a total of 10 d or up to discharge, whichever is sooner
Society of Maternal–Fetal Medicine[18]	Oral or intravenous dexamethasone 6 mg daily for up to 10 d	Intramuscular dexamethasone 6 mg every 12 h for 4 doses followed by oral or IV Dexamethasone 6 mg daily up to a total of 10 d
Saad et al.[15]	Oral or intravenous methylprednisolone 32 mg once a day or in divided doses, for 10 d or up to discharge, whichever is sooner	Intramuscular dexamethasone 6 mg every 12 h for 4 doses followed by switching to oral or intravenous methylprednisolone 32 mg once a day to complete a total of 10 d or up to discharge, whichever is sooner

associated with COVID-19.[21–23] However, in critically ill patients, therapeutic heparin was not shown to increase survival to hospital discharge or affect the number of days for respiratory organ support.[24] Based on the current data, multiple professional societies and guidelines recommend prophylactic doses of anticoagulation unless contraindicated. The National Institutes of Health (NIH) COVID-19 Treatment Guidelines recommend that pregnant patients hospitalized for severe COVID-19 receive prophylactic dose anticoagulation.[25] SMFM recommends prophylactic unfractionated heparin or low-molecular-weight heparin (LMWH) in critically ill or mechanically ventilated pregnant women.[18] RCOG recommends all pregnant and recently pregnant women to be assessed for risk of venous thromboembolism (VTE) and receive thromboprophylaxis with LMWH.[17] The risk of bleeding and benefits of VTE prophylaxis must be carefully weighed in each case. Currently, there is not enough evidence to recommend therapeutic anticoagulation in the absence of proven VTE.

Remdesivir

Remdesivir is an inhibitor of the viral RNA-dependent RNA polymerase and it inhibits SARS-CoV-2 replication in vitro.[26] In an international, multicenter, double-blind, randomized, placebo-controlled trial of 1062 nonpregnant patients hospitalized with COVID-19 with evidence of lower respiratory tract infection, IV remdesivir (for 10 days or until hospital discharge or death) was superior to placebo in shortening the time to recovery.[27] Remdesivir was approved by the Food and Drug Administration

(FDA) for use in adults and children (aged $\geq$12 years and weighing $\geq$40 kg) hospitalized with COVID-19. Safety data from the manufacture label of remdesivir states that there are insufficient data to evaluate for a drug-associated risk of major birth defects, miscarriage, or adverse maternal or fetal outcomes when used in pregnant patients.[28] Data for the use of Remdesivir in pregnant women with COVID-19 are extremely limited. In a study by Burwick and colleagues, 67 hospitalized pregnant patients (82% were $\geq$24-week gestation) with COVID-19 were treated on a compassionate use basis with remdesivir.[29] Among pregnant women, 93% of those on mechanical ventilation were extubated, 93% recovered, and 90% were discharged, and remdesivir was generally well tolerated.[29] Aside from this study, published data on outcomes and adverse events for remdesivir use in pregnant women with COVID-19 mostly come from smaller case series and case reports and are overall limited.

Tocilizumab

Tocilizumab is a monoclonal antibody against the interleukin-6 receptor, and it has been shown to improve outcomes in patients with severe COVID-19 pneumonia in some studies.[30–33] Tocilizumab is currently available under FDA emergency use authorization for the treatment of COVID-19. Tocilizumab crosses the placenta and data describing tocilizumab for use in pregnant patients with COVID-19 are scarce. The use for the treatment of COVID-19 in pregnancy is not currently recommended given limited data. Further study is necessary to confirm the benefit-risk profile of tocilizumab use among pregnant women.

Noninvasive Ventilation

The goal oxygen saturation for nonpregnant patients with COVID-19 is 92%. For pregnant patients, SMFM recommends a target of 95%.[18] Patients that do not require immediate intubation, high flow nasal cannula is an appealing alternative. Pacheco colleagues recommend the initiation of 50 to 60 L per minute (LPM) with 100% Fio_2 and then subsequent weaning of Fio_2 down to 40% to 50% followed by a decrease in flow by 5 to 10 LPM every 4 to 6 hours.[34] Noninvasive ventilation such as bilevel positive airway pressure (BIPAP) tends to be avoided in pregnancy because of an increased risk of aspiration due to decreased esophageal sphincter tone and increased abdominal pressure.[35]

Mechanical Ventilation

There are limited data regarding the management of mechanical ventilation for pregnant patients. In general, ventilatory strategies in pregnant patient are similar to nonpregnant patients but with some key differences, especially in ARDS. In general, the $Paco_2$ should be aimed at a pregnancy-specific hypocapnia.[36] However, a severe respiratory alkalosis should be avoided as it leads to uterine vasoconstriction.[37] Hyperoxia in ARDS is avoided, but for the pregnant patient, the goal is an oxygen saturation of at least 95% and Pao_2 of at least 70 mm Hg to allow for adequate fetal oxygenation.[35] In the nonpregnant patient, standard ARDS therapy also involves low tidal volume ventilation. If lung pathology constrains the use of low tidal volume ventilation, then permissive hypercapnia may be tolerated as it is not contraindicated in pregnancy; mild hypercapnia 50 to 60 mm Hg is general acceptable.[36] However, if hypercapnia is greater than 60 mm Hg there is a potential of fetal acidemia shifting the fetal oxyhemoglobin dissociation curve to the right.[36,38] ARDSnet protocol recommends a goal plateau pressure of less than 30 cmH2O but given the reduction in chest wall compliance a higher plateau pressure greater than 30 cmH2O may be appropriate; especially because transpulmonary pressures may not be elevated.[39] Therefore, esophageal pressure monitoring may be helpful.[36]

Sedation

Critically ill patients on a ventilator need some form of analgesia and/or sedation. The 2018 Clinical Practice Guidelines for the Management of Pain, Agitation/Sedation, Delirium, Immobility, and Sleep Disruption in Adult Patients in the ICU (PADIS) suggest using the analgesia-first approach to spare and/or minimize the use of both opioids and sedatives.[40] When sedation is needed, the guideline recommends using light sedation (vs deep sedation) in critically ill, mechanically ventilated patients using established assessment tools such as the Richmond Agitation and Sedation Scale.[40] There are some situations in which deeper sedation is targeted, such as patients with severe hypoxemia, severe ARDS, and patients who are receiving neuromuscular blocking agents.

There is limited evidence to guide decisions regarding sedation and analgesia in critically ill pregnant patient. In general, commonly used agents for sedation and paralysis are safe in pregnancy.[41] Analgesic medications such as fentanyl, hydromorphone, and morphine are considered safe in pregnancy.[42] However, if used in pregnant patients close to the delivery time, neonatologists should be alerted as the neonate may develop signs of neonatal abstinence syndrome.[42] For sedation, the PADIS guideline suggests using either propofol or dexmedetomidine over benzodiazepines for sedation in critically ill mechanically ventilated adults.[40] There is no clear evidence that propofol causes congenital anomalies or adverse pregnancy outcomes.[42] Moreover, although Dexmedetomidine crosses the placenta there is no evidence that it is teratogenic.[42] If benzodiazepines are used the association between in utero benzodiazepine exposure and congenital malformations are conflicting. Similar to opiates, if used close to the delivery time, neonatologists should be alerted as the neonate may require additional support.[42]

Paralysis

Paralytics are recommended for ventilated patients with moderate to severe ARDS to facilitate lung-protective ventilation.[43] They can be used for persistent ventilator dyssynchrony, to enable proning, and to limit high plateau pressures.[43] When indicated cisatracurium is the preferred neuromuscular blocker and may be used during pregnancy.[42]

Prone Positioning

The prone positioning in severe acute respiratory distress syndrome (PROSEVA) trial has shown that in mechanically ventilated patients with ARDS, early application of prolonged prone-positioning sessions increases the rate of successful extubation and decreases mortality.[44] With regards to the management of ARDS due to COVID-19, international treatment guidelines of critically ill adults with COVID-19 by the Surviving Sepsis Campaign panel suggest prone ventilation in moderate to severe ARDS for 12 to 16 hours.[43] However, data on pregnant patients are lacking as they were excluded from the PROSEVA trial. There are several case reports reporting successful prone ventilation in both nonventilated and ventilated pregnant patients with severe ARDS.[45–49] Proning pregnant patients is more challenging owing to the large gravid uterus but is feasible with padding using pillows and blankets above and below the gravid uterus (**Fig. 2**). This method offloads the uterus and avoids aortocaval compression.[36]

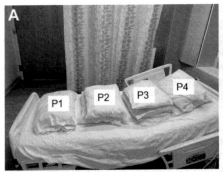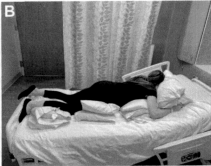

Fig. 2. (A) Suggested support pillow location for prone positioning during pregnancy. P1: pillows supporting shins/knees, P2: pillows supporting maternal pelvis, P3: pillows supporting maternal chest, P4: pillows supporting maternal head. (Note: head of bed elevated 10–20°). (B) 33-week pregnant patient in the prone position with gravid abdomen supported between P2 and P3

Inhaled Pulmonary Vasodilators

Inhaled nitric oxide (iNO) is a selective pulmonary vasodilator that reduces the pulmonary artery pressure and increases arterial oxygenation in patients with severe ARDS.[50] While the antiviral property of iNO has been well described,[51–55] the role of iNO in the management of hypoxia due to COVID-19 remains unclear. The Surviving Sepsis Campaign panel recommends against the routine use of iNO in mechanically ventilated patients with COVID-19 ARDS but suggests a trial of iNO as a rescue strategy in mechanically ventilated adults with COVID-19, severe ARDS, and hypoxemia despite optimizing ventilation and other rescue strategies.[43] Data on iNO use in pregnant patients with COVID-19 are scarce. Safaee Fakhr and colleagues treated 6 pregnant patients meeting criteria for severe or critical COVID-19 with twice daily high-dose (160–200 ppm) nitric oxide via mask. They reported an increase in systemic oxygenation with each administration session and it was well-tolerated without acute adverse events.[56] Further studies and trials are needed to elucidate the potential benefits of iNO therapy in patients with COVID-19.

Venous-Venous Extracorporeal Membrane Oxygenation

Information on venous-venous extracorporeal membrane oxygenation (VV-ECMO) in pregnancy is limited. Nonetheless, pregnancy is not a contraindication.[18] A systematic review by Naoum and colleagues of critically ill pregnant patients that underwent VV-ECMO showed 80.2% survived with the most common complication being maternal bleeding.[57] Since the pandemic there have been many case reports of pregnant patients with COVID-19 ARDS and the use of VV-ECMO.[58–60] The decision to place patients on VV-ECMO should be undertaken with a multidisciplinary team approach with members from critical care, cardiothoracic surgery, obstetrics/maternal–fetal medicine (MFM), and neonatology. Indications for VV-ECMO in the hypoxic pregnant patient should follow as per Extracorporeal Life Support Organization (ELSO) guidelines.[18] If patients worsen despite standard ARDS management, VV-ECMO should be considered in patients with severe ARDS with Pao_2/Fio_2 (P/F) ratios less than 80 for more than 6 hours, less than 50 for more than 3 hours, or a pH less than 7.25 with $Paco_2$ greater than 60 for more than 6 hours.[61] Cannulation site is affected by the stage of pregnancy. If the uterus fundus is at the level of the umbilicus femoral cannulation may be difficult.[41] Therefore, the preferred cannulation method is a single dual lumen catheter in the right internal jugal vein; however, their smaller size may not match adequate flow needs due to the increased cardiac output of pregnancy. Once initiated, the management of the ECMO circuit and weaning should follow ELSO protocols.[61] However, if the patient were to give birth on ECMO there is an increased risk of hemorrhage. Therefore, an ECMO strategy without anticoagulation could be considered as some reports have shown it to be safe.[62,63]

Fetal Monitoring

Fetal monitoring should be viewed as yet another measure of maternal hemodynamics. Fetal monitoring provides a noninvasive means of ensuring placental perfusion, as well as serving as a proxy for fetal oxygenation and acid–base status.[64] The key drivers to ensuring adequate placental perfusion are maternal hemodynamic stability, maternal oxygenation, volume status, and acid–base status.[41,65,66] There are little data to guide on the use of fetal monitoring in the critically ill pregnant patient; as such, a multidisciplinary team including MFM/high-risk obstetrics, critical care, neonatology, and nursing should be used to determine the frequency, duration, and location of monitoring. Many variables are considered in making the decision to perform fetal monitoring; however, gestational age and maternal acuity should be atop the list.[67]

The term "fetal viability" is often used when considering initiating fetal monitoring. At most centers, 22 weeks is the lowest threshold to consider a fetus viable, with most centers not recommending neonatal intervention until 24 weeks. The decision to initiate fetal monitoring should be based on balancing the family's expectation/desires for neonatal outcomes and the clinical situation.[68] As such, fetal monitoring should not be performed until a joint neonatology/MFM consultation has occurred. With advances in neonatal care and improved access to neonatal ICU, neonatal survival rates have progressively improved over time in the 22–24-week periviable period.[68]

In the critically ill previable parturient, fetal heart auscultation at daily to weekly intervals is appropriate to confirm the pregnancy remains present; however, before viability, management plans should not deviate because of fetal status. Once the fetus is viable, fetal monitoring should be used to not only assure fetal health but also as yet another hemodynamic parameter to ensure placental perfusion.[69] The frequency of fetal monitoring needs to be individualized, and flexible, based on maternal acuity and decompensation. Recognizing practice vary by institution, a minimum of daily monitoring is recommended for the critically ill. Often, until maternal stability has been established or in the mechanically ventilated or ECMO patient, continuous monitoring is recommended.[67]

Timing of Delivery

The decision to proceed with delivery in the critically ill parturient needs to be balanced with (1) potential benefit toward maternal status and (2) risk of prematurity. In the setting of reassuring fetal monitoring and maternal stability, delivery is seldom recommended. In cases whereby ventilation cannot be optimized, consideration for delivery is appropriate to improve respiratory mechanics.[70] Decision making around delivery needs to include critical care medicine, neonatology, MFM, and obstetrics anesthesia. Delivery location should be prioritized to a labor and delivery suite; however, if delivery in the critical care setting is needed, multidisciplinary advanced planning is critical to ensure all resources are available for both the mother and neonate. In our practice, delivery in the ICU should be limited to perimortem cesarean delivery or whereby maternal/fetal status does not allow for any delay. Therefore, while in the ICU preparations should be made for imminent delivery in case of emergency (**Box 1**).

Box 1
Recommended obstetric and neonatal supplies for delivery in adult ICU

Maternal
    Cesarean Delivery Kit
    Vaginal Delivery Kit (if plan to deliver in ICU)
    Uterotonic Medications[a] (Pitocin, Misoprostol, Methylergometrine)
    Uterine Balloon[a]

Neonatal
    Baby Warmer
    Neonatal Code Cart
    Oxygen Blender
    Neonatal Transport Isolette

[a] Available to treat unexpected postpartum hemorrhage

As mentioned above, any parturient with a viable fetus should receive a course of glucocorticoids for fetal lung maturity if critical status presents before 34 weeks gestation.[71] Based on expert opinion from the current pandemic, the following should be considered in terms of timing of delivery. From the point of viability to 31w6d, delivery should be reserved for cases whereby maternal status continues to rapidly deteriorate or when fetus status is nonreassuring despite interventions. Beyond 32 weeks, delivery should be strongly considered in cases requiring mechanical ventilation or ECMO, after a course of glucocorticoids for fetal lung maturity. If maternal status deteriorates beyond 34 weeks, delivery is recommended.[67] It is important to note that mode of delivery (cesarean vs induction of labor) should be determined by standard obstetrics principles if both maternal and fetus status allow.[66,67,70]

Maternal cardiac arrest should prompt decision for urgent (less than 5 minutes) perimortem cesarean delivery. A perimortem cesarean delivery should be performed wherever the arrest occurred; as such, preparing for delivery in the critical care setting is highly recommended. This delivery is performed to maximize maternal resuscitative efforts, most notably, improving cardiac return by decompressing the inferior vena cava of the gravid uterus allowing for more effective CPR.[72]

Postpartum

Despite delivery occurring, pregnancy physiology continues for many weeks postpartum.[8] Irrespective of gestational age at the time of delivery, there is a physiologic autotransfusion from the utero-placental unit into maternal circulation resulting in increased visceral perfusion and flow. This autotransfusion results in increased pulmonary pressures and the resultant increased risk of pulmonary edema.[8,73] In addition, an increase in catecholamines and fluid shifts during the postpartum period make the lungs particularly vulnerable to capillary leak.[73]

The other significant consideration during the postpartum state is the increased risk of VTE. The increased thrombogenic state continues for up to 12 weeks postpartum, with the first 6 weeks carrying the highest risk of thromboembolism.[74] With the added risk associated with severe COVID-19, the postpartum critically ill patient should be considered high risk for thromboembolism and appropriate prophylaxis should be administered. As mentioned earlier, adjusted risk-based prophylactic dosing is recommended in critically ill patients, this recommendation still holds true for the postpartum patient.[66,75]

Lastly, lactation issues often arise in critically ill postpartum patients, and COVID-19 is no exception. The benefits of breastfeeding are well established, and every effort should be made to support this activity if it is consistent with the patient's wishes. In addition to the well-known benefits of breastfeeding, breast milk from postpartum patients with COVID-19 has been shown to contain both anti–SARS-CoV-2 IgA and IgG, providing passive immunity to the vulnerable newborn.[76] Consultation with MFM, lactation, pharmacy, and neonatology should occur to confirm medication compatibility with breastfeeding. Providing assistance with pumping or hand expression of milk by nursing staff, lactation, or family is critical to ensure adequate milk production and continue supply.[77]

SUMMARY

The pregnant patient is at increased risk for severe COVID-19 disease. Although there are limited data, management should focus on the early identification of critically ill patient for triage to the ICU. Standard therapy includes medical management with steroids and maintenance of an oxygenation saturation of at least 95%. The deteriorating patient requires special consideration with the application of therapies such as proning, sedation/analgesia, paralysis, and VV-ECMO. Furthermore, particular attention to fetal monitoring, timing of delivery, and preparation for postpartum issues are essential.

DISCLOSURE

The authors have no financial conflicts of interest to disclose

REFERENCES

1. Zambrano LD, Ellington S, Strid P, et al. Update: characteristics of symptomatic women of reproductive age with laboratory-confirmed SARS-CoV-2 infection by pregnancy status - United States, January 22-October 3, 2020. MMWR Morb Mortal Wkly Rep 2020;69(44):1641–7.
2. Ko JY, DeSisto CL, Simeone RM, et al. Adverse pregnancy outcomes, maternal complications, and severe illness among US delivery Hospitalizations with and without a coronavirus disease 2019 (COVID-19) Diagnosis. Clin Infect Dis 2021;73(Suppl 1):S24–31.
3. Pierce-Williams RAM, Burd J, Felder L, et al. Clinical course of severe and critical coronavirus disease 2019 in hospitalized pregnancies: a United States cohort study. Am J Obstet Gynecol MFM 2020;2(3):100134.
4. Easter SR, Gupta S, Brenner SK, et al. Outcomes of critically ill pregnant women with COVID-19 in the United States. Am J Respir Crit Care Med 2021;203(1):122–5.
5. Allotey J, Stallings E, Bonet M, et al. Clinical manifestations, risk factors, and maternal and perinatal outcomes of coronavirus disease 2019 in pregnancy: living systematic review and meta-analysis. BMJ 2020;370. https://doi.org/10.1136/bmj.m3320. m3320.
6. Panagiotakopoulos L, Myers TR, Gee J, et al. SARS-CoV-2 infection among hospitalized pregnant women: Reasons for admission and pregnancy Characteristics - Eight U.S. Health care centers, March 1-may 30, 2020. MMWR Morb Mortal Wkly Rep 2020;69(38):1355–9.
7. Galang RR, Newton SM, Woodworth KR, et al. Risk factors for illness Severity among pregnant women with confirmed severe acute respiratory syndrome

coronavirus 2 infection-Surveillance for emerging Threats to mothers and Babies Network, 22 state, local, and Territorial health Departments, 29 March 2020-5 March 2021. Clin Infect Dis 2021;73(Suppl 1):S17–23.

8. Ouzounian JG, Elkayam U. Physiologic changes during normal pregnancy and delivery. Cardiol Clin 2012;30(3):317–29.

9. Wastnedge EAN, Reynolds RM, van Boeckel SR, et al. Pregnancy and COVID-19. Physiol Rev 2021;101(1):303–18.

10. Hegewald MJ, Crapo RO. Respiratory physiology in pregnancy. Clin Chest Med 2011;32(1):1–13.

11. Donders F, Lonnee-Hoffmann R, Tsiakalos A, et al. ISIDOG recommendations Concerning COVID-19 and pregnancy. Diagnostics (Basel) 2020;10(4). https://doi.org/10.3390/diagnostics10040243.

12. Committee on Obstetric P. Committee Opinion No. 713. Antenatal corticosteroid therapy for fetal maturation. Obstet Gynecol 2017;130(2):e102–9.

13. American College of O, Gynecologists' Committee on Practice B-O. Practice Bulletin No. 171: management of preterm labor. Obstet Gynecol 2016;128(4): e155–64.

14. Saccone G, Berghella V. Antenatal corticosteroids for maturity of term or near term fetuses: systematic review and meta-analysis of randomized controlled trials. BMJ 2016;355:i5044. https://doi.org/10.1136/bmj.i5044.

15. Saad AF, Chappell L, Saade GR, et al. Corticosteroids in the management of pregnant patients with coronavirus disease (COVID-19). Obstet Gynecol 2020; 136(4):823–6.

16. Group RC, Horby P, Lim WS, et al. Dexamethasone in hospitalized patients with Covid-19. N Engl J Med 2021;384(8):693–704.

17. Gynaecologists RCoOa. Coronavirus (COVID-19) infection In Pregnancy - Version 14. 2021;

18. Halscott TV, J and the SMFM COVID-19 Task Force. Management considerations for pregnant patients with COVID-19. 2020;

19. Heit JA, Kobbervig CE, James AH, et al. Trends in the incidence of venous thromboembolism during pregnancy or postpartum: a 30-year population-based study. Ann Intern Med 2005;143(10):697–706.

20. Pomp ER, Lenselink AM, Rosendaal FR, et al. Pregnancy, the postpartum period and prothrombotic defects: risk of venous thrombosis in the MEGA study. J Thromb Haemost 2008;6(4):632–7.

21. Malas MB, Naazie IN, Elsayed N, et al. Thromboembolism risk of COVID-19 is high and associated with a higher risk of mortality: a systematic review and meta-analysis. Eclinicalmedicine 2020;29:100639. https://doi.org/10.1016/j.eclinm.2020.100639.

22. Bikdeli B, Madhavan MV, Jimenez D, et al. COVID-19 and thrombotic or thromboembolic disease: Implications for Prevention, Antithrombotic therapy, and follow-up: JACC state-of-the-Art review. J Am Coll Cardiol 2020;75(23):2950–73.

23. Middeldorp S, Coppens M, van Haaps TF, et al. Incidence of venous thromboembolism in hospitalized patients with COVID-19. J Thromb Haemost 2020;18(8): 1995–2002.

24. Investigators R-C, Investigators AC-a, Investigators A, et al. Therapeutic anticoagulation with heparin in critically ill patients with Covid-19. N Engl J Med 2021;385(9):777–89.

25. COVID-19 Treatment Guidelines Panel. Coronavirus disease 2019 (COVID-19) treatment guidelines. National Institutes of Health. Available at: https://www.covid19treatmentguidelines.nih.gov/. Accessed September 29 2021.

26. Wang M, Cao R, Zhang L, et al. Remdesivir and chloroquine effectively inhibit the recently emerged novel coronavirus (2019-nCoV) in vitro. Cell Res 2020;30(3): 269–71.

27. Beigel JH, Tomashek KM, Dodd LE, et al. Remdesivir for the treatment of Covid-19 - Final report. N Engl J Med 2020;383(19):1813–26.

28. Veklury (remdesivir). [package insert]. Gilead Sciences, Inc.; 2021.

29. Burwick RM, Yawetz S, Stephenson KE, et al. Compassionate Use of remdesivir in pregnant women with severe Covid-19. Clin Infect Dis 2020. https://doi.org/10.1093/cid/ciaa1466.

30. Salama C, Han J, Yau L, et al. Tocilizumab in patients hospitalized with Covid-19 pneumonia. N Engl J Med 2021;384(1):20–30.

31. Somers EC, Eschenauer GA, Troost JP, et al. Tocilizumab for treatment of mechanically ventilated patients with COVID-19. Clin Infect Dis 2021;73(2):e445–54.

32. Horby P, Staplin N, Haynes R, et al. Tocilizumab in COVID-19 therapy: who benefits, and how? - Authors' reply. Lancet 2021;398(10297):300.

33. Investigators R-C, Gordon AC, Mouncey PR, et al. Interleukin-6 receptor Antagonists in critically ill patients with Covid-19. N Engl J Med 2021;384(16): 1491–502.

34. Pacheco LD, Saad AF, Saade G. Early acute respiratory support for pregnant patients with coronavirus disease 2019 (COVID-19) infection. Obstet Gynecol 2020; 136(1):42–5.

35. Schwaiberger D, Karcz M, Menk M, et al. Respiratory failure and mechanical ventilation in the pregnant patient. Crit Care Clin 2016;32(1):85–95.

36. Tolcher MC, McKinney JR, Eppes CS, et al. Prone positioning for pregnant women with hypoxemia due to coronavirus disease 2019 (COVID-19). Obstet Gynecol 2020;136(2):259–61.

37. Lapinsky SE. Acute respiratory failure in pregnancy. Obstet Med 2015;8(3): 126–32.

38. Campbell LA, Klocke RA. Implications for the pregnant patient. Am J Respir Crit Care Med 2001;163(5):1051–4.

39. Lapinsky SE, Posadas-Calleja JG, McCullagh I. Clinical review: ventilatory strategies for obstetric, brain-injured and obese patients. Crit Care 2009;13(2):206.

40. Devlin JW, Skrobik Y, Gelinas C, et al. Clinical practice guidelines for the Prevention and management of Pain, Agitation/sedation, Delirium, Immobility, and Sleep Disruption in adult patients in the ICU. Crit Care Med 2018;46(9):e825–73.

41. Oxford-Horrey C, Savage M, Prabhu M, et al. Putting it all Together: clinical considerations in the care of critically ill obstetric patients with COVID-19. Am J Perinatol 2020;37(10):1044–51.

42. Pacheco LD, Saade GR, Hankins GD. Mechanical ventilation during pregnancy: sedation, analgesia, and paralysis. Clin Obstet Gynecol 2014;57(4):844–50.

43. Alhazzani W, Moller MH, Arabi YM, et al. Surviving Sepsis Campaign: guidelines on the management of critically ill adults with coronavirus disease 2019 (COVID-19). Crit Care Med 2020;48(6):e440–69.

44. Guerin C, Reignier J, Richard JC, et al. Prone positioning in severe acute respiratory distress syndrome. N Engl J Med 2013;368(23):2159–68.

45. Kenn S, Weber-Carstens S, Weizsaecker K, et al. Prone positioning for ARDS following blunt chest trauma in late pregnancy. Int J Obstet Anesth 2009;18(3): 268–71.

46. Samanta S, Samanta S, Wig J, et al. How safe is the prone position in acute respiratory distress syndrome at late pregnancy? Am J Emerg Med 2014;32(6): 687 e1–3.

47. Schnettler WT, Al Ahwel Y, Suhag A. Severe acute respiratory distress syndrome in coronavirus disease 2019-infected pregnancy: obstetric and intensive care considerations. Am J Obstet Gynecol MFM 2020;2(3):100120.

48. Vibert F, Kretz M, Thuet V, et al. Prone positioning and high-flow oxygen improved respiratory function in a 25-week pregnant woman with COVID-19. Eur J Obstet Gynecol Reprod Biol 2020;250:257–8.

49. Pozos CKP DT, Deloya TE, Perez NOR, et al. Severe acute respiratory distress syndrome in pregnancy. Review of the literature and two cases report. Med Crit 2019;33(4):209–14.

50. Rossaint R, Falke KJ, Lopez F, et al. Inhaled nitric oxide for the adult respiratory distress syndrome. N Engl J Med 1993;328(6):399–405.

51. Akaike T, Maeda H. Nitric oxide and virus infection. Immunology 2000;101(3):300–8.

52. Colasanti M, Persichini T, Venturini G, et al. S-nitrosylation of viral proteins: molecular bases for antiviral effect of nitric oxide. IUBMB Life 1999;48(1):25–31.

53. Saura M, Zaragoza C, McMillan A, et al. An antiviral mechanism of nitric oxide: inhibition of a viral protease. Immunotechnology 1999;10(1):21–8.

54. Garren MR, Ashcraft M, Qian Y, et al. Nitric oxide and viral infection: Recent developments in antiviral therapies and Platforms. Appl Mater Today 2021;22. https://doi.org/10.1016/j.apmt.2020.100887.

55. Keyaerts E, Vijgen L, Chen L, et al. Inhibition of SARS-coronavirus infection in vitro by S-nitroso-N-acetylpenicillamine, a nitric oxide donor compound. Int J Infect Dis 2004;8(4):223–6.

56. Safaee Fakhr B, Wiegand SB, Pinciroli R, et al. High concentrations of nitric oxide Inhalation therapy in pregnant patients with severe coronavirus disease 2019 (COVID-19). Obstet Gynecol 2020;136(6):1109–13.

57. Naoum EE, Chalupka A, Haft J, et al. Extracorporeal life support in pregnancy: a systematic review. J Am Heart Assoc 2020;9(13):e016072.

58. Hou L, Li M, Guo K, et al. First successful treatment of a COVID-19 pregnant woman with severe ARDS by combining early mechanical ventilation and ECMO. Heart Lung 2021;50(1):33–6.

59. Larson SB, Watson SN, Eberlein M, et al. Survival of pregnant coronavirus patient on extracorporeal membrane oxygenation. Ann Thorac Surg 2021;111(3):e151–2.

60. Barrantes JH, Ortoleva J, O'Neil ER, et al. Successful treatment of pregnant and postpartum women with severe COVID-19 associated acute respiratory distress syndrome with extracorporeal membrane oxygenation. Asaio J 2021;67(2):132–6.

61. Badulak J, Antonini MV, Stead CM, et al. Extracorporeal membrane oxygenation for COVID-19: Updated 2021 guidelines from the extracorporeal life support Organization. Asaio j 2021;67(5):485–95.

62. Fina D, Matteucci M, Jiritano F, et al. Extracorporeal membrane oxygenation without systemic anticoagulation: a case-series in challenging conditions. J Thorac Dis 2020;12(5):2113–9.

63. Kurihara C, Walter JM, Karim A, et al. Feasibility of Venovenous extracorporeal membrane oxygenation without systemic anticoagulation. Ann Thorac Surg 2020;110(4):1209–15.

64. ACOG Practice Bulletin No. 106: Intrapartum fetal heart rate monitoring: nomenclature, interpretation, and general management principles. Obstet Gynecol 2009;114(1):192–202.

65. Meschia G. Fetal oxygenation and maternal ventilation. Clin Chest Med 2011; 32(1):15–9.
66. Crozier TME. General care of the pregnant patient in the intensive care Unit. Semin Respir Crit Care Med 2017;38(2):208–17.
67. Rose CH, Wyatt MA, Narang K, et al. Timing of delivery with coronavirus disease 2019 pneumonia requiring intensive care unit admission. Am J Obstet Gynecol MFM 2021;3(4):100373.
68. Obstetric care consensus No. 6: periviable birth. Obstet Gynecol 2017;130(4): e187–99.
69. Poon LC, Yang H, Kapur A, et al. Global interim guidance on coronavirus disease 2019 (COVID-19) during pregnancy and puerperium from FIGO and allied partners: Information for healthcare professionals. Int J Gynaecol Obstet 2020; 149(3):273–86.
70. Lapinsky SE. Management of acute respiratory failure in pregnancy. Semin Respir Crit Care Med 2017;38(2):201–7.
71. Roberts D, Brown J, Medley N, et al. Antenatal corticosteroids for accelerating fetal lung maturation for women at risk of preterm birth. Cochrane Database Syst Rev 2017;3:CD004454.
72. Oxford CM, Ludmir J. Trauma in pregnancy. Clin Obstet Gynecol 2009;52(4): 611–29.
73. Chen L, Jiang H, Zhao Y. Pregnancy with COVID-19: management considerations for care of severe and critically ill cases. Am J Reprod Immunol 2020;84(5): e13299.
74. Kamel H, Navi BB, Sriram N, et al. Risk of a thrombotic event after the 6-week postpartum period. N Engl J Med 2014;370(14):1307–15.
75. Susen S, Tacquard CA, Godon A, et al. Prevention of thrombotic risk in hospitalized patients with COVID-19 and hemostasis monitoring. Crit Care 2020; 24(1):364.
76. Pace RM, Williams JE, Jarvinen KM, et al. Characterization of SARS-CoV-2 RNA, Antibodies, and Neutralizing capacity in milk produced by women with COVID-19. mBio 2021;(1):12. https://doi.org/10.1128/mBio.03192-20.
77. Dauphinee JD, Amato K, Kiehl E. Support of the breast-feeding mother in critical care. AACN Clin Issues 1997;8(4):539–49.

Extracorporeal Membrane Oxygenation in COVID-19

Manuel Tisminetzky, MD[a], Bruno L. Ferreyro, MD[a,b], Eddy Fan, PhD[a,b,c,d],*

KEYWORDS

- ARDS • ECMO • COVID-19 • Prone positioning

KEY POINTS

- COVID-19-related ARDS has a similar clinical presentation, course, and outcome as ARDS due to other risk factors.
- Ventilatory strategies and adjuvant therapies for COVID-19 should follow similar evidence-based principles as for non-COVID-19 ARDS.
- Extracorporeal membrane oxygenation (ECMO) is an intervention used in patients with severe ARDS that cannot achieve adequate gas exchange despite optimization of lung-protective ventilation.
- Current evidence suggests that the efficacy, clinical outcomes, and complications of ECMO in COVID-19-related ARDS are similar to non-COVID-19 ARDS.
- In this review, we summarize the rationale, evidence, and complications of venovenous ECMO support in severe ARDS secondary to COVID-19.

INTRODUCTION

At the end of 2019 an outbreak of pneumonia caused by a novel severe acute respiratory syndrome-coronavirus 2 (SARS-CoV-2) was discovered in the city of Wuhan, China.[1] Although most cases of COVID-19 present with mild symptoms including fever, cough, and myalgia, a substantial number of patients develop acute hypoxemic respiratory failure and acute respiratory distress syndrome (ARDS).[2,3] Resembling other etiologies of ARDS, the treatment of severe presentations of COVID-19 frequently involves invasive mechanical ventilation and, in most severe cases, extracorporeal membrane oxygenation (ECMO).[4]

---

[a] Department of Medicine, Division of Respirology, Sinai Health System and University Health Network, 585 University Avenue, 9-MaRS-9013, Toronto, Ontario M5G2G2, Canada; [b] Institute of Health Policy, Management and Evaluation, Dalla Lana School of Public Health, University of Toronto, 155 College Street, 4th Floor, Toronto, ON M5T 3M6, Canada; [c] Toronto General Hospital Research Institute, 200 Elizabeth Street, Toronto, ON M5G 2C4, Canada; [d] Interdepartmental Division of Critical Care Medicine, University of Toronto, 204 Victoria Street, 4th Floor, Room 411, Toronto, Ontario M5B 1T8, Canada
* Corresponding author. Interdepartmental Division of Critical Care Medicine, Toronto General Hospital, 585 University Avenue, 9-MaRS-9013, Toronto, Ontario M5G2G2, Canada.
E-mail address: eddy.fan@uhn.ca

Crit Care Clin 38 (2022) 535–552
https://doi.org/10.1016/j.ccc.2022.01.004
0749-0704/22/© 2022 Elsevier Inc. All rights reserved.

criticalcare.theclinics.com

ECMO constitutes a costly and resource-intense treatment of severe ARDS.[5] In the context of the COVID-19 pandemic and with an increasing number of patients requiring admission to an intensive care unit (ICU) worldwide, the appropriateness of use of such treatments as ECMO has been the focus of some discussions.[6] This review describes the role of venovenous (VV) ECMO in patients with COVID-19-related ARDS.

EXTRACORPOREAL MEMBRANE OXYGENATION FOR ACUTE RESPIRATORY DISTRESS SYNDROME: RATIONALE AND HISTORY

ARDS is associated with high morbidity and mortality caused by direct or indirect lung injury leading to multiorgan dysfunction.[7,8] Mechanical ventilation remains the cornerstone of support for this syndrome, with the main goal to unload the respiratory muscles, providing adequate gas exchange while the lungs recover from the original insult.[9] Although mechanical ventilation is a life-saving intervention, it can also lead to ventilator-induced lung injury through different mechanisms.[10] The fundamental principle of lung-protective ventilation is to allow for adequate gas exchange while preventing ventilator-induced lung injury.[11,12] In the most severe cases, lung-protective ventilation alone may be insufficient to achieve such goals and adjuvant strategies are needed. In this setting, ECMO can provide gas exchange bypassing the lungs allowing for a reduction in the intensity of mechanical ventilation.[13]

The most frequent configuration used in this context (VV-ECMO) consists of a drainage cannula that withdraws deoxygenated blood from a central vein (eg, femoral vein), a mechanical pump coupled with an oxygenator, and a return cannula that restores oxygenated blood to the circulation through another central vein (eg, internal jugular vein).[13]

ECMO is not a novel technology and its successful application in a setting of acute respiratory failure was first described in the early 1970s. However, its use remained restricted to neonatal and pediatric patients for decades.[14,15] Following technological advances, a new window of opportunity for ECMO in adults with acute respiratory failure opened during the influenza A (H1N1) pandemic in 2009. During this time, ECMO was used in adults with severe ARDS as a salvage therapy.[16] Despite increasing enthusiasm and use, it remained unclear whether it was associated with a survival benefit.[17]

Also in 2009, the Conventional Ventilatory Support Versus Extracorporeal Membrane Oxygenation for Severe Adult Respiratory Failure (CESAR) trial compared the efficacy, safety, and cost-effectiveness of standard of care in mechanical ventilation with VV-ECMO.[18] There was a significant increase in survival without disability in the group randomized to referral for ECMO consideration. Importantly, only 70% of the conventional treatment group received lung-protective ventilation in this pragmatic trial. Furthermore, only 76% of the patients allocated to the ECMO group actually received ECMO. The main conclusion of this trial was that referring patients to a center of excellence capable of providing ECMO improved outcome, but it could not prove that ECMO by itself was responsible for this.[19]

To help address this gap, the ECMO to Rescue Lung Injury in Severe ARDS (EOLIA) trial randomized patients with severe ARDS to receive treatment with VV-ECMO or conventional mechanical ventilation. The trial was stopped early for futility, with 60-day mortality of 35% in the ECMO group and 46% in the control group.[20] Although this difference was not statistically significant, a number of secondary outcomes and a post-hoc analyses favoured ECMO. In addition, a post hoc Bayesian analysis concluded that the posterior probability of a mortality benefit with ECMO was high even when using a strongly skeptical prior distribution.[21] Finally, the benefit of VV-

ECMO on mortality in patients with severe ARDS is supported by individual patient data, study level, and network meta-analyses.[12,22–24]

COVID-19-RELATED ACUTE RESPIRATORY DISTRESS SYNDROME: IS IT REALLY DIFFERENT?

The definition of ARDS encompasses clinical and radiologic criteria along with the presence of typical risk factors for direct or indirect lung injury.[25,26] Clinical and biologic heterogeneity within ARDS is therefore implied and has been topic of extensive research.[27–30] Since the beginning of the pandemic, the overwhelming number of patients with COVID-19 admitted to ICUs around the globe allowed clinicians and researchers to appreciate this clinical heterogeneity and in consequence, treatment strategies based on different clinical features were suggested.[31] As more data emerged through the course of the pandemic, the characterization of COVID-19-related ARDS as a distinct entity was challenged.

Indeed, the current body of clinical, physiologic, and pathologic data seems to support the notion that this disease, although exhibiting some heterogeneity, has common features to ARDS secondary to other risk factors.[32–34] Accordingly, it is reasonable to apply the best evidence-based recommendations, particularly with respect to ventilatory strategies and adjutants to mechanical ventilation.[32,34]

Venovenous Extracorporeal Membrane Oxygenation in COVID-19-Related Acute Respiratory Distress Syndrome: Old and New Challenges

The role of VV-ECMO as a strategy for severe ARDS in the context of the COVID-19 pandemic exhibits old and new challenges. Given the increasing number of patients requiring ICU admission and ventilatory support, the role of ECMO was again brought to the attention of clinicians and the public at the same time, leading to a detailed description of patients' trajectories.[35–41] Furthermore, debate on whether ARDS secondary to COVID-19 is a different entity also led to questioning the role of VV-ECMO support in this context, and whether the existing evidence could be applied. Finally, increasing concerns about ICU capacity and strain led to discussions about the appropriateness of ECMO as a highly technical intervention and to whether resources should be directed toward this intervention.[42,43]

Extracorporeal Membrane Oxygenation in COVID-19-Related Acute Respiratory Distress Syndrome: Clinical Outcomes

The literature surrounding the experience and outcomes of ECMO in patients with COVID-19 has transitioned from mainly anecdotical reports to large single and multicenter analyses **(Table 1)**. At the beginning of the pandemic, preliminary reports from China raised concerns highlighting increased mortality of COVID-19-related ARDS when compared with ARDS secondary to other risk factors.[6] The appropriateness of using a treatment that requires a highly specialized and technical team and a higher level of care at the bedside in the context of increased system strain was brought to the center of discussion.[6,44,45]

In a pooled analysis, Henry and Lippi[6] described that among 17 patients that required ECMO early in the pandemic mortality was 94%. However, mortality in the non-ECMO group was also considerably high, the sample was rather small, and data regarding baseline characteristics were missing. Huang and colleagues[46] found similar results and suggested using ECMO only for younger patients without preexisting diseases, but these data were also derived from a small case series. Thus, these

Table 1
Studies reporting outcomes in patients on ECMO for COVID-19 ARDS

Study	Study Design	Sample Size On ECMO (Total)	Mean Age	Mean Pao$_2$/Fio$_2$ Ratio	Included Patients and Time Period	Mortality (%)	Median days on ECMO	Main Complications
Barbaro et al,[49] 2020	Cohort study	1035 (1035)	49	72	Patients included in the ELSO registry From January 16th–May 1st 2020	37.4	14	Hemorrhagic stroke 6% Hemolysis 13%
Charlton et al, 2020	Cohort study	34 (34)	46	86	Severe COVID-19 ARDS Supported with ECMO April 1st–May 31st 2020	47	13	Not reported
Cousin et al, 2020	Cohort study	30 (30)	57	69 (n = 27)	Severe COVID-19 ARDS Supported with ECMO for at least 48 h March 9th–May 6th 2020	53.3	11	Acute kidney injury 50% Deep venous thrombosis 10% Pulmonary embolism 6.7% Hemorrhagic stroke 10% Major bleeding 43% Bloodstream infection 13%
Falcoz et al,[47] 2020	Cohort study	17 (17)	56	71	Adults meeting EOLIA criteria March 3rd–April 1st 2020	35	9	Thrombotic 29% Bleeding 35% VAP 59% AKI 70%
Guihaire et al, 2020	Cohort study	24 (24)	49	67	Severe COVID-19 ARDS Supported with ECMO March 23rd–May 5th 2020	29	19	Pulmonary hemorrhage 17% Pulmonary embolism 25% Hemorrhagic stroke 4%

						ECMO: 94 in ECMO: 71 non-ECMO	Not reported	Not reported
Henry and Lippi,[6] 2020	Review (pooled analysis)	17 (234)	56	Not reported	Not reported			
Jackel et al, 2020	Cohort study	15 (15)	61	64	Severe COVID-19 ARDS or influenza A/B infection Supported with ECMO October 2010 and June 2020	51.4	11	Renal-replacement therapy 33% Circuit change 33%
Jang et al, 2020	Cohort study	19 (19) 3 received VA-ECMO	63	92	Severe COVID-19 ARDS Supported with ECMO February 1st–April 30th 2020	52.6	17	Not reported
Mustafa et al,[63] 2020	Cohort study	40 (40)	48	69	Severe respiratory failure caused by COVID-19 March 17th–July 17th 2020	15	30	Not reported
Schmidt et al,[39] 2020	Cohort study	83 (492)	49	60	Adults with COVID-19 ARDS supported with VA or VV ECMO March 17th–July 17th 2020	31	20	Hemolysis 13% Pulmonary embolism 19% Massive hemorrhage 42% Hemorrhagic stroke 5% Oronasal bleeding 24% VAP 87% Cannula infection 23%
Shih et al, 2020	Cohort study	37 (37)	51	95	Severe COVID-19 ARDS March 1st–June 28th 2020	43.2	17	VAP 19% Bloodstream infection 11% Hemorrhagic stroke 8% Bleeding 32% Circuit malfunction 5%

(continued on next page)

Table 1
(continued)

Study	Study Design	Sample Size On ECMO (Total)	Mean Age	Mean Pao₂/Fio₂ Ratio	Included Patients and Time Period	Mortality (%)	Median days on ECMO	Main Complications
Takeda et al, 2020	Cohort study	26 (26)	71	70	Severe COVID-19 ARDS Supported with ECMO February 15th–March 15th 2020	38.5	Not reported	Not reported
Yang et al, 2020	Cohort study	21 (59)	58	60	Severe COVID-19 ARDS January 8th–March 31st 2020	57.1	9	Catheter site bleeding 9% Hemorrhagic stroke 4% Renal-replacement therapy 38% VAP 28%
Zayat et al, 2020	Cohort study	17 (17)	57	<100 not reported as a mean	Severe COVID-19 ARDS March 1st–April 20th 2020	47.1	Not reported	Not reported
Zhang et al, 2020	Cohort study	43 (43)	46	67	Severe COVID-19 ARDS Supported with ECMO March 3rd–May 2nd 2020	32.6	13	Acute kidney injury 50% Deep venous thrombosis 10% Pulmonary embolism 7% Hemorrhagic stroke 10% Bleeding leading to transfusion 43% Bloodstream infection 13%

Study	Study type	No. enrolled			Inclusion criteria			Complications
Akhtar et al, 2021	Cohort study	18 (18)	47	Not reported	Severe COVID-19 ARDS Supported with ECMO	22	17	Renal-replacement therapy 56% Thromboembolic disease 56% Hemorrhagic stroke 11% Gastrointestinal bleeding 11%
Diaz et al,[37] 2021	Cohort study	94 (94)	48	87	Age ≥15 y COVID-19 ARDS Supported with ECMO March 3rd–August 31st 2020	38.8	16	Pulmonary embolism 2% Hemorrhagic stroke 13% Pneumothorax 14% Thromboembolic disease 22% Bleeding 39% VAP 51% Infection 71%
Lebreton et al,[40] 2021	Cohort study	288 (302) 11 received VA-ECMO and 3 VA-V-ECMO	52	61	Severe COVID-19 ARDS Supported with ECMO Admitted to any ICU in greater Paris March 8th–June 3rd 2020	54	14	Renal-replacement therapy 43% Pulmonary embolism 18% Hemorrhagic stroke 12% Pneumothorax 9% Bleeding 43% VAP 85%
Ramanathan et al,[55] 2021	Systematic review and meta-analysis	1896 (1896)	51 (n = 491)	68	Cohort study studies or randomised clinical trials examining ECMO in adults with COVID-19 ARDS December 1st 2019–January 10th 2020	35.7 (n = 1737)	16 (n = 1711)	Acute kidney injury 35% Mechanical 27% Infectious 10%

(continued on next page)

Table 1
(continued)

Study	Study Design	Sample Size On ECMO (Total)	Mean Age	Mean Pao₂/Fio₂ Ratio	Included Patients and Time Period	Mortality (%)	Median days on ECMO	Main Complications
Rabie et al, 2021	Cohort study	307 (307)	45	60	Adult patients of 19 ECMO centers March 1st–September 30th 2020	42	15	Infections 70% Major bleeding 24% Renal-replacement therapy 32% Pulmonary embolism 5%
Riera et al,[50] 2021	Cohort study	319 (319)	53	76	Severe COVID-19 ARDS Supported with ECMO	1st wave 41.1 2nd wave 60.1	17	Pneumonia 50% Acute kidney injury 26% Vascular thrombosis 16% Circuit clotting 37% Hemorrhagic shock 14%
Roedl et al, 2021	Cohort study	20 (223)	Not reported	Not reported	Adults admitted to ICU with COVID-19 February 1st– June 3rd 2020	65	Not reported	Not reported

Study	Study type				Inclusion criteria			Complications
Shaefi et al,[51] 2021	Target trial	130 (1297)	49 (ECMO) 58 (non-ECMO)	80 (ECMO) 90 (non-ECMO)	Diagnosis of COVID-19 Age ≥18 y Admitted to an ICU capable of offering VV ECMO Pao_2/Fio_2 <100 mm Hg From March 1st–July 1st 2020	34.6 Non-ECMO: 47	16	AKI 22% Pneumothorax 13% Pulmonary embolism 2% Deep vein thrombosis 18% Hemorrhagic stroke 4% Systemic bleeding 25% Bacterial pneumonia 35%

Search strategy: We performed a search in PubMed for articles published in English language between December 2019 and September 2021, using combinations of the terms "COVID-19," "Extracorporeal membrane oxygenation," and "Acute respiratory distress syndrome." We determined relevance based on content, focusing on studies including at least 15 participants. We also manually retrieved articles from references. Finally, we also searched for relevant reports at the ELSO registry Web site: www.elso.org.

Abbreviations: AKI, acute kidney injury; DVT, deep venous thrombosis; ELSO, Extracorporeal Life Support Organization; Pao_2/Fio_2, ratio of arterial oxygen partial pressure to fractional inspired oxygen; PE, pulmonary embolism; VAP, ventilator-associated pneumonia.

initial descriptions of ECMO for patients with severe COVID-19 were difficult to interpret and to translate into meaningful clinical recommendations.

In contrast, a prospective cohort study that included 17 patients on ECMO because of COVID-19 ARDS showed that 60-day mortality was significantly lower (35%) than the previous reports.[47] Schmidt and colleagues[39] reported a retrospective cohort of 83 patients placed on ECMO for COVID-19 ARDS comparing their results with those of the EOLIA trial. Despite having a greater severity of hypoxemia in their cohort, these patients had a similar 90-day mortality.[39] Based in part on these results, the Extracorporeal Life Support Organization advocated for the use of ECMO in specialized centers only.[48,49]

A retrospective cohort study that included 319 patients on ECMO from 24 ICUs in Spain and Portugal reported similar results (mortality 35%). This study suggested a significant higher mortality during the second wave, which may be explained by patient-level (age, time on ventilator before cannulation) and center level characteristics.[40,50] Finally, a systematic review and meta-analysis of 1896 patients from 22 studies reported a pooled in-hospital mortality of 37%, similar to those from randomized trials and systematic reviews in patients without COVID-19.[18,22,23]

Although encouraging, none of these studies had a comparative non-ECMO control group. Therefore, Shaefi and colleagues[51] emulated a target trial comparing mechanically ventilated patients with severe hypoxemia who received and those who did not receive ECMO within 7 days of ICU admission. Patients with severe hypoxia who received ECMO had a lower mortality compared with those who did not (35% vs 47%), similar estimates as observed in the EOLIA trial.[20] Despite known limitations, well-conducted observational research has an important role in understanding the efficacy of this intervention, given the lack of feasibility for another randomized trial.

Extracorporeal Membrane Oxygenation in COVID-19: Patient Selection

Patient selection for VV-ECMO in patients with COVID-19 should follow the same guiding principles as for ARDS from other causes (**Fig. 1**).[52] Before initiation of ECMO is considered, referring centers should ensure conventional management has been optimized, including lung-protective ventilation, adequate level of positive end-expiratory pressure, prone positioning, and consideration of deep sedation/neuromuscular paralysis. If all these strategies fail or when lung-protective ventilation cannot be achieved (ie, a need for injurious ventilation), ECMO should be considered in

Patient Selection Criteria for ECMO Consideration			
Severity of Disease		Mechanical Ventilation Optimized	Patient Related Characteristics
Oxygenation	**Ventilation**	FiO2 ≥80%	Age ≤50 y
PaO2/FiO2 <50 mmHg for >3 h	pH <7.25 + PaCO2 ≥60 mmHg + RR 35/min for >6h	PEEP ≥10 cmH2O VT ≤6ml/kg (PBW) Plateau Pressure ≤32 cmH2O Prone positioning Neuromuscular blockade	Absence of comorbidities affecting short-term recovery Invasive Mechanical Ventilation ≤7d Adequate vascular access Absence of distributive Shock Low risk of hemorrhagic complications
OR			
PaO2/FiO2 <80 mmHg for >6h			

Fig. 1. Patient selection criteria for VV-ECMO in patients with COVID-19 ARDS. Fio$_2$, fraction of inspired oxygen; Paco$_2$, arterial partial pressure of carbon dioxide; Pao$_2$/Fio$_2$ ratio of arterial oxygen partial pressure to fractional inspired oxygen; PBW, predicted body weight; PEEP, positive end-expiratory pressure; RR, respiratory rate; VT, tidal volume.

the absence of factors associated with poor benefit, such as advanced age, comorbidities, multiorgan dysfunction, and prolonged duration of invasive mechanical ventilation.[52,53] Although patient selection focuses on time from initiation of invasive ventilation to ECMO cannulation, increasing awareness of time on noninvasive respiratory support (eg, high-flow oxygen, noninvasive ventilation) before intubation is being raised as a potential predictor of outcome and a key parameter for adequate patient selection.[37]

THE COURSE OF EXTRACORPOREAL MEMBRANE OXYGENATION SUPPORT IN PATIENTS WITH COVID-19: PATIENT TRAJECTORIES

During the COVID-19 pandemic, many centers experienced increased demands for ECMO, even in those with previous long-standing experience.[39,40] This accentuated the multiple clinical trajectories that exist among these patients once they are initially placed on ECMO (**Fig. 2**). Certain patients exhibit lung recovery shortly after cannulation, and liberation from ECMO is quickly and successfully achieved. This group meets the foundational criteria and expectation when starting this treatment: ECMO as a bridge to recovery. At the other end of the spectrum, certain patients undergo prolonged treatment on ECMO without significant lung recovery, introducing unique clinical and ethical challenges. For these patients, ECMO can still be a bridge to recovery, but other trajectories are also possible, including discussions about lung transplantation candidacy or transitioning to palliative care.[54] Decision-making by patients and families/caregivers is influenced by the spectrum of clinical trajectories. Given the prolonged time that certain patients can be on ECMO (median time up to 30 days, see **Table 1**), this can also lead to important challenges for decision-making by policy makers, particularly during a pandemic where ICU beds and human resources are scarce.[42]

THE COURSE OF EXTRACORPOREAL MEMBRANE OXYGENATION SUPPORT IN PATIENTS WITH COVID-19: COMPLICATIONS

During the course of ICU stay, patients on ECMO can suffer a range of complications, which can be life-threatening. These are categorized as the typical complications

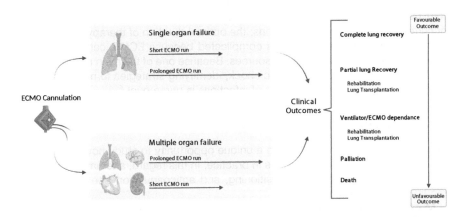

Fig. 2. Clinical trajectories for patients on VV-ECMO with COVID-19. Patients on ECMO may present single or multiple organ failure, which affects the duration of ECMO run and consequently clinical outcomes. The spectrum of clinical outcomes varies from complete lung recovery to death.

observed because of prolonged critical illness, ECMO-specific complications, and those specific to COVID-19.

Acute renal failure with or without need for renal-replacement therapy was consistently reported as one of the most frequent complications.[40,50,55] Whether this is solely related to the severity of COVID-19 infection or to ECMO support is unclear. Potential mechanisms by which ECMO can contribute to kidney failure include hemolysis, secondary infections, and major bleeding.[56]

Major bleeding was frequently reported and often associated with worse outcome in patients with COVID-19-related ARDS supported with ECMO.[57] These complications are not usually associated with an identifiable coagulopathy and independent of heparin use. Clinically important bleeding in the largest cohorts was reported in 35% to 43% of the patients, with frequent sources being oronasal, cannula-related, and hemothorax.[37,39,40,47] In a French study, major bleeding requiring transfusions was significantly higher in patients that died but only 4% of the patients died of hemorrhagic shock.[40] A study conducted in Chile reported a surprisingly high rate of intracranial hemorrhage (13%), doubling what was published in the COVID-19 Extracorporeal Life Support Organization report.[37,49] This could be explained by the lack of protocols to control relative changes in $Paco_2$ early after cannulation, which was shown to be associated with an increased incidence of neurologic complications.[58] In face of these complications, recommendations for anticoagulation strategies and target were highly variable during the pandemic.[47,59] Indeed, the optimal strategy for anticoagulation during ECMO remains one of the areas where further research is warranted.

Thromboembolic complications have also been described in these patients, including deep vein thrombosis, pulmonary embolism, or circuit thrombosis.[60] Underlying mechanisms include endothelial dysfunction, platelet activation, and disseminated intravascular coagulation.[61] This increased risk persists despite the use of different degrees of anticoagulation.[37,40,50]

Infectious complications have been reported in up to 37% of patients receiving ECMO for COVID-19.[49] Ventilator-associated pneumonia was the most frequent source, followed by bloodstream infections, and *Staphylococcus aureus* the most commonly cultured organism.[49,55] Optimization of antimicrobial therapy in the context of extracorporeal life-support poses unique challenges because of the scarce literature describing pharmacokinetic and dosing requirements during ECMO.[62] In the occurrence of bloodstream infections, the optimal duration of therapy and the definition of adequate source control is complicated because ECMO cannulas could be perceived as persistent infectious sources. Because one of the main reported causes of death in this population is septic shock, identifying strategies to maximize source control and appropriate treatments of infections is paramount.[4]

NOVEL TECHNIQUES AND VARIATIONS IN PRACTICE

The COVID-19 pandemic was also a unique opportunity to study novel approaches, adjuvant treatments, and variations in practice. In this regard, alternative cannulation techniques, the use of prone positioning, and anticoagulation-free runs of ECMO require special attention.

Mustafa and colleagues[63] retrospectively collected data from 40 patients with COVID-19 ARDS supported on ECMO in two hospitals in Chicago. They used a single-access, dual-stage right atrium-to-pulmonary-artery cannula, with drainage of blood from the right atrium lumen (decreasing right-sided preload), and oxygenated blood is returned into the pulmonary artery. Their strategy included a focus on earlier discontinuation of mechanical ventilation and rehabilitation. By the time of the publication, all patients were successfully weaned off invasive mechanical ventilation, 80% had been decannulated, 73% had been discharged from hospital, and overall mortality was 15%.[63] These results may be associated with early mobilization, reduced need for sedation, and right ventricle support. The later might have been critical because right ventricular dysfunction is a frequently reported cause of death in patients with COVID-19 ARDS.[64]

The pandemic also raised awareness of the use of prone positioning, including increased use in nonintubated patients and during VV-ECMO.[65–68] In a report by Schmidt and colleagues,[39] prone positioning was used in up to 81% of patients on VV ECMO and the authors suggested that this might have contributed to improve survival rates. Similar results were reported by Guervilly and colleagues,[69] suggesting prone positioning while on ECMO is associated with increased liberation from ECMO and survival. Finally, a recent study reported that the rate of complications was low (6%) and only 2% of proned patients needed to be supinated to resolve the complication.[70] Although this finding is reassuring, prone positioning during ECMO should be performed in experienced centers.[70]

Titrating systemic anticoagulation to prevent clot formation while avoiding bleeding complications is one of the main challenges of ECMO management. Because of the scarce high-quality data, there is practice variation among centers particularly regarding the best method to monitor anticoagulation and the need for antithrombin supplementation.[71] Furthermore, an international survey from 50 different countries showed that up to 3% of the centers did not routinely prescribe anticoagulation for patients on VV ECMO.[72] To investigate the feasibility and safety of this approach, Kurihara and colleagues[73] compared 38 patients that received systemic anticoagulation with 36 patients that received thromboprophylaxis. The group of patients who received systemic anticoagulation had higher rates of gastrointestinal bleeding, received more blood transfusions, and had higher rates of oxygenator dysfunction. Although done at a single center and with a small sample size, results were consistent with previous reports.[74] Given that hemorrhagic complications contribute to morbidity and mortality associated to ECMO, an anticoagulation-free approach is appealing, and could be an opportunity for future research.

SUMMARY AND FUTURE DIRECTIONS

Despite early reports suggesting COVID-19-related ARDS should warrant distinct management, current evidence suggests that similar management principles to non-COVID-19 ARDS should be applied. These include lung-protective ventilation and the use of adjuvant treatments when appropriate. Data from large cohorts and observational studies emulating clinical trials suggest that the efficacy and outcomes of ECMO in the context of severe COVID-19 is similar to ARDS because of other risk factors. The spectrum of patients' trajectories range from short ECMO runs with full lung recovery to prolonged ECMO support with significant organ dysfunction. Typical complications, such as bleeding and thromboembolic events, are frequent in patients who receive treatment with ECMO, often presenting as life-threatening. Ongoing and future research will help understand whether alternative approaches for ECMO cannulation, prone positioning, and variations in anticoagulation practices can improve the safety and efficacy of this intervention. The ongoing pandemic poses a unique opportunity to improve the understanding of the strengths and limitations of this resource-intensive intervention. Finally, enhanced collaboration among centers locally, nationally, and internationally is key for rapidly generating an important body of clinical evidence.

CLINICS CARE POINTS

- COVID-19-related ARDS resembles ARDS caused by other risk factors in its clinical presentation and outcomes.
- Evidence-based principles of lung-protective ventilation and adjuvant therapies, such as ECMO, for the management of ARDS should be applied similarly for severe COVID-19.
- Emerging evidence in the field currently suggests that the role of ECMO in the management of COVID-19-related ARDS is comparable with non-COVID-19 ARDS, and patient selection should follow similar principles.
- Frequent complications of ECMO include acute kidney failure, major bleeding, thromboembolic events, and secondary infections.
- The dramatically high number of patients requiring ECMO worldwide for COVID-19 ARDS poses an opportunity to study variations in practice, such as different cannulation techniques, prone positioning, and alternatives in the use of anticoagulation.

DISCLOSURE

Dr B.L. Ferreyro is supported by a Vanier Canada Graduate Scholarship. Dr E. Fan reports personal fees from ALung Technologies, Aerogen, Baxter, Boehringer-Ingelheim, GE Healthcare, MC3 Cardiopulmonary, and Vasomune outside the submitted work.

REFERENCES

1. Zhou F, Yu T, Du R, et al. Clinical course and risk factors for mortality of adult inpatients with COVID-19 in Wuhan, China: a retrospective cohort study. Lancet 2020;395(10229):1054–62.
2. Huang C, Wang Y, Li X, et al. Clinical features of patients infected with 2019 novel coronavirus in Wuhan, China. Lancet 2020;395(10223):497–506.
3. Wang D, Hu B, Hu C, et al. Clinical characteristics of 138 hospitalized patients with 2019 novel coronavirus–infected pneumonia in Wuhan, China. Jama 2020;323(11):1061–9.
4. Blazoski C, Baram M, Hirose H. Outcomes of extracorporeal membrane oxygenation in acute respiratory distress syndrome due to COVID-19: the lessons learned from the first wave of COVID-19. J Cardiovasc Surg 2021;36(7):2219–24.
5. Abrams D, Ferguson ND, Brochard L, et al. ECMO for ARDS: from salvage to standard of care? Lancet Respir Med 2019;7(2):108–10.
6. Henry BM, Lippi G. Poor survival with extracorporeal membrane oxygenation in acute respiratory distress syndrome (ARDS) due to coronavirus disease 2019 (COVID-19): pooled analysis of early reports. J Crit Care 2020;58:27–8.
7. Herridge MS, Chu LM, Matte A, et al. The RECOVER Program: disability risk groups and 1-year outcome after 7 or more days of mechanical ventilation. Am J Resp Crit Care 2016;194(7):831–44.
8. Herridge MS, Tansey CM, Matté A, et al. Functional disability 5 years after acute respiratory distress syndrome. N Engl J Med 2011;364(14):1293–304.
9. Goligher EC, Ferguson ND, Brochard LJ. Clinical challenges in mechanical ventilation. Lancet 2016;387(10030):1856–66.
10. Vasques F, Duscio E, Cipulli F, et al. Determinants and prevention of ventilator-induced lung injury. Crit Care Clin 2018;34(3):343–56.
11. Sorbo LD, Goligher EC, McAuley DF, et al. Mechanical ventilation in adults with acute respiratory distress syndrome. Summary of the experimental evidence

for the clinical practice guideline. Ann Am Thorac Soc 2017;14(Supplement_4): S261–70.

12. Aoyama H, Uchida K, Aoyama K, et al. Assessment of therapeutic interventions and lung protective ventilation in patients with moderate to severe acute respiratory distress syndrome: a systematic review and network meta-analysis. Jama Netw Open 2019;2(7):e198116.

13. Brodie D, Bacchetta M. Extracorporeal membrane oxygenation for ARDS in adults. N Engl J Med 2011;365(20):1905–14.

14. Hill JD, O'Brien TG, Murray JJ, et al. Prolonged extracorporeal oxygenation for acute post-traumatic respiratory failure (shock-lung syndrome): use of the Bramson membrane lung. N Engl J Med 1972;286(12):629–34.

15. Bartlett RH, Gazzaniga AB, Jefferies MR, et al. Extracorporeal membrane oxygenation (ECMO) cardiopulmonary support in infancy. Trans - Am Soc Artif Intern Organs 1976;22:80–93.

16. Brodie D. The evolution of extracorporeal membrane oxygenation for adult respiratory failure. Ann Am Thorac Soc 2018;15(Supplement_1):S57–60.

17. Pham T, Combes A, Rozé H, et al. Extracorporeal membrane oxygenation for pandemic influenza A(H1N1)-induced acute respiratory distress syndrome. Am J Resp Crit Care 2013;187(3):276–85.

18. Peek GJ, Mugford M, Tiruvoipati R, et al. Efficacy and economic assessment of conventional ventilatory support versus extracorporeal membrane oxygenation for severe adult respiratory failure (CESAR): a multicentre randomised controlled trial. Lancet 2009;374(9698):1351–63.

19. Zwischenberger JB, Lynch JE. Will CESAR answer the adult ECMO debate? Lancet 2009;374(9698):1307–8.

20. Combes A, Hajage D, Capellier G, et al. Extracorporeal membrane oxygenation for severe acute respiratory distress syndrome. N Engl J Med 2018;378(21): 1965–75.

21. Goligher EC, Tomlinson G, Hajage D, et al. Extracorporeal membrane oxygenation for severe acute respiratory distress syndrome and posterior probability of mortality benefit in a post hoc Bayesian analysis of a randomized clinical trial. Jama 2018;320(21):2251.

22. Munshi L, Walkey A, Goligher E, et al. Venovenous extracorporeal membrane oxygenation for acute respiratory distress syndrome: a systematic review and meta-analysis. Lancet Respir Med 2019;7(2):163–72.

23. Combes A, Peek GJ, Hajage D, et al. ECMO for severe ARDS: systematic review and individual patient data meta-analysis. Intensive Care Med 2020;46(11): 2048–57.

24. Sud S, Friedrich JO, Adhikari NKJ, et al. Comparative effectiveness of protective ventilation strategies for moderate and severe acute respiratory distress syndrome. A network meta-analysis. Am J Resp Crit Care 2021;203(11):1366–77.

25. Force ADT, Ranieri VM, Rubenfeld GD, et al. Acute respiratory distress syndrome: the Berlin definition. Jama 2012;307(23):2526–33.

26. Thompson BT, Chambers RC, Liu KD. Acute respiratory distress syndrome. N Engl J Med 2017;377(6):562–72.

27. Fan E, Brodie D, Slutsky AS. Acute respiratory distress syndrome: advances in diagnosis and treatment. Jama 2018;319(7):698–710.

28. Sinha P, Calfee CS. Phenotypes in acute respiratory distress syndrome. Curr Opin Crit Care 2019;25(1):12–20.

29. Calfee CS, Delucchi K, Parsons PE, et al. Subphenotypes in acute respiratory distress syndrome: latent class analysis of data from two randomised controlled trials. Lancet Respir Med 2014;2(8):611–20.

30. Khan YA, Fan E, Ferguson ND. Precision medicine and heterogeneity of treatment effect in therapies for acute respiratory distress syndrome. Chest 2021. https://doi.org/10.1016/j.chest.2021.07.009.

31. Gattinoni L, Chiumello D, Caironi P, et al. COVID-19 pneumonia: different respiratory treatments for different phenotypes? Intensive Care Med 2020;46(6):1099–102.

32. Goligher EC, Ranieri VM, Slutsky AS. Is severe COVID-19 pneumonia a typical or atypical form of ARDS? And does it matter? Intensive Care Med 2021;47(1):83–5.

33. Tobin MJ. Pondering the atypicality of ARDS in COVID-19 is a distraction for the bedside doctor. Intensive Care Med 2021;47(3):361–2.

34. Fan E, Beitler JR, Brochard L, et al. COVID-19-associated acute respiratory distress syndrome: is a different approach to management warranted? Lancet Respir Med 2020;8(8):816–21.

35. Hoyler MM, Kumar S, Thalapallil R, et al. VV-ECMO usage in ARDS due to COVID-19: clinical, practical and ethical considerations. J Clin Anesth 2020;65:109893.

36. Abrams D, Lorusso R, Vincent JL, et al. ECMO during the COVID-19 pandemic: when is it unjustified? Crit Care 2020;24(1):507.

37. Diaz RA, Graf J, Zambrano JM, et al. Extracorporeal membrane oxygenation for COVID-19–associated severe acute respiratory distress syndrome in Chile: a nationwide incidence and cohort study. Am J Resp Crit Care 2021;204(1):34–43.

38. Lorusso R, Combes A, Coco VL, et al. ECMO for COVID-19 patients in Europe and Israel. Intensive Care Med 2021;47(3):344–8.

39. Schmidt M, Hajage D, Lebreton G, et al. Extracorporeal membrane oxygenation for severe acute respiratory distress syndrome associated with COVID-19: a retrospective cohort study. Lancet Respir Med 2020;8(11):1121–31.

40. Lebreton G, Schmidt M, Ponnaiah M, et al. Extracorporeal membrane oxygenation network organisation and clinical outcomes during the COVID-19 pandemic in Greater Paris, France: a multicentre cohort study. Lancet Respir Med 2021. https://doi.org/10.1016/s2213-2600(21)00096-5.

41. Fernando SM, Mathew R, Slutsky AS, et al. Media portrayals of outcomes after extracorporeal membrane oxygenation. J Intern Med 2021;181(3):391–4.

42. Dao B, Savulescu J, Suen JY, et al. Ethical factors determining ECMO allocation during the COVID-19 pandemic. Bmc Med Ethics 2021;22(1):70.

43. Enumah ZO, Carrese J, Choi CW. The ethics of extracorporeal membrane oxygenation: revisiting the principles of clinical bioethics. Ann Thorac Surg 2021;112(1):61–6.

44. Yang X, Yu Y, Xu J, et al. Clinical course and outcomes of critically ill patients with SARS-CoV-2 pneumonia in Wuhan, China: a single-centered, retrospective, observational study. Lancet Respir Med 2020;8(5):475–81.

45. MacLaren G, Fisher D, Brodie D. Preparing for the most critically ill patients with COVID-19. Jama 2020;323(13):1245–6.

46. Huang S, Xia H, Wu Z, et al. Clinical data of early COVID-19 cases receiving extracorporeal membrane oxygenation in Wuhan, China. J Clin Anesth 2020;68:110044.

47. Falcoz PE, Monnier A, Puyraveau M, et al. Extracorporeal membrane oxygenation for critically ill patients with COVID-19–related acute respiratory distress syndrome: worth the effort? Am J Resp Crit Care 2020;202(3):460–3.

48. Shekar K, Badulak J, Peek G, et al. Extracorporeal Life Support Organization coronavirus disease 2019 interim guidelines: a consensus document from an international group of interdisciplinary extracorporeal membrane oxygenation providers. Asaio J 2020;66(7):707–21.

49. Barbaro RP, MacLaren G, Boonstra PS, et al. Extracorporeal membrane oxygenation support in COVID-19: an international cohort study of the Extracorporeal Life Support Organization registry. Lancet 2020;396(10257):1071–8.

50. Riera J, Roncon-Albuquerque R, Fuset MP, et al. Increased mortality in patients with COVID-19 receiving extracorporeal respiratory support during the second wave of the pandemic. Intensive Care Med 2021;1–4. https://doi.org/10.1007/s00134-021-06517-9.

51. Shaefi S, Brenner SK, Gupta S, et al. Extracorporeal membrane oxygenation in patients with severe respiratory failure from COVID-19. Intensive Care Med 2021;47(2):208–21.

52. Bullen EC, Teijeiro-Paradis R, Fan E. How I do it: how I select which ARDS patients should be treated with venovenous extracorporeal membrane oxygenation. Chest 2020;158(3):1036–45.

53. Bartlett RH, Ogino MT, Brodie D, et al. Initial ELSO guidance document: ECMO for COVID-19 patients with severe cardiopulmonary failure. Asaio J 2020;66(5):472–4.

54. Cypel M, Keshavjee S. When to consider lung transplantation for COVID-19. Lancet Respir Med 2020;8(10):944–6.

55. Ramanathan K, Shekar K, Ling RR, et al. Extracorporeal membrane oxygenation for COVID-19: a systematic review and meta-analysis. Crit Care 2021;25(1):211.

56. Legrand M, Bell S, Forni L, et al. Pathophysiology of COVID-19-associated acute kidney injury. Nat Rev Nephrol 2021;1–14. https://doi.org/10.1038/s41581-021-00452-0.

57. Cavayas YA, Sorbo L del, Fan E. Intracranial hemorrhage in adults on ECMO. Perfusion 2018;33(1_suppl):42–50.

58. Cavayas YA, Munshi L, Sorbo L del, et al. The early change in PaCO2 after extracorporeal membrane oxygenation initiation is associated with neurological complications. Am J Resp Crit Care 2020;0(ja):1525–35.

59. Gaisendrees C, Walter SG, Elderia A, et al. Adequate anticoagulation and ECMO therapy in COVID-19 patients with severe pulmonary embolism. Perfusion 2021;36(6):575–81.

60. Ripoll B, Rubino A, Besser M, et al. Observational study of thrombosis and bleeding in COVID-19 VV ECMO patients. Int J Artif Organs 2021. https://doi.org/10.1177/0391398821989065. 039139882198906.

61. Asakura H, Ogawa H. Overcoming bleeding events related to extracorporeal membrane oxygenation in COVID-19. Lancet Respir Med 2020;8(12):e87–8.

62. Abdul-Aziz MH, Roberts JA. Antibiotic dosing during extracorporeal membrane oxygenation: does the system matter? Curr Opin Anaesthesiol 2020;33(1):71–82.

63. Mustafa AK, Alexander PJ, Joshi DJ, et al. Extracorporeal membrane oxygenation for patients with COVID-19 in severe respiratory failure. Jama Surg 2020;155(10):990–2.

64. Creel-Bulos C, Hockstein M, Amin N, et al. Acute cor pulmonale in critically ill patients with Covid-19. N Engl J Med 2020;382(21):e70.

65. Garcia B, Cousin N, Bourel C, et al. Prone positioning under VV-ECMO in SARS-CoV-2-induced acute respiratory distress syndrome. Crit Care 2020;24(1):428.

66. Oujidi Y, Bensaid A, Melhoaui I, et al. Prone position during ECMO in patients with COVID-19 in Morocco: case series. Ann Med Surg 2021;69:102769.

67. Telias I, Katira BH, Brochard L. Is the prone position helpful during spontaneous breathing in patients with COVID-19? JAMA 2020. https://doi.org/10.1001/jama.2020.8539.

68. Guérin C, Reignier J, Richard JC, et al. Prone positioning in severe acute respiratory distress syndrome. N Engl J Med 2013;368(23):2159–68.

69. Guervilly C, Prud'homme E, Pauly V, et al. Prone positioning and extracorporeal membrane oxygenation for severe acute respiratory distress syndrome: time for a randomized trial? Intensive Care Med 2019;45(7):1040–2.

70. Giani M, Martucci G, Madotto F, et al. Prone positioning during venovenous extracorporeal membrane oxygenation in acute respiratory distress syndrome. A multicenter cohort study and propensity-matched analysis. Ann Am Thorac Soc 2021;18(3):495–501.

71. Chlebowski MM, Baltagi S, Carlson M, et al. Clinical controversies in anticoagulation monitoring and antithrombin supplementation for ECMO. Crit Care 2020;24(1):19.

72. Protti A, Iapichino GE, Nardo MD, et al. Anticoagulation management and antithrombin supplementation practice during veno-venous extracorporeal membrane oxygenation. Anesthesiology 2020;132(3):562–70.

73. Kurihara C, Walter JM, Karim A, et al. Feasibility of venovenous extracorporeal membrane oxygenation without systemic anticoagulation. Ann Thorac Surg 2020;110(4):1209–15.

74. Krueger K, Schmutz A, Zieger B, et al. Venovenous extracorporeal membrane oxygenation with prophylactic subcutaneous anticoagulation only: an observational study in more than 60 patients. Artif Organs 2017;41(2):186–92.

Acute Neurologic Complications of COVID-19 and Postacute Sequelae of COVID-19

Neha S. Dangayach, MD, MSCR, FAAN, FNCS[a,b,*],
Virginia Newcombe, MD, PhD[c], Romain Sonnenville, MD, PhD[d,e]

KEYWORDS

- Neurologic complications • Long-COVID • Cerebrovascular complications
- Neuro-COVID

KEY POINTS

- Neurologic complications of COVID-19 are common. They can occur in patients with mild to severe COVID-19.
- Cerebrovascular complications, such as acute ischemic stroke, are seen in about 1.5% of all patients with COVID-19, whereas cerebral sinus venous thrombosis is rare, and intracerebral hemorrhage can occur as a consequence of therapeutic anticoagulation or because of hemorrhagic transformation of acute ischemic stroke. Stroke systems of care must be adapted to provide the same high-quality care for patients with COVID-19 to uphold time is brain by providing rapid access to testing and personal protective equipment.
- Coma and prolonged disorders of consciousness may be seen in patients with COVID-19 as a consequence of viral infection, as prolonged use of sedative drips and delayed metabolism of these medications are due to hepatorenal dysfunction. Delirium is common in COVID-19. Compliance with the intensive care unit liberation bundle or the A2F bundle was lower than during the first and second waves of COVID-19, and lack of family visitation may have been an important contributor to increased incidence of delirium.
- Neurologic complications in postacute sequelae of COVID-19 range from persistent fatigue, headaches, brain fog, depression, anxiety, postural orthostatic tachycardia even in patients with mild disease to an overlap with postintensive care syndrome in intensive care unit survivors, highlighting the need for long-term follow-up.

[a] Neurocritical Care Division, Department of Neurosurgery, Icahn School of Medicine at Mount Sinai, 1 Gustave L, Levy Place, New York, NY 10029, USA; [b] Department of Neurology, Icahn School of Medicine at Mount Sinai, 1 Gustave L, Levy Place, New York, NY 10029, USA; [c] University Division of Anaesthesia, Department of Medicine, University of Cambridge, Box 93, Addenbrooke's Hospital, Hills Road, Cambridge CB2 0QQ, United Kingdom; [d] Department of Intensive Care Medicine, AP-HP, Hôpital Bichat-Claude Bernard, 46 Rue Henri Huchard, Paris Cedex F-75877, France; [e] Université de Paris, INSERM UMR 1148, Team 6, Paris F-75018, France
* Corresponding author. 1 Gustave L. Levy Place, Annenberg 8-42 B, New York, NY 10029.
E-mail address: neha.dangayach@mountsinai.org

Crit Care Clin 38 (2022) 553–570
https://doi.org/10.1016/j.ccc.2022.03.002
0749-0704/22/© 2022 Elsevier Inc. All rights reserved.

criticalcare.theclinics.com

ACUTE NEUROLOGIC COMPLICATIONS OF COVID-19 AND POSTACUTE SEQUELAE OF COVID-19

Three hundred forty million people have suffered from the novel coronavirus, severe acute respiratory syndrome coronavirus 2 (SARS-CoV-2 [COVID-19]), across the world at the time of publication, and 5.57 million deaths have occurred since the beginning of the pandemic.[1] COVID-19 is a multisystem viral sepsis syndrome that can affect different organ systems with symptoms ranging from mild to life threatening.[2] Neurologic complications are commonly described and may occur as direct or indirect consequences of the viral infection, complications of treatment, or, in some cases, may be incidental associations. These insults do not just occur in the acute phases, with ongoing sequelae occurring and/or persisting for weeks to months after the initial infection, often as part of a syndrome known as postacute sequelae of COVID-19 (PASC) or long-COVID.[3–8] Critically ill patients have a higher likelihood of neurologic complications than patients with mild COVID-19.[3,4]

The recognition and diagnosis of these neurologic complications are challenging, particularly in the context of overstrained medical systems, where an underrecognition or delays in diagnosis of neurologic complications may contribute to poor outcomes.[5]

In this review, the authors highlight acute neurologic complications of COVID-19 as well as neurologic manifestations of PASC.

In the first section of this review, the authors discuss overall epidemiology, pathophysiology, and risk factors for neurologic manifestations followed by a discussion of specific neurologic manifestations.

EPIDEMIOLOGY

The risk of neurologic manifestations increases with hospitalization and higher severity of COVID-19 infection, although even patients with mild initial disease may have neurologic sequelae. These include non-life-threatening but debilitating symptoms ranging from anosmia, dysgeusia, fatigue, malaise, headaches to stroke, encephalitis, and Guillain-Barre syndrome (GBS), among others (**Table 1**).

The understanding of the neurologic complications of COVID-19 comes mainly from observational studies. **Table 1** summarizes neurologic complications described in some of the larger cohort studies of hospitalized patients. In a systematic review and meta-analysis (n = 13,480 patients and a third of these patients with severe COVID-19), the most common neurologic manifestations were myalgia (22%), dysgeusia (20%), anosmia (18%), headache (12%), dizziness (11%), encephalopathy (9.4%), and stroke (2.5%). Myalgia, elevated creatine kinase and lactate dehydrogenase, and acute stroke were significantly more common in severe cases.[6,7]

RISK FACTORS FOR ACUTE NEUROPSYCHIATRIC COMPLICATIONS AND POSTACUTE SEQUELAE OF COVID-19

Older patients, multiple comorbidities, Hispanic patients, south Asian, black, and mixed ethnicity patients, and patients with preexisting neurologic disorders have a higher risk of developing neurologic complications of acute COVID-19. Additional risk factors for PASC include age greater than 40 years, white ethnicity, and female sex.[8] A systematic review identified the following risks for neuropsychiatric consequences of PASC[9]

- For depression and/or anxiety (seen in 20%–40% of survivors): Women, those with infected family members, postinfectious physical symptoms, severe infection, elevated inflammatory markers, prior psychiatric diagnoses

Table 1
Summary of neurologic manifestations in cohort studies

Study	Varatharaj et al	Meppiel et al	Frontera et al	Chou et al
No. of patients with neurologic complications	153	222	606	2439/3054
Encephalopathy, %	23	30	51	51
Stroke, %	62	26 (ischemic strokes)	14	3
Seizures/status epilepticus	Not reported	9.5%	12%	1%
Acute inflammatory central nervous system syndromes, %	9	9.5	0	1
PNS disease	5%	6.8%	Not reported	6%
Other	Neuropsychiatric disorders 23/125 patients	Not reported	Hypoxic brain injury 11%	Coma 17%

- For posttraumatic stress disorder (PTSD) (20%–30% of survivors): Women, younger age, critically ill, past psychiatric history, obesity, type 2 diabetes mellitus, autoimmune disorders
- For cognitive issues, such as memory loss, concentration difficulties, difficulties with multitasking, processing speed (20%–30% of survivors): Delirium, older age

PATHOPHYSIOLOGY

COVID-19 can be thought of as having the following phases, which include an early viremic phase during which patients may remain asymptomatic for the first 48 to 72 hours followed by a prothrombotic, inflammatory phase, followed by an immune dysregulatory state (**Fig. 1, Table 2**).[10]

The COVID-19 spike protein attaches to the ACE2 receptor on various organs and activates an inflammatory cascade. It also attaches to the ACE2 receptor on endothelium and activates a prothrombotic state.[11] By binding to ACE2, the SARS-CoV-2 virus may damage vascular endothelial cells by inhibiting mitochondrial function and endothelial nitric oxide synthetase activity, leading to secondary cardiovascular and cerebrovascular effects.[12] It is possible that because the density and concentration of ACE2 receptors are limited in the central nervous system (CNS), direct viral invasion may be a rare phenomenon. Consistent with this, viral particles have been identified very rarely in the brain in autopsy studies. Whether this is a consequence of low viral invasion or that by the time these patients died they had progressed from the early viremic to the inflammatory or prothrombotic state is not known.[7,13,14] Acute demyelinating encephalomyelitis (ADEM).

Inflammation

In an autopsy series, microglial activation, microglial nodules and neuronophagia, was observed in most of the brains. They were thought to not result from direct viral infection of brain parenchyma, but more likely from systemic inflammation, perhaps with synergistic contribution from hypoxia/ischemia.[7,13]

A postmortem study (n = 43) found that neuropathologic changes in patients with COVID-19 seem to be mild, with pronounced neuroinflammatory changes in the

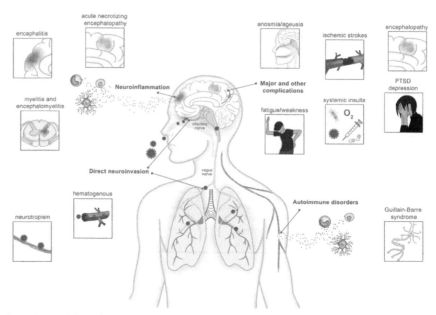

Fig. 1. Potential mechanisms and complications of neuroCOVID. (*From* Newcombe VFJ, Dangayach NS, Sonneville R. Neurological complications of COVID-19. Intensive Care Med. 2021;47(9):1021-1023. https://doi.org/10.1007/s00134-021-06439-6; with permission)

Table 2
Mechanism of injury and clinical examples of neurologic complications

Mechanism/Cause	Example
Direct viral invasion into the CNS	• Infectious encephalitis, meningitis, myelitis
Parainfectious, immune-mediated	• ADEM • Transverse myelitis • Guillain-Barré syndrome
Neurologic complications of systemic disease	• Hypercoagulability → ischemic stroke • Hypoxic respiratory failure → hypoxic brain injury • Sepsis → encephalopathy/delirium
Exacerbation of baseline neurologic disorder	• Epilepsy: increased seizure frequency/status epilepticus • Multiple sclerosis flare
Treatment-associated neurologic complications	• Anticoagulation → CNS hemorrhages • Steroids & paralytic medications → critical illness neuropathy/myopathy • Sedatives → delirium/encephalopathy
Thrombotic complications	• Stroke: arterial and venous
Associated with critical illness	• Postintensive care syndrome
Unclear	• Long-COVID

brainstem being the most common finding. There was no evidence for CNS damage directly caused by SARS-CoV-2.[14] Inflammation around blood vessels but not viral particles in a study that included n = 8 postmortem samples suggests that COVID-19 is associated with endotheliopathy and microvascular injury.[15] Patients with coma or prolonged disorders of consciousness (DOC) may have a higher systemic inflammatory burden as compared with patients who do not have coma or DOC.[16]

Prothrombotic

COVID-19 is thought to be an endotheliopathy and triggers a prothrombotic state. Of note, patients with COVID-19 acute respiratory distress syndrome (ARDS) had a higher level of various prothrombotic factors and thrombotic events, as compared with non-COVID-19 patients.[17]

Treatment Effects

Severely ill patients with COVID-19 are at a high risk of encephalopathy and intensive care–acquired weakness. These neurologic consequences were much higher than expected in these patients and likely explained by the prolonged needs for sedation, immobilization, and social isolation, increasing the risk of delirium and postintensive care syndrome (PICS). Although some of these factors may have been related to the severity of the underlying illness, others were likely due to the decreased compliance with the A2F bundle due to concerns for staff safety, shortage of personal protective equipment (PPE), medications, and limitations of family visitation.[18,19]

SPECTRUM OF NEUROLOGIC COMPLICATIONS

Neurologic complications can be broadly categorized under cerebrovascular disease, CNS inflammatory disease, demyelinating disease, encephalopathy, peripheral neuropathy, taste/smell disorders, and other.[20]

Fig. 2 describes a few potential ways of classifying neurologic complications of COVID-19.

NEURODIAGNOSTIC STUDIES, NEUROMONITORING

Early diagnosis of neurologic complications in patients with COVID-19 will rely on focused bedside neurologic examinations. Such focused clinical examinations can then guide a judicious utilization of imaging and electrophysiologic studies. However,

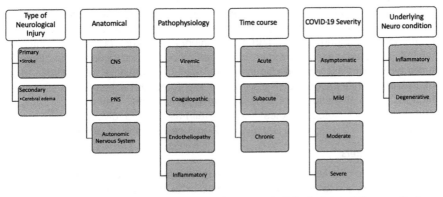

Fig. 2. Classifying neurologic complications of COVID-19. PNS, Peripheral Nervous System.

the pandemic has posed specific challenges in this clinical neuromonitoring with a reduction in both frequency of clinical examinations and compliance of bundles of care, which include choice and depth of sedation and choice of pain control when patient numbers are high.

Imaging Findings

Critically ill patients with COVID-19 may not be stable hemodynamically or from a ventilation/oxygenation perspective to tolerate lying flat for several minutes in an MRI scanner. Performing computed tomographic (CT) scans in such patients suspected of having neurologic complications may be the first step in diagnosis. Given the risk of cerebrovascular complications in these patients, it may be pertinent to perform vessel imaging for the arterial and venous systems at the same time as the CT or MRI session.

Common imaging findings described in patients with severe COVID-19 have included leukoencephalopathy, ischemia/infarction with patterns of large vessel occlusion, leptomeningeal enhancement, encephalitis, hemorrhage in locations not typical for hypertension (lobar and/or cortical, which raises the question of whether it is secondary to anticoagulation), and perfusion abnormalities.[21] Another key finding in patients with coma/DOC has been microhemorrhages.[22] In another case series, 25/ 115 hospitalized patients with COVID-19 had cerebral microbleeds documented on MRI, often with concomitant leukoencephalopathy. These were most common in patients with more severe respiratory illness.[23]

Other findings have included findings typical for posterior reversible encephalopathy syndrome, hypoxic ischemic encephalopathy.[24] In a retrospective multicenter study (n = 64), MRI abnormalities have included leptomeningeal enhancement in 17% and encephalitis in 13%; 46% of MRI studies was normal.[25]

Cerebrospinal Fluid Studies and Biomarkers

Pleocytosis is usually not seen in cerebrospinal fluid (CSF) of patients with COVID-19. Studies have demonstrated that CSF findings could range from being inflammatory to the only abnormality being an elevated protein. In a case-control study that included n = 18 CSF samples from patients with COVID-19, the investigators described an absence of pleocytosis as well as an absence of increased proinflammatory markers or cytokines (IL-6, ferritin, or D-dimer). They also found that in non-COVID-19 stroke patients and COVID-19 stroke patients there was a similar increase in proinflammatory cytokines (IL-6, TNFα, IL-12p70).[26]

In a small case series of patients with moderate to severe COVID-19, an unusual pattern of marked CSF inflammation emerged, in which soluble markers of neuroinflammation (neopterin, β2-microglobulin, and immunoglobulin G index), blood-brain barrier integrity (albumin ratio), and axonal injury (CSF neurofilament light chain protein[NfL]) was increased. However, white cell response and other immunologic features typical of CNS viral infections were absent.[27] In patients with COVID-19 with neurologic manifestations, CSF pleocytosis was found to be associated with parainfectious or postinfectious encephalitis and polyradiculitis. Elevations in anti-GD1b and anti-Caspr2 autoantibodies[28] and myelin-associated glycoprotein[29] may be seen raising the possibility of SARS-CoV-2–induced secondary autoimmunity.

Serum Biomarkers

Serum markers of brain injury including neurofilament light (NFL), glial fibrillary acidic protein (GFAP), and total Tau have been found to be increased in a severity-dependent manner in hospitalized patients, with elevations persisting at 4-month follow-up.[29] In these patients, elevations in NFL and GFAP were associated with elevations of proinflammatory cytokines, as well as autoantibodies. Another case-control study that included plasma samples from n = 57 patients at less than 48 hours of COVID-19 hospitalization, and 20 matched controls investigated levels of 6 brain injury molecules (BIMs), 2 endothelial injury molecules (EIMs), and chemokines/cytokines. Three BIMs: MAP2, NSE, and S100B; 2 EIMs: sICAM1 and sVCAM1; and 7 chemokines and cytokines: GRO, IL10, sCD40L, IP10, IL1Ra, MCP1, and TNFα, were significantly (P<.05) elevated in the COVID-19 cohort compared with controls.[30]

In summary, pleocytosis is not seen in CSF of patients with COVID-19 with encephalopathy, but protein levels can be elevated with oligoclonal bands. Elevated plasma and CSF levels of cytokines, GFAP, and NFL in COVID-19 are thought to reflect a proinflammatory systemic and brain response that involves microglial activation and subsequent neuronal damage.[27] Further evidence for inflammatory mechanisms comes from imaging findings, which showed meningeal enhancement and diffuse white matter abnormalities as well as microhemorrhages.[13] It should be noted that several of these biomarkers are not being measured routinely as part of clinical care, and further understanding of when, how high, and the meaning of elevations is required before use in clinical practice.

NON-LIFE-THREATENING BUT POTENTIALLY DISTRESSING SYMPTOMS
Anosmia/Dysgeusia

A meta-analysis of 83 studies involving more than 27,000 patients reported that olfactory dysfunction occurs in 48% of cases.[31] Olfactory bulb involvement was described on postmortem brain MRI earlier in the pandemic.[32] Most patients recover from anosmia and dysgeusia.[33–35]

Whether this high incidence of anosmia will be seen in patients with other COVID-19 variants remains to be seen.

Headache

Headache is a common symptom of COVID-19. A meta-analysis that included n = 3598 patients showed that headache was present in 11% to 14% of patients infected with COVID-19.[36] Earlier studies from China reported a lower incidence of headache at about 6.5% to 8%.[37–39] In a cohort study of n = 47 patients with COVID-19, 64% had headaches. Bilateral headache localization was reported by 94% of patients; headache severity was determined as severe in 53%, and constant headaches with median period of 15 days occurred in 15% of cases.[40]

LIFE-THREATENING NEUROLOGIC COMPLICATIONS
Stroke

There have been several cohort studies and meta-analyses describing the risk of stroke and outcomes in patients with COVID-19. Before the COVID-19 pandemic, it was already known that sepsis and related inflammation can trigger strokes.[41,42]

In one of the earlier reports of stroke in COVID-19, which included n = 108,571 patients with COVID-19, acute stroke occurred in 1.4% (95% confidence interval: 1.0–1.9). The investigators compared the risk of stroke in patients with COVID-19 with those with influenza and concluded that more patients with COVID-19 suffer from stroke as compared with patients with influenza (0.9%).[43]

The first cases of large vessel occlusion were described in young, asymptomatic, or mild COVID-19 cases. Subsequent studies have shown that the average age of patients with COVID-19 with stroke may be slightly lower than the average age in non-

COVID-19 stroke patients, but stroke is not as common in young patients (<50 years of age). Also, COVID-19 stroke patients tend to have a higher comorbidity burden.[44–46] Mechanisms of stroke can vary from thromboembolic, large-artery atherosclerosis, COVID-19–associated myocarditis, to arrhythmias, cryptogenic.[24,47] In a review that included n = 46 studies with 129,491 patients, COVID-19 stroke patients were younger, tend to be men, and have an increased stroke severity, compared with stroke patients in the prepandemic period. The investigators found no difference in rates of intravenous thrombolysis but found that patients with COVID-19 were more likely to undergo thrombectomy.[48,49] Stroke systems of care had to be adapted to COVID-19–related staff safety, PPE, and staff shortages. The American Heart Association released a statement to provide guidance to health systems to provide expeditious access to thrombectomy.[49]

Mortality in patients with stroke and COVID-19 is higher than in non-COVID-19 patients with a similar stroke burden.[48] A multicenter study from n = 31 centers in the United States that included n = 230 stroke patients found that only 33% of them were younger than 60 years of age. Of the patients, 102/203 (50%) had poor outcomes with an observed mortality of 38.8% (35/219).[50] The in-hospital mortality for COVID-19 stroke patients was about 38.1% and for intracerebral hemorrhage (ICH) was 58.3%.[50]

Good outcome has been reported for patients who develop malignant cerebral edema concurrent with COVID-19, and so infection should not be used to exclude patients from this potentially life-saving surgery.[51]

Hemorrhagic Stroke

Intracerebral hemorrhage
ICH is less common than ischemic stroke after COVID-19, comprising approximately 20% of strokes, and its incidence ranges from 0.2% to 0.86%.[52,53] This rate is higher than the worldwide incidence of ICH, which is 24.6/100,000 person-years or 0.02% per person-year.[54] In patients with COVID-19 with stroke, less than 20% have ICH.[55] The pooled incidence of ICH in a systematic review was 0.7% in patients with COVID-19 that included n = 23 studies and n = 148 COVID-19 ICH patients.[56]

In a study that analyzed data from Vizient Clinical Data Base comparing n = 559 patients with ICH-COVID-19 and 23,378 non-COVID-19 ICH controls from 194 hospitals, patients with ICH-COVID-19 had a longer hospital stay (21.6 vs 10.5 days), a longer intensive-care stay (16.5 vs 6.0 days), and a higher in-hospital death rate (46.5% vs 18.0%). Patients with COVID-19 with ICH or subarachnoid hemorrhage (SAH) were more likely to be a racial or ethnic minority, diabetic, and obese and to have higher rates of death and longer hospital length of stay when compared with controls.[57] A patient level pooled meta-analysis that included n = 139 patients with ICH with COVID-19, the investigators found that the ICH in these patients had different characteristics compared with ICH not associated with COVID-19, including frequent lobar location (67%) and multifocality (36%), a high rate of anticoagulation, and high mortality.[58] In a systematic review,[59] older age, non-Caucasian race, respiratory failure requiring mechanical ventilation, and therapeutic anticoagulation were identified as risk factors for ICH.[60]

Subarachnoid hemorrhage
In a study where the investigators analyzed data from the Vizient database comparing COVID-19 SAH cases versus non-COVID-19 SAH controls, there were 212 SAH-COVID patients and 5029 controls from 119 hospitals. The hospital (26.9 vs 13.4 days) and intensive-care (21.9 vs 9.6 days) length of stays and in-hospital death rate (42.9% vs 14.8%) were higher in the SAH-COVID cohort than in controls.[57] In another cohort study that included data from 62 health care facilities using the Cerner

deidentified COVID-19 data set, there were n = 86 (0.1%) and n = 376 (0.2%) patients with SAH among 85,645 patients with COVID-19 and 197,073 patients without COVID-19, respectively. The investigators found that there was no increase in the risk of SAH in patients with COVID-19 but higher mortality probably driven by systemic complications (31.4% vs 12.2%).[61]

Cerebral sinus venous thrombosis
In a case series from New York City at the height of the COVID-19 pandemic's first wave (March through May 2020), cerebral sinus venous thrombosis (CSVT) was diagnosed in 12 of 13,500, for a frequency of 0.088 per million as compared with CSVT in the general population is 5 per million annually.[62] In a systematic review of n = 34,331 patients with COVID-19, the estimated frequency of CSVT was 0.08%.[63] The superior sagittal and transverse sinuses were the most common sites for acute CVST.[64] CSVT and vaccine induced thrombocytopenia (VITT) are discussed later in this review.[64]

Extracorporeal membrane oxygenation and neurologic complications
In a systematic review on neurologic complications in extracorporeal membrane oxygenation (ECMO) for patients with COVID-19 that included n = 1322 patients from case series and retrospective cohort studies, the prevalence of intracranial hemorrhage (ICH), ischemic stroke, and hypoxic ischemic brain injury was 5.9% (n = 78), 1.1% (n = 15), and 0.3% (n = 4), respectively. The overall mortality of the 1296 ECMO patients in the 10 studies that reported death was 36% (n = 477), and the mortality of the subset of patients who had a neurologic event was 92%.[65]

In a multicenter case-control study of ECMO patients, the investigators included 29/142 (20%) patients with ICH versus 4/68 (6%) non-COVID-19 patients with ICH on ECMO. Half of the patients with COVID-19 had a clinically significant ICH and a third of them suffered in-hospital mortality. The overall intensive care unit (ICU) mortality in the presence of ICH of any severity was 88%. This study showed a 6-fold increased adjusted risk for ICH and a 3.5-fold increased incidence of ICH in patients with COVID-19 on ECMO, versus non-COVID-19 patients.[66] In another study that included ARDS patients on ECMO comparing COVID-19 versus non-COVID-19 patients, ICH was detected in 10% of patients with ARDS. Despite statistically higher rates of antiplatelet therapy and therapeutic anticoagulation in patients with COVID-19, there was a similar rate of ICH in patients with ARDS owing to COVID-19 compared with other causes of ARDS.[67]

Delirium/encephalopathy
In a systematic review that included n = 48 studies with 11,553 patients with COVID-19 from 13 countries, the pooled prevalence, incidence, and mortalities for delirium in patients with COVID-19 were 24.3%, 32.4%, and 44.5%, respectively.[68]

In a hospitalized cohort of patients with COVID-19 of n = 419, about 80% of them were diagnosed with a neurologic complication anytime from presentation to later during their hospitalization, and 30% of these patients had encephalopathy.[69] In addition, these patients often require longer ventilation with prolonged sedation and paralysis than used in many common ICU conditions.

In a cohort study that included patients with severe COVID-19, 84% patients were found to have neurologic symptoms, mainly delirium.[70] In a subsequent study (n = 140 patients), 70% developed agitation during ICU stay. In addition, more than half (17/28) of the patients had MRI abnormalities, and more than half (18/28) had an inflammatory CSF profile. Electroencephalogram showed only nonspecific findings.[71]

Delirium was present in 55% patients in the COVID-D cohort study of n = 2088 critically ill patients with COVID-19. Mechanical ventilation, use of restraints, benzodiazepine, opioid, and vasopressor infusions, and antipsychotics were each associated with a higher risk of delirium the next day, whereas family visitation (in person or virtual) was associated with a lower risk of delirium.[19]

Coma/encephalitis

Among patients with COVID-19 with a disorder of consciousness (DoC), coma, serum inflammatory markers were higher as compared with patients with COVID-19 without coma.[72] After cessation of sedatives, patients with severe respiratory failure secondary to COVID-19 may have a prolonged period of unconsciousness, which may be weeks before complete recovery.[73] In a prospective, longitudinal study, consecutive critically ill patients with COVID-19 with a DoC unexplained by sedation or structural brain injury, who underwent a brain MRI, were enrolled. In addition to structural imaging, the investigators performed a resting state functional MRI and diffusion MRI to evaluate functional and structural connectivity, as compared with healthy controls and patients with DoC resulting from severe traumatic brain injury. Of the 12 patients included in this study, one died shortly after enrollment, and the rest recovered consciousness between 0 and 25 days after stopping all sedatives.[74] Given the long length of recovery time seen, caution is advised when prognosticating in these patients.

POSTINTENSIVE CARE SYNDROME AND POSTACUTE SEQUELAE OF COVID-19

PICS has been described as the unintended consequences of critical care with new or worsening impairments in the physical, cognitive, or mental health domains.[75,76]

In a single-center, observational cohort study, 294 of 622 patients, including both COVID-19 and non-COVID-19 patients (median age, 64 years; 36% women); 16% and 13% of these patients reported probable PTSD, 29% and 20% probable anxiety, and 32% and 24% probable depression at 1 and 3 months after hospital discharge, respectively. The investigators found a similar risk of neuropsychiatric consequences in both COVID-19 and non-COVID-19 hospitalized patients, concluding that there is a need for long-term follow-up for hospitalized patients during this pandemic to focus on the needs of both of these cohorts.[69]

Of COVID-19 survivors, 90% suffered from impairments to one or more PICS domains in a prospective cohort from New York City.[77] At 3 months of follow-up, 87.5% (28/32) had not regained their baseline level of daily activities in a cohort study of COVID-19 ICU survivors, and 40% patients had impairments in multiple domains.[78]

Similar problems can be seen in all those who require critical care. PICS is a common constellation of physical, psychological, and cognitive problems experienced by those who have been in critical care, with holistic rehabilitation programs required for each component.[79]

Patients and caregivers should be educated to monitor for persistent symptoms (**Fig. 3**) and followed up in a multidisciplinary fashion to address the needs of patients with PASC. Dedicated COVID-19 centers may not be widely available in all countries; however, awareness of such centers, along with the ability to follow up via telehealth, may have help to bridge the gap in meeting the needs of COVID-19 survivors. Studies have shown that about half of the patients with COVID-19 will develop PASC.[80] Similar to acute COVID-19, PASC could also include multisystem manifestations. Recognizing that COVID-19 survivors will have multisystem needs, COVID-19 survivors need to be followed up in multidisciplinary clinics. For critical care survivors, impairments in different domains (physical, cognitive, behavioral) have long been characterized as PICS. Clinics developed for survivors of critical illness offer a model to address PASC survivorship for both acute and nonhospitalized patients with COVID-19 for

Common PASC / long COVID symptoms

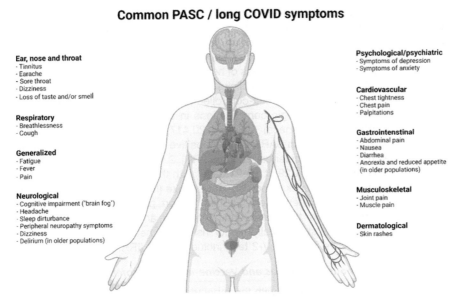

Ear, nose and throat
- Tinnitus
- Earache
- Sore throat
- Dizziness
- Loss of taste and/or smell

Respiratory
- Breathlessness
- Cough

Generalized
- Fatigue
- Fever
- Pain

Neurological
- Cognitive impairment ('brain fog')
- Headache
- Sleep dirturbance
- Peripheral neuropathy symptoms
- Dizziness
- Delirium (in older populations)

Psychological/psychiatric
- Symptoms of depression
- Symptoms of anxiety

Cardiovascular
- Chest tightness
- Chest pain
- Palpitations

Gastrointensinal
- Abdominal pain
- Nausea
- Diarrhea
- Anorexia and reduced appetite
  (in older populations)

Musculoskeletal
- Joint pain
- Muscle pain

Dermatological
- Skin rashes

Fig. 3. Common PASC symptoms. (*From* Newcombe VFJ, Dangayach NS, Sonneville R. Neurological complications of COVID-19. Intensive Care Med. 2021;47(9):1021-1023. https://doi.org/10.1007/s00134-021-06439-6; with permission)

better understanding the trajectory, clustering of symptoms as well as providing an opportunity to pool data to inform survivorship trajectories. A multidisciplinary program of care should include access to rehabilitation services, social work and welfare support, pharmacy, subspecialty care via direct inclusion or targeted referrals, and structured peer support program with trained moderators; coordination with primary care is essential.[73]

PASC clinics also offer research opportunities that should be harnessed to inform knowledge of survivorship trajectories after SARS-CoV-2 infection, and to improve service innovation and delivery.[81] Although resources for follow-up and rehabilitation will vary between and within countries, awareness and innovations like telehealth may help bridge the gap in meeting the needs of COVID-19 survivors. Symptom assessment could be performed between 4 and 6 weeks and at 12 weeks after discharge, along with screening for neuropsychiatric symptoms in addition to follow-up for other organ system involvement, for example, pulmonary, hematological, along with early referral for ongoing clinical trials, and for physical, occupational, and cognitive therapy.[82]

NEUROLOGIC COMPLICATIONS OF VACCINES

There are several approved COVID-19 vaccines being used in different parts of the world. Different systems are used in different parts of the world to track and report adverse events owing to vaccines for, for example, in the United States, the Vaccine Adverse Events Reporting Systems (VAERS), in the United Kingdom, Coronavirus Yellow Card reporting Web site (https://coronavirus-yellowcard.mhra.gov.uk/).

Any patient or health care provider can report side effects of vaccines through the Centers for Disease Control and Prevention (CDC) through VAERS; patients, providers, and manufacturers can also report complications to the Food and Drug Administration Adverse Event Reporting System. The most common neurologic symptoms included dizziness, headache, pain, muscle spasms, myalgia, and paresthesias, which are expected to occur as acute, transient effects of the vaccination. Rare cases of tremor, diplopia, tinnitus, dysphonia, seizures, and reactivation of herpes zoster have been reported. In order of reporting frequency in 2021, there are facial palsy, GBS, stroke, transverse myelitis, and acute disseminated encephalomyelitis in the VAERS database.[83] Transient episodes of headaches, myalgias, and fatigue were reported in about 5% of participants in clinical trials.[84]

From the United Kingdom, in a self-controlled case series study to investigate hospital admissions from neurologic complications in the 28 days after a first dose of ChAdOx1nCoV-19 (AstraZeneca) (n = 20,417,752) or BNT162b2 (Pfizer) (n = 12,134,782), and after an SARS-CoV-2–positive test (n = 2,005,280), there was an increased risk of GBS (incidence rate ratio [IRR], 2.90 at 15 to 21 days after vaccination) and Bell palsy (IRR, 1.29 at 15–21 days) with the AstraZeneca vaccine.[85]

There was an increased risk of hemorrhagic stroke (IRR, 1.38 at 15–21 days) with Pfizer vaccine. Another independent Scottish cohort provided further support for the association between the AstraZeneca vaccine and GBS (IRR, 2.32 at 1–28 days). There was a substantially higher risk of all neurologic outcomes in the 28 days after a positive SARS-CoV-2 test, including GBS (IRR, 5.25).[85]

Cerebral Sinus Venous Thrombosis and Vaccine-Induced Thrombocytopenia

The initial 12 US cases of CVST with thrombocytopenia after Ad26.COV2.S vaccination were reported as serious events.[86] In the United Kingdom, up to 12 January 2022, the Medicines and Healthcare Products Regulatory Agency (MHRA) had received Yellow Card reports of 435 cases of major thromboembolic events with concurrent thrombocytopenia following vaccination with COVID-19 Vaccine AstraZeneca. Forty-nine of the 435 reports have been reported after a second dose. Of the 435 reports, 217 occurred in women, and 214 occurred in men aged from 18 to 93 years. The overall case fatality rate was 18% with 76 deaths, 6 of which occurred after the second dose. CSVT was reported in 157 cases (average age, 46 years), and 278 had other major thromboembolic events (average age, 54 years) with concurrent thrombocytopenia. The estimated number of first doses of COVID-19 Vaccine AstraZeneca administered in the United Kingdom by 12 January was 24.9 million, and the estimated number of second doses was 24.2 million. There is some evidence that the reported incidence rate is higher in women compared with men, although this is not seen across all age groups, and the difference remains small. The overall incidence of thromboembolic events with concurrent low platelets after second doses was 2.0 cases per million doses. Considering the different numbers of patients vaccinated with COVID-19 Vaccine AstraZeneca in different age groups, the data indicate that there is a lower reported incidence rate in younger adult age groups following the second dose compared with the older groups (1.0 per million doses in those aged 18–49 years compared with 2.1 per million doses in those aged 50 years and over). The scientific review concluded that there is a possible link between CVST without low platelets and COVID-19 Vaccine AstraZeneca.

Current advice from the US and UK governmental agencies, the CDC and MHRA, respectively, has been that the benefit of the vaccination outweighs the risk, and this appears to be accurate from a neurologic standpoint. In order to establish causality, clinical case definitions must be established, for example, via the Brighton collaboration guidelines for conditions recognized to be associated with vaccination and proactive clinician-led definitions in emergent conditions (such as VITT). In assessing causality, tools such as the WHO GACVS or Bradford Hill criteria,[87] may be used; however, the authors additionally propose criteria that classify associated neurologic or neuropsychiatric events into probable, possible, and unlikely cases, considering the temporal relationship, individual risk factors, and the likelihood of an alternative cause. In such cases as the urgent SARS-CoV-2 vaccination campaign in which ongoing randomized controlled clinical trials may be unfeasible and/or unethical, epidemiologic methods of causality assessment, such as triangulation, may be used.[87]

SUMMARY

Neurologic manifestation of acute COVID-19 and PASC is common in hospitalized patients with COVID-19. Having a high clinical suspicion to screen, diagnose, and treat life-threatening neurologic complications (such as acute ischemic stroke or ICH) is needed to help frontline providers leverage existing resources appropriately. Systems of health care delivery need to be optimized to prepare for the long-term needs of COVID-19 survivors with periodic screening for neuropsychiatric manifestations and providing multidisciplinary support to help rehabilitate these patients. Adapting existing systems to help uphold the paradigm that time is brain, address barriers for implementing evidence-based bundles for liberation from the ICU can help prevent and treat acute neurologic complications, and perhaps, may help reduce the burden of PASC in ICU survivors. Patients with mild COVID-19 also remain at risk of PASC. Educating these patients to self-monitor their symptoms, increasing awareness about local multidisciplinary COVID-19 centers, engaging primary care can help patients with PASC return to their baseline.

CLINICS CARE POINTS

- Although patients with any severity of COVID-19 can suffer from neurologic complications, the incidence of these complications is much higher in patients with severe COVID-19. Early diagnosis of neurologic complications in patients with COVID-19will rely on focused bedside neurologic examinations. Such focused clinical examinations can then guide a judicious utilization of imaging and electrophysiologic studies. Stroke occurs in about 1.5% of all patients with COVID-19, and these stroke patients were younger, tend to be men, and have an increased stroke severity and worse outcomes compared with stroke patients in the prepandemic period.

- Hemorrhagic stroke may be seen in patients with COVID-19 on therapeutic anticoagulation, on extracorporeal membrane oxygenation, or spontaneously. The pattern of ICH in these patients had different characteristics compared with intracerebral hemorrhage not associated with COVID-19, including frequent lobar location (67%) and multifocality (36%), a high rate of anticoagulation, and high mortality.

- Status epilepticus, new-onset seizures, and encephalitis occur rarely in patients with COVID-19.

- Delirium may be present in more than half of the patients with severe COVID-19. There are several challenges to the implementation of the evidence-based intensive care unit liberation in these patients, including mechanical ventilation, use of restraints and benzodiazepine, opioid, and vasopressor infusions, and antipsychotics; limitations on family visitation have been associated with a higher risk of delirium.

- Patients and caregivers should be educated to monitor for persistent symptoms and followed up in a multidisciplinary fashion to address the needs of patients with postacute sequelae of COVID-19. Systems of health care delivery need to be optimized to prepare for the long-term needs of COVID-19 survivors with periodic screening for neuropsychiatric manifestations and providing multidisciplinary support to help rehabilitate these patients.

DISCLOSURE

The authors have no relevant conflicts of interest.

REFERENCES

1. WHO Coronavirus (COVID-19) dashboard. WHO coronavirus (COVID-19) dashboard with vaccination data. Available at. https://covid19.who.int/. Accessed December 9, 2021.
2. Wiersinga WJ, Rhodes A, Cheng AC, et al. Pathophysiology, transmission, diagnosis, and treatment of coronavirus disease 2019 (COVID-19): a review. JAMA 2020;324(8):782–93.
3. Liotta EM, Batra A, Clark JR, et al. Frequent neurologic manifestations and encephalopathy-associated morbidity in Covid-19 patients. Ann Clin translational Neurol 2020;7(11):2221–30.
4. Mao L, Jin H, Wang M, et al. Neurologic manifestations of hospitalized patients with coronavirus disease 2019 in Wuhan, China. JAMA Neurol 2020;77(6): 683–90.
5. Newcombe VFJ, Dangayach NS, Sonneville R. Neurological complications of COVID-19. *Intensive care medicine* 2021. https://doi.org/10.1007/S00134-021-06439-6. Published online].
6. Yassin A, Nawaiseh M, Shaban A, et al. Neurological manifestations and complications of coronavirus disease 2019 (COVID-19): a systematic review and meta-analysis. BMC Neurol 2021;(1):21. https://doi.org/10.1186/S12883-021-02161-4.
7. Thakur KT, Miller EH, Glendinning MD, et al. COVID-19 neuropathology at Columbia University Irving Medical Center/New York Presbyterian Hospital. Brain 2021;144(9):2696–708.
8. Group PCC, Evans RA, McAuley H, et al. Physical, cognitive and mental health impacts of COVID-19 following hospitalisation – a multi-centre prospective cohort study. medRxiv 2021;22:21254057. https://doi.org/10.1101/2021.03.22.21254057.
9. Nakamura ZM, Nash RP, Laughon SL, et al. Neuropsychiatric complications of COVID-19. Curr Psychiatry Rep 2021;23(5):1–9.
10. Fotuhi M, Mian A, Meysami S, et al. Neurobiology of COVID-19. J Alzheimer's Dis 2020;76(1):3–19.
11. Boldrini M, Canoll P, psychiatry RKJ. Undefined. How COVID-19 affects the brain. JAMA Psychiatry 2021;78(6):682–3. https://doi.org/10.1001/jamapsychiatry.2021.0500. Available at. jamanetwork.com. Published online 2021.
12. Lei Y, Zhang J, Schiavon CR, et al. SARS-CoV-2 spike protein impairs endothelial function via downregulation of ACE 2. Circ Res 2021;128:1323–6.
13. Solomon T. Neurological infection with SARS-CoV-2 — the story so far. Nat Rev Neurol 2021;17(2):1.
14. Matschke J, Lütgehetmann M, Hagel C, et al. Neuropathology of patients with COVID-19 in Germany: a post-mortem case series. Lancet Neurol 2020;19(11): 919–29.
15. Lee MH, Perl DP, Nair G, et al. Microvascular injury in the brains of patients with covid-19. N Engl J Med 2021;384(5):481–3.
16. Boehme AK, Doyle K, Thakur KT, et al. Disorders of consciousness in hospitalized patients with COVID-19: the role of the systemic inflammatory response syndrome. Neurocrit Care 2021. https://doi.org/10.1007/s12028-021-01256-7. Published online June 28].
17. Helms J, Tacquard C, Severac F, et al. High risk of thrombosis in patients with severe SARS-CoV-2 infection: a multicenter prospective cohort study. Intensive Care Med 2020;46(6):1089–98.

18. Khan SH, Lindroth H, Perkins AJ, et al. Delirium incidence, duration and severity in critically ill patients with COVID-19. medRxiv 2020. https://doi.org/10.1101/2020.05.31.20118679. PG-2020.05.31.20118679.

19. Pun BT, Badenes R, Heras La Calle G, et al. Prevalence and risk factors for delirium in critically ill patients with COVID-19 (COVID-D): a multicentre cohort study. Lancet Respir Med 2021;9(3):239–50.

20. Sullivan BN, Fischer T. Age-associated neurological complications of COVID-19: a systematic review and meta-analysis. Front Aging Neurosci 2021;13:374.

21. Newcombe VFJ, Dangayach NS, Sonneville R. Neurological complications of COVID-19. Intensive Care Med 2021;47(9):1021–3.

22. Hernandez-Fernandez F, Sandoval Valencia H, Barbella-Aponte RA, et al. Cerebrovascular disease in patients with COVID-19: neuroimaging, histological and clinical description. Brain 2020;143(10):3089–103.

23. Agarwal S, Jain R, Dogra S, et al. Cerebral microbleeds and leukoencephalopathy in critically ill patients with COVID-19. Stroke 2020;51(9):2649–55.

24. Lin E, Lantos JE, Strauss SB, et al. Brain imaging of patients with COVID-19: findings at an academic institution during the height of the outbreak in New York City. AJNR Am J neuroradiology 2020;41(11):2001–8.

25. Kremer S, Lersy F, Anheim M, et al. Neurologic and neuroimaging findings in patients with COVID-19: a retrospective multicenter study. Neurology 2020;95(13):e1868–82.

26. Garcia MA, Barreras Pv, Lewis A, et al. Cerebrospinal fluid in COVID-19 neurological complications: neuroaxonal damage, anti-SARS-Cov2 antibodies but no evidence of cytokine storm. J Neurol Sci 2021;427:117517.

27. Edén A, Kanberg N, Gostner J, et al. CSF biomarkers in patients with COVID-19 and neurologic symptoms: a case series. Neurology 2021;96(2):e294–300.

28. Guilmot A, Maldonado Slootjes S, Sellimi A, et al. Immune-mediated neurological syndromes in SARS-CoV-2-infected patients. J Neurol 2021;268(3):751–7.

29. Needham E, Ren A, Digby R, et al. Brain injury in COVID-19 is associated with autoinflammation and autoimmunity. medRxiv 2021;19:2021.

30. Savarraj J, Park ES, Colpo GD, et al. Brain injury, endothelial injury and inflammatory markers are elevated and express sex-specific alterations after COVID-19. J Neuroinflammation 2021;18(1):1–12.

31. Saniasiaya J, Islam MA, Abdullah B. Prevalence of olfactory dysfunction in coronavirus disease 2019 (COVID-19): a meta-analysis of 27,492 patients. Laryngoscope 2021;131(4):865–78.

32. Coolen T, Lolli V, Sadeghi N, et al. Early postmortem brain MRI findings in COVID-19 non-survivors. Neurology 2020;95(14):e2016–27.

33. Eliezer M, Hamel AL, Houdart E, et al. Loss of smell in patients with COVID-19: MRI data reveal a transient edema of the olfactory clefts. Neurology 2020;95(23):e3145–52.

34. Paderno A, Mattavelli D, Rampinelli V, et al. Olfactory and gustatory outcomes in COVID-19: a prospective evaluation in nonhospitalized subjects. otolaryngology-head and neck surgery. J Am Acad Otolaryngology 2020;163(6):1144–9.

35. Lechien JR, Chiesa-Estomba CM, de Siati DR, et al. Olfactory and gustatory dysfunctions as a clinical presentation of mild-to-moderate forms of the coronavirus disease (COVID-19): a multicenter European study. Eur Arch Otorhinolaryngology 2020;277(8):2251–61.

36. do Nascimento IJB, Cacic N, Abdulazeem HM, et al. Novel coronavirus infection (COVID-19) in humans: a scoping review and meta-analysis. J Clin Med 2020;9(4). https://doi.org/10.3390/JCM9040941.

37. Tian S, Hu N, Lou J, et al. Characteristics of COVID-19 infection in Beijing. J Infect 2020;80(4):401–6.
38. Huang C, Wang Y, Li X, et al. Clinical features of patients infected with 2019 novel coronavirus in Wuhan, China. Lancet (London, England) 2020;395(10223): 497–506.
39. Seth V, Kushwaha S. Headache due to COVID-19: a disabling combination. Headache 2020;60(10):2618–21.
40. Rocha-Filho PAS, Magalhães JE. Headache associated with COVID-19: frequency, characteristics and association with anosmia and ageusia. Cephalalgia 2020;40(13):1443–51.
41. Boehme AK, Luna J, Kulick ER, et al. Influenza-like illness as a trigger for ischemic stroke. Ann Clin translational Neurol 2018;5(4):456–63.
42. Boehme AK, Ranawat P, Luna J, et al. Risk of acute stroke after hospitalization for sepsis: a case-crossover study. Stroke 2017;48(3):574–80.
43. Merkler A, Parikh N, Mir S, et al. Risk of ischemic stroke in patients with coronavirus disease 2019 (COVID-19) vs patients with influenza. JAMA Neurol 2020. Published Online.
44. Majidi S, Fifi JT, Ladner TR, et al. Emergent large vessel occlusion stroke during New York City's covid-19 outbreak: clinical characteristics and paraclinical findings. Stroke 2020;51(9):2656–63.
45. Oxley TJ, Mocco J, Majidi S, et al. Large-vessel stroke as a presenting feature of Covid-19 in the young. N Engl J Med 2020;382(20):e60.
46. Fridman S, Bullrich MB, Jimenez-Ruiz A, et al. Stroke risk, phenotypes, and death in COVID-19: systematic review and newly reported cases. Neurology 2020; 95(24):E3373–85.
47. Yaghi S, Ishida K, Torres J, et al. SARS-CoV-2 and stroke in a New York healthcare system. Stroke 2020;51(7):2002–11.
48. Katsanos AH, Palaiodimou L, Zand R, et al. Changes in stroke hospital care during the COVID-19 pandemic: a systematic review and meta-analysis. Stroke 2021;52(11):3651–60. Published online].
49. Lyden P. Temporary emergency guidance to US stroke centers during the covid-19 pandemic on behalf of the AHA/ASA Stroke Council leadership running title: temporary emergency guidance to US stroke centers. Stroke 2020. https://doi.org/10.1161/STROKEAHA.120.030023.
50. Siegler JE, Cardona P, Arenillas JF, et al. Cerebrovascular events and outcomes in hospitalized patients with COVID-19: the SVIN COVID-19 multinational registry. Int J Stroke 2021;16(4):437–47.
51. Liang JW, Reynolds AS, Reilly K, et al. COVID-19 and decompressive hemicraniectomy for acute ischemic stroke. Stroke 2020;51(9):E215–8.
52. Requena M, Olivé-Gadea M, Muchada M, et al. COVID-19 and stroke: incidence and etiological description in a high-volume center. J Stroke Cerebrovasc Dis 2020;29(11). https://doi.org/10.1016/J.JSTROKECEREBROVASDIS.2020.105225.
53. Dogra S, Jain R, Cao M, et al. Hemorrhagic stroke and anticoagulation in COVID-19. J Stroke Cerebrovasc Dis 2020;29(8). https://doi.org/10.1016/J.JSTROKECEREBROVASDIS.2020.104984.
54. Margos NP, Meintanopoulos AS, Filioglou D, et al. Intracerebral hemorrhage in COVID-19: a narrative review. J Clin Neurosci 2021;89:271–8.
55. Mishra S, Choueka M, Wang Q, et al. Intracranial hemorrhage in COVID-19 patients. J stroke Cerebrovasc Dis 2021;30(4). https://doi.org/10.1016/J.JSTROKECEREBROVASDIS.2021.105603.

56. Cheruiyot I, Sehmi P, Ominde B, et al. Intracranial hemorrhage in coronavirus disease 2019 (COVID-19) patients. Neurol Sci 2021. https://doi.org/10.1007/s10072-020-04870-z/.

57. Ravindra VM, Grandhi R, Delic A, et al. Impact of COVID-19 on the hospitalization, treatment, and outcomes of intracerebral and subarachnoid hemorrhage in the United States. PloS one 2021;16(4). https://doi.org/10.1371/JOURNAL.PONE.0248728.

58. Beyrouti R, Best JG, Chandratheva A, et al. Characteristics of intracerebral haemorrhage associated with COVID-19: a systematic review and pooled analysis of individual patient and aggregate data. J Neurol 2021;268:3105–15. https://doi.org/10.1007/s00415-021-10425-9.

59. Daly SR, Nguyen Av, Zhang Y, et al. The relationship between COVID-19 infection and intracranial hemorrhage: a systematic review. Brain Hemorrhages 2021;2(4):141–50.

60. Melmed KR, Cao M, Dogra S, et al. Risk factors for intracerebral hemorrhage in patients with COVID-19. J Thromb Thrombolysis 2021;51(4):953–60.

61. Qureshi AI, Baskett WI, Huang W, et al. Subarachnoid hemorrhage and COVID-19: an analysis of 282,718 patients. World Neurosurg 2021;151:e615–20.

62. Al-Mufti F, Amuluru K, Sahni R, et al. Cerebral venous thrombosis in COVID-19: a New York metropolitan cohort study. AJNR Am J neuroradiology 2021;42(7):1196–200.

63. Baldini T, Asioli GM, Romoli M, et al. Cerebral venous thrombosis and severe acute respiratory syndrome coronavirus-2 infection: a systematic review and meta-analysis. Eur J Neurol 2021;28(10):3478–90.

64. Abdalkader M, Shaikh SP, Siegler JE, et al. Cerebral venous sinus thrombosis in COVID-19 patients: a multicenter study and review of literature. J Stroke Cerebrovasc Dis 2021;30(6). https://doi.org/10.1016/J.JSTROKECEREBROVASDIS.2021.105733.

65. Kannapadi Nv, Jami M, Premraj L, et al. Neurological complications in COVID-19 patients with ECMO support: a systematic review and meta-analysis. Heart Lung Circ 2021;31(2):292–8.

66. Seeliger B, Doebler M, Hofmaenner DA, et al. Intracranial hemorrhages on extracorporeal membrane oxygenation: differences between covid-19 and other viral acute respiratory distress syndrome. Crit Care Med 2022. https://doi.org/10.1097/CCM.0000000000005441.

67. Lang CN, Dettinger JS, Berchtold-Herz M, et al. Intracerebral hemorrhage in COVID-19 patients with pulmonary failure: a propensity score-matched registry study. Neurocrit Care 2021;34(3):739–47.

68. Pranata R, Huang I, Lim MA, et al. Delirium and mortality in coronavirus disease 2019 (COVID-19) - a systematic review and meta-analysis. Arch Gerontol Geriatr 2021;95. https://doi.org/10.1016/J.ARCHGER.2021.104388.

69. Liotta EM, Batra A, Clark JR, et al. Frequent neurologic manifestations and encephalopathy-associated morbidity in Covid-19 patients. Ann Clin translational Neurol 2020;7(11):2221–30.

70. Helms J, Kremer S, Merdji H, et al. Neurologic features in severe SARS-CoV-2 infection. N Engl J Med 2020;382(23):2268–70.

71. Helms J, Kremer S, Merdji H, et al. Delirium and encephalopathy in severe COVID-19: a cohort analysis of ICU patients. Crit Care (London, England) 2020;24(1). https://doi.org/10.1186/S13054-020-03200-1.

72. Boehme A, Doyle K, Thakur K, et al. Undefined disorders of consciousness in hospitalized patients with covid-19: the role of the systemic inflammatory

response syndrome. Springer; 2021. Available at. https://link.springer.com/article/10.1007/s12028-021-01256-7. Accessed August 1, 2021.

73. Abdo WF, Broerse CI, Grady BP, et al. Prolonged unconsciousness following severe COVID-19. Neurology 2021;96(10):e1437–42.

74. Fischer D, Snider SB, Barra ME, et al. Disorders of consciousness associated with COVID-19: a prospective, multimodal study of recovery and brain connectivity. Neurology 2021;98(3):e315–25.

75. Hosey MM, Needham DM. Survivorship after COVID-19 ICU stay. Nat Rev Dis Primers 2020;6(1). https://doi.org/10.1038/S41572-020-0201-1.

76. Vlake JH, van Bommel J, Hellemons ME, et al. Intensive care unit-specific virtual reality for psychological recovery after ICU treatment for COVID-19; a brief case report. Front Med 2021;7. https://doi.org/10.3389/FMED.2020.629086.

77. Martillo M, Dangayach N, Tabacof L, et al. Postintensive care syndrome in survivors of critical illness related to coronavirus disease 2019: cohort study from a New York City critical care recovery clinic. Crit Care Med 2021;49(9):1427–38. Available at. https://journals.lww.com/ccmjournal/Abstract/9000/Postintensive_Care_Syndrome_in_Survivors_of.95305.aspx. Accessed July 31, 2021.

78. Rousseau AF, Minguet P, Colson C, et al. Post-intensive care syndrome after a critical COVID-19: cohort study from a Belgian follow-up clinic. Ann Intensive Care 2021;11(1):1–9.

79. O'Sullivan O. Long-term sequelae following previous coronavirus epidemics. Clin Med (London, England) 2021;21(1):E68–70.

80. Groff D, Sun A, Ssentongo AE, et al. Short-term and long-term rates of postacute sequelae of SARS-CoV-2 infection: a systematic review. JAMA Netw Open 2021; 4(10):e2128568.

81. Parker AM, Brigham E, Connolly B, et al. Addressing the post-acute sequelae of SARS-CoV-2 infection: a multidisciplinary model of care. Lancet Respir Med 2021;9(11):1328.

82. Nalbandian A, Sehgal K, Gupta A, et al. Post-acute COVID-19 syndrome. nature.com. 2021. Available at. https://www.nature.com/articles/s41591-021-01283-z. Accessed December 18, 2021.

83. Goss AL, Samudralwar RD, Das RR, et al. ANA investigates: neurological complications of COVID-19 vaccines. Ann Neurol 2021;89(5):856.

84. Beatty AL, Peyser ND, Butcher XE, et al. Analysis of COVID-19 vaccine type and adverse effects following vaccination key points + supplemental content. JAMA Netw Open 2021;4(12):2140364.

85. Patone M, Handunnetthi L, Saatci D, et al. Neurological complications after first dose of COVID-19 vaccines and SARS-CoV-2 infection. Nat Med 2021;27(12): 2144–53.

86. Siegler JE, Klein P, Yaghi S, et al. Cerebral vein thrombosis with vaccine-induced immune thrombotic thrombocytopenia. Stroke 2021;52(9):3045–53.

87. Butler M, Tamborska A, Wood GK, et al. Considerations for causality assessment of neurological and neuropsychiatric complications of SARS-CoV-2 vaccines: from cerebral venous sinus thrombosis to functional neurological disorder. J Neurol Neurosurg Psychiatry 2021;92(11):1144–51.

Severe COVID-19 and Multisystem Inflammatory Syndrome in Children in Children and Adolescents

Check for updates

Allison M. Blatz, MD[a], Adrienne G. Randolph, MD, MS[b,c],*

KEYWORDS

• Pediatrics • Multisystem inflammatory syndrome • MIS-C • COVID-19

KEY POINTS

- Severe lung disease due to SARS-CoV-2 is uncommon in children and occurs mostly in children with underlying risk factors such as obesity, chronic lung disease, and other underlying conditions.
- Severe, acute COVID-19 can also present in children as severe CNS disease and rarely as acute myocarditis.
- Multisystem inflammatory syndrome in children (MIS-C) is a newly recognized disorder characterized by systemic hyperinflammation and multisystem involvement and appears to be a post-infectious complication of SARS-CoV-2.
- Usual treatment of critically ill MIS-C patients involves prompt initiation of immune modulation with IVIG and/or corticosteroids.

INTRODUCTION

Severe complications related to COVID-19 are fortunately uncommon in children and adolescents. Acute COVID-19 affects mostly children with underlying chronic conditions. A new disorder emerged early in the pandemic called multisystem inflammatory syndrome in children (MIS-C) that seems to be a postinfectious complication of SARS-CoV-2.[1] Children and adolescents with MIS-C have hyperinflammation and multiple organ system involvements. About half have cardiovascular involvement which can be life-threatening. The diagnostic criteria for these 2 conditions have some overlap, making differential diagnosis challenging in some cases. This review focuses on these 2 severe complications related to SARS-CoV-2 infection in children and adolescents

[a] Department of Pediatrics, Division of Infectious Diseases, Children's Hospital of Philadelphia, 3401 Civic Center Boulevard, Philadelphia, PA 19104, USA; [b] Department of Anesthesiology, Critical Care and Pain Medicine, Division of Critical Care, Boston Children's Hospital, 300 Longwood Avenue, Bader 634, Boston, MA 02115, USA; [c] Department of Anaesthesia and Pediatrics, Harvard Medical School, Boston, MA 02115, USA
* Corresponding author.
E-mail address: adrienne.randolph@childrens.harvard.edu

Crit Care Clin 38 (2022) 571–586
https://doi.org/10.1016/j.ccc.2022.01.005
0749-0704/22/© 2022 Elsevier Inc. All rights reserved.

criticalcare.theclinics.com

admitted to the ICU, including their presentation, epidemiology, diagnosis, and evaluation. We then review therapeutic strategies for each.

SEVERE, ACUTE PEDIATRIC COVID-19
Definition

The great majority of children infected with SARS-CoV-2 will be asymptomatic or develop mild COVID-19. However, some children present with severe or critical COVID-19, and this review focuses on those patients. There are multiple acute presentations for severe COVID-19 requiring ICU admission. Most commonly, children present with acute hypoxic respiratory failure.[2] Other children develop central nervous system (CNS) pathology and/or complications relating to a hypercoagulable state such as thrombosis.[3,4]

Epidemiology

Most children with severe acute COVID-19 admitted to the ICU have one or more underlying medical conditions. Teenagers with obesity and/or metabolic syndrome are at increased risk and may present more similarly to adults with COVID-19 acute respiratory distress syndrome (ARDS).[5] Infants, those with the history of prematurity and those with immune compromise are also at higher risk of severe disease.[2,6,7]

Incidence of pediatric hospitalization for severe COVID-19 has ranged from 0.1 to 1.4 per 100,000 per week during the pandemic, with a recent increase with the predominance of the B.1.617.2 (Delta) variant.[8,9] that is likely due to its higher transmissibility. Fewer than 2% of pediatric COVID-19 cases require intensive care admission and almost all will survive with supportive care. Recent data from the CDC estimate the rate of myocarditis due to COVID-19 at 0.146%; however, it is 16 times higher than for those without COVID-19.[10]

Diagnostic Criteria

Children and adolescents suspected of having acute COVID-19 should be tested for SARS-CoV-2 with either a PCR or an antigen test from a respiratory specimen. While both tests are highly specific, the PCR test is much more sensitive.[11] In patients with negative testing, retesting should be considered if there is high suspicion such as during a household outbreak. If testing is confirmed negative, alternate diagnoses are likely.

Pathogenesis

Children are exposed to SARS-CoV-2 just as adults are—through droplets. Many children are asymptomatic. In those that do develop symptoms, onset is typically 5 to 7 days after viral exposure, peaking 7 to 14 days after exposure.

Clinical Manifestations

Respiratory: Pulmonary symptoms in pediatric patients hospitalized in the pediatric intensive care unit (PICU) can range from mild hypoxemia, status asthmaticus, to ARDS. COVID-19 ARDS presents similarly in children as it does in adults, though it is less severe in most pediatric patients.[12] Children are less likely to require invasive mechanical ventilation for acute respiratory failure than adults and they have shorter durations of hospital stay. Presentation is usually with gradual onset of symptoms, though may be acute in onset in those with underlying complex conditions.

Cardiovascular: Cardiovascular involvement is less common than pulmonary involvement. Critically ill patients can develop shock, acute myocarditis, and acute cardiac dysfunction.[2,5]

Neurologic: Severe neurologic involvement in children related to SARS-CoV-2 is rare, but can manifest with both peripheral and CNS symptoms, including severe encephalopathy, stroke, direct CNS infection, fulminant cerebral swelling, Guillain–Barré syndrome, or a demyelinating syndrome.[13] Patients cannulated for extracorporeal membrane oxygenation (ECMO) for ARDS are at risk of cerebral hemorrhage as a secondary complication. A recent multi-center U.S. public health surveillance registry showed that preexisting neurologic conditions were at higher risk of developing CNS complications from COVID-19, Recommended Initial Evaluation including the exacerbation of an underlying seizure disorder.[4]

Hematologic: Patients with severe, acute COVID-19 are often hypercoagulable. This can lead to deep venous thrombus and/or pulmonary embolus as a presenting symptom or complication of acute COVID-19. Teenagers are more likely than younger children to develop thrombotic events.[3]

Laboratory and Imaging Abnormalities

Baseline laboratory studies may demonstrate lymphopenia and neutrophilia, mild acute kidney injury, and/or mild hepatitis. Inflammatory markers are usually modestly elevated.

In the setting of acute respiratory failure due to COVID-19, children develop hypoxia. Chest imaging frequently shows bilateral, diffuse pulmonary infiltrates.

Children with symptoms of cardiovascular shock may have elevated lactate or other markers of end-organ perfusion. Troponin will be elevated in the setting of acute myocarditis. Brain natriuretic peptide (BNP) or pro-BNP may be high in the setting of decreased cardiac function. Echocardiogram can demonstrate decreased function or show signs of pulmonary hypertension, depending on pulmonary disease.

Neurologic manifestations are more likely to be found by physical examination rather than laboratory studies. Imaging findings vary based on the presenting syndrome.[4] These can include delirium, confusion, obtundation, inability to walk, and seizures.

Children may be hypercoagulable with an increased D-dimer, especially in the setting of a thrombus. Other coagulation laboratories may also be prolonged, and thrombocytopenia may develop.

Recommended Initial Evaluation

Initial evaluation of children with critical illness is guided by the presentation and is similar to the evaluation of acute respiratory disease from other causes (eg, chest radiograph, blood gas, continuous pulse oximetry). Patients should be screened for hypercoagulopathy and markers of inflammation should be followed. If any neurologic deficits are present on examination, expedited CNS imaging is indicated with computed tomography (CT), or magnetic resonance imaging (MRI).

MULTISYSTEM INFLAMMATORY SYNDROME IN CHILDREN
Background

In April 2020, case series emerged from the UK, Italy, and later from the US describing children admitted to the hospital for persistent fever, diffuse inflammation, and shock that seemed similar to Kawasaki disease (KD) or toxic shock syndrome (TSS) which are described in **Table 1**.[14–17] These patients presented differently than most children with KD; they were older, had markedly increased frequency of cardiovascular shock and most had gastrointestinal symptoms. Children presented approximately 1 month after surges of COVID-19 cases in the general population in a region, so it was

Table 1
Criteria for diagnosis of Kawasaki disease and Toxic Shock Syndrome (TSS)

Kawasaki Disease	Toxic Shock Syndrome due to *Staphylococcal* spp.
Persistent fever ≥ 5 d that is otherwise unexplained	Must meet all 5 criteria below to be considered probable and is confirmed if desquamation occurs 2 wk later:
4 to 5 (complete) or 2 to 3 (incomplete) clinical criteria below: • Eyes: Conjunctival injection that is bilateral • Mouth: mucous membrane changes (eg, cracked lips, fissures, strawberry tongue) • Hands or feet: erythema, swelling, periungual desquamation. • Skin: Rash • Neck: Cervical lymphadenopathy	• Fever • Diffuse macular erythroderma • Hypotension • 3 or more organs involved • Negative microbial testing for other causes

Data from McCrindle BW, Rowley AH, Newburger JW, et al. Diagnosis, Treatment, and Long-Term Management of Kawasaki Disease: A Scientific Statement for Health Professionals From the American Heart Association. *Circulation.* 2017;135(17):e927-e999. https://doi.org/10.1161/CIR. 0000000000000484; and Staphylococcus aureus | Red Book 2021 | Red Book Online | AAP Point-of-Care-Solutions. Accessed October 8, 2021. https://redbook.solutions.aap.org/chapter.aspx?sectionid=247326921&bookid=2591.

suspected to be a postinfectious complication.[18] MIS-C has now emerged in many countries across the world, and national and international public health registries have been tracking this life-threatening disease. Early identification and aggressive treatment strategies have become the standard of care, aimed at decreasing the risk of fatal and long-term cardiovascular sequelae.

Diagnostic Criteria

In mid-May of 2020, the U.S. Centers for Disease Control and Prevention (CDC) developed diagnostic criteria for MIS-C as did the World Health Organization (WHO).[19] There are similarities and differences in these criteria, which are listed in **Table 2**.[20] In the UK, the term "Pediatric Inflammatory Multisystem Syndrome Temporally related to COVID-19" (PIMS-TS) is used to describe the syndrome.[21]

It is important to highlight that children diagnosed with MIS-C must have fever, evidence of inflammation, at least 2 organs involved, no other active infection that could explain their condition, and a plausible epidemiologic link to SARS-CoV-2 through a positive laboratory test (PCR, antigen or antibody) or confirmed exposure. MIS-C is a clinical diagnosis based on symptomology and laboratory features. The CDC definition requires hospitalization, which is used to define the disease as severe, whereas the WHO definition does not.[19]

Differential Diagnosis

Sepsis is the most common condition to be ruled out before diagnosing a patient with MIS-C. Bacterial pathogens must be screened for using blood and other cultures or rapid testing (**Table 3**). In particular, TSS from *Staphylococcus aureus* or *Streptococcus* spp. should be considered (see **Table 1**) given the acute presentation of shock, fever, diffuse inflammation, hepatitis, and skin changes such as erythroderma. Rocky Mountain Spotted Fever due to *Rickettsia rickettsiae* should be another

Table 2
U.S. Centers for Disease Control and Prevention (CDC) versus World Health Organization (WHO) Diagnostic criteria for Multisystem Inflammatory Syndrome in Children (MIS-C) and adolescents with differences highlighted in bold

Criteria	CDC	WHO
Age	< 21 y	< 20 y
Fever	≥ 1 d	≥ 3 d
Inflammation	Elevated CRP, PCT, ESR, fibrinogen, D-dimer, ferritin, lactate, LDH, IL-6, elevated neutrophils, decreased lymphocytes, decreased albumin	Elevated CRP, PCT, ESR
Multisystem Involvement	≥ 2 of the following: Cardiac (eg, shock, elevated troponin, elevated BNP, abnormal echocardiogram, arrhythmia)	≥ 2 of the following: Cardiac dysfunction, pericarditis, valvulitis, or coronary abnormalities (including echocardiographic findings or elevated troponin/BNP); AND/OR Hypotension or shock
	Hematologic (eg, coagulopathy)	Evidence of coagulopathy (prolonged PT or PTT; elevated D-dimer)
	Gastrointestinal (eg, abdominal pain, vomiting, diarrhea, elevated liver enzymes, ileus, gastrointestinal bleeding)	Acute gastrointestinal symptoms (diarrhea, vomiting, or abdominal pain)
	Dermatologic (eg, erythroderma, mucositis, other rashes)	Rash, bilateral nonpurulent conjunctivitis, or mucocutaneous inflammation signs (oral, hands, or feet)
	Respiratory (eg, pneumonia, ARDS, pulmonary embolism) Renal (eg, acute kidney injury, renal failure) Neurologic (eg, seizure, stroke, aseptic meningitis)	
Association with SARS-CoV-2	Positive by RT-PCR, serology, or antigen test or exposure to a suspected/confirmed COVID-19 case within the 4 wk prior to the onset of symptoms	Positive by RT-PCR, serology, or antigen test or likely contact with patients with COVID-19
Alternative diagnoses*	No alternative plausible diagnoses	No other obvious microbial cause of inflammation including bacterial sepsis and staphylococcal or streptococcal toxic shock syndromes
Severity	Requires hospitalization	

Data from Royal College of Pediatrics and Child Health. Guidance: Pediatric Multisystem Inflammatory Syndrome Temporally Associated with COVID-19. Published online May 2020. Accessed September 26, 2021. https://www.rcpch.ac.uk/sites/default/files/2020-05/COVID-19-Paediatric-multisystem-%20inflammatory%20syndrome-20200501.pdf; and Centers for Disease Control. Information for Healthcare Providers about Multisystem Inflammatory Syndrome in Children (MIS-C) | CDC. Published 2020. Accessed October 23, 2020. https://www.cdc.gov/mis-c/hcp/.

Table 3
Overall differences between severe COVID-19 and Multisystem Inflammatory Syndrome in Children (MIS-C) in the national comparative study from the Overcoming COVID-19 public health surveillance registry

Severe Acute COVID-19	MIS-C
Much more likely (70%–80%) to affect children with underlying conditions (obesity, type 1 diabetes mellitus, prematurity, immune compromise)	Much more likely (70%–80%) to affect previously healthy children
More pulmonary involvement and acute respiratory failure	More cardiac dysfunction with 40%–50% requiring vasopressors
Milder systemic inflammation	Severe systemic inflammation
Children 0–4 years old and older teenagers are more likely to be affected	Peak incidence is in children 6–12 years old

Data from Feldstein LR, Tenforde MW, Friedman KG, et al. Characteristics and Outcomes of US Children and Adolescents With Multisystem Inflammatory Syndrome in Children (MIS-C) Compared With Severe Acute COVID-19. *JAMA.* 2021;325(11):1074–1087. https://doi.org/10.1001/JAMA. 2021.2091.

consideration in certain geographic areas in the summertime, especially in patients with hyponatremia, thrombocytopenia, and a palmar rash. Overlap exists in the diagnosis of MIS-C and KD, and approximately 40% of patients with MIS-C will meet diagnostic criteria for KD (see **Table 1**).[18]

Approximately 30% of patients with MIS-C will have a positive respiratory test for SARS-CoV-2.[5] Inflammation and coagulopathy can be features of both acute COVID-19 and MIS-C, and multiorgan involvement is common in critically ill patients with acute COVID-19. The definition of MIS-C is broad, and it is likely that some patients diagnosed with MIS-C have acute COVID-19, especially in those with cardiorespiratory involvement (see **Table 3**). A comparison of children and adolescents with the 2 diagnoses showed that patients with MIS-C were overall more inflamed with higher C-reactive protein (CRP) and neutrophil to lymphocyte ratio (NLR), that thrombocytopenia (<150,000 platelets per microliter) was more common in MIS-C, and patients with acute COVID-19 tended to be more often 0 to 4 or 13 to 17 years of age.[5] In addition, those with acute COVID-19 were much more likely to have underlying medical conditions, whereas the majority of patients with MIS-C were previously healthy.[22]

Epidemiology

As of October 4th, 2021, there were 5217 cases of MIS-C reported to US state public health departments.[23] Additionally, many hundreds of cases have been reported in the United Kingdom, continental Europe, and South America.[24–27] There are also MIS-C case reports in the literature from Africa and Asia.[28,29]

Overall population incidence estimates for MIS-C range from 2 per 100,000 children in New York State to 3 per 10,000 individuals less than 21 years of age infected with SARS-CoV-2.[30,31] Incidence after a diagnosis of MIS-C is difficult to determine as so many children are asymptomatic with their initial infection thus not tested. By definition, children with MIS-C are hospitalized, and over two-thirds require admission to the ICU.[32]

The most common age of onset is 6 to 12 years of age, though there are case reports spanning from the neonatal period to early adulthood.[5,22,30,31] Black and

Hispanic children are overly represented in multiple cohorts, as are males.[5,7,30,33] Most children with MIS-C were previously healthy. Some studies report an elevated prevalence of obesity among patients with MIS-C.[5,34] There is evidence that some children have an underlying genetic predisposition to hyperinflammation that likely explains their MIS-C.[32,35]

A similar clinical syndrome also exists in adults: Multisystem Inflammatory Syndrome in Adults (MIS-A). It is hypothesized that this is also a postinfectious phenomenon that occurs from a dysregulated immune response to SARS-CoV-2. The CDC diagnostic criteria for MIS-A are as follows:

1) a severe illness requiring hospitalization in a person aged $\geq$21 years;
2) a positive test result for current or previous SARS-CoV-2 infection;
3) severe dysfunction of one or more extrapulmonary organ systems;
4) laboratory evidence of severe inflammation;
5) absence of severe respiratory illness.[36]

The major difference between the criteria for MIS-A versus MIS-C, aside from age, is that the presence of pulmonary symptoms excludes MIS-A, whereas a patient can have pulmonary symptoms as part of multisystem involvement in MIS-C. Given the biphasic course of acute COVID-19 in adults, this criterion exists as to not confuse MIS-A with the hyperinflammatory phase of acute COVID-19. MIS-A is much rarer than MIS-C with only 221 cases described in the literature as of September 2021. Most cases were in younger adults (median age = 21 years).[37] Clinical evaluation and treatment strategies are similar to those for MIS-C.

Pathogenesis

The pathogenesis of MIS-C is poorly understood though is hypothesized to be a delayed, overactive immune response to infection with SARS-CoV-2 given its temporal association to SARS-CoV-2 infections in the population (**Fig. 1**). It typically develops 3 to 6 weeks after exposure to SARS-CoV-2. The initial SARS-CoV-2 infection may go undetected due to no or mild symptoms. Much research aims to elucidate the precise pathogenesis of MIS-C. Both the innate and adaptive immune systems are thought to be overly activated[38,39] One theory hypothesizes that the SARS-CoV-2 spike protein can act as a "superantigen," activating both T- and B-cells, leading to the hyperinflammatory state and a subsequent cytokine storm, and similar to the staphylococcal endotoxin B implicated in TSS.[40]

Clinical Manifestations

MIS-C presents with fever and systemic inflammation that leads to the involvement of multiple organ systems, including the cardiovascular, gastrointestinal, neurologic, and mucocutaneous systems (**Table 4**). Involvement can present as follows:

Fever: Children must have persistent fever to meet the criteria for MIS-C. Length of fever before presentation varies but is usually present for at least 24 to 48 hours and most commonly 3 days or more.[18]

Cardiovascular: Acutely, children can present with cardiovascular instability, decreased cardiac function, arrhythmias including heart block, or myocarditis.[41] Approximately 50% to 80% of children present with shock and approximately half require vasoactive support.[17,18] More than 80% of cases have cardiovascular involvement.[18] Severity of these symptoms range from mild, fluid-responsive shock, shock requiring vasoactive agents, to complete cardiovascular collapse requiring extracorporeal support.

Daily MIS-C Cases and COVID-19 Cases Reported to CDC (7-Day Moving Average)

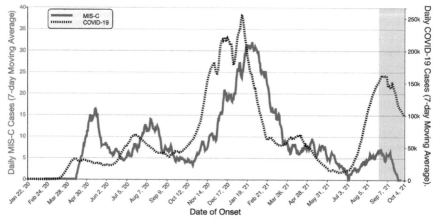

Fig. 1. Daily cases of Multisystem Inflammatory Syndrome in Children (MIS-C) in the U.S. reported to the Centers for Disease Control and Prevention (CDC) from the state public health departments in relation to reported pediatric cases of COVID-19. (*From* The Centers for Disease Control & Prevention https://covid.cdc.gov/covid-data-tracker/#mis-national-surveillance (Accessed 10/9/2021).)

A finding of major concern in MIS-C is the development of a coronary artery aneurysm (CAA) resulting from severe, diffuse inflammation. CAAs in MIS-C are defined as a Z score ≥ 2.5 in the proximal right coronary artery or proximal left anterior descending coronary artery. The exact mechanism of CAA development is unclear. Multicenter case series suggest that CAA occurs in between 8% and 14% of cases of MIS-C.[5,42] The majority of these CAAs resolve within 30 days of hospital admission; therefore, most are unlikely to be vasculitis similar to what is identified in patients with KD,[5] Even in severe MIS-C, CAA in the great majority of patients with MIS-C is likely to resolve by 3 to 6 months after diagnosis and treatment.[43] Longer term outcomes of these CAAs related to MIS-C are under study.

Respiratory: Respiratory symptoms are common in patients diagnosed with MIS-C, reported in about one-third to one-half of patients in a national cohort.[5,22] These range from mild tachypnea and hypoxemia to respiratory failure with pulmonary infiltrates. Lower respiratory symptoms are more common in severe, acute COVID-19 than in MIS-C (62% vs 43%, respectively).[5] Some of the respiratory involvement may be

Table 4	
Frequency of organ system involvement in patients with Multisystem Inflammatory Syndrome in Children (MIS-C) in published surveillance studies	
Gastrointestinal	**80%–90%[5]**
Mucocutaneous	74%–83%[47,48]
Cardiovascular	66.7%–86.5%[5,22]
Hematologic	47.5%[5]
Respiratory	36.5%[5]
Neurologic	12.2%[4,5]

cardiogenic and other patients who have positive respiratory testing for SARS-CoV-2 may be misclassified and have acute COVID-19 with multisystem involvement and hyperinflammation.

Gastrointestinal: Studies report that up to 90% of patients with MIS-C have gastrointestinal symptoms.[5,44] Symptoms include severe abdominal pain with or without emesis, peritonitis, mesenteric lymphadenopathy, and diffuse secretory diarrhea.[45] Abdominal pain has been so severe that cases have been mistaken for acute appendicitis. Terminal ileitis and diffuse colitis have also been observed.

Mucocutaneous: Rashes in MIS-C are variable, and there is not a pathognomonic presentation in MIS-C. More than half of children with MIS-C have a polymorphous exanthem. There have been a variety of lesions described, including maculopapular lesions, annular plaques, and morbilliform eruptions with coalescing papules.[46,47] Most common rash locations include anterior and posterior trunk and extremities. Erythroderma has also been described, along with facial, palmar, and sole erythema and edema. Additionally cracked, dry, erythematous lips are often present. Nonexudative conjunctivitis has also been well-described (see **Table 4**). Younger children are more likely to have mucocutaneous findings.[48]

Neurologic: CNS involvement can include mild to severe acute encephalopathy, stroke, demyelinating lesions, fulminant cerebral edema, headache, delirium, impaired consciousness, inability to walk or crawl, and neck pain. A recent multicenter study reported that 12% of MIS-C cases had neurologic involvement. CNS findings were generally mild and transient but 8% of patients had severe involvement.[4] Case reports describe head imaging findings that range from normal to mild, diffuse cerebral swelling. Evaluations of cerebral spinal fluid have demonstrated a range of symptoms from normal CSF parameters to pleocytosis that can mimic acute bacterial or viral meningitis. Neurologic dysfunction is more common in MIS-C than in severe COVID-19.

Hematologic: Patients may present with deep venous thrombosis, pulmonary embolus, or coagulopathy. A recent multicenter, retrospective cohort study identified thrombi in 6.5% of patients with MIS-C and found MIS-C to be an independent risk factor for thrombotic events, with most thrombi occurring in children 12 years and over.[3]

Laboratory and Imaging Abnormalities

Multiple laboratory abnormalities are described in MIS-C. Inflammation is required, but other findings need not be present to make a diagnosis. Common laboratory findings are summarized in **Box 1**. Polymerase chain reaction (PCR) or antigen testing for SARS-CoV-2 is positive in about 30% of reported cases. Most patients are positive for antibody (IgG) testing, and those who are antibody negative should be investigated fully to identify alternate diagnoses. In those patients who are PCR positive, often the cycle threshold from a SARS-CoV-2 PCR is high, indicating a lower viral load and a later stage of infection, though the utility of this test remains controversial.[49]

Cardiac studies are frequently abnormal. Case series describe a variety of EKG findings, including normal sinus rhythm, sinus tachycardia, heart block, and non–specific ST-wave abnormalities.[41,42] An echocardiogram may show decreased left ventricular systolic function with an ejection fraction of less than 55%. Myocardial deformation parameters (such as global longitudinal strain) can be present even with persevered ejection fraction. CAAs are seen in approximately 8% of patients, especially in delayed or very severe presentation.[41,42]

Recommended Initial Evaluation

Initial evaluation should be performed as shown in **Table 3**. A thorough patient history should be obtained, with a focus on the presence of fever, close contact with an

---

Box 1
Common laboratory and diagnostic test abnormalities identified in children presenting with Multisystem Inflammatory Syndrome in Children (MIS-C)[a]

Inflammatory markers: Elevated CRP, PCT, or ESR. Cytokine panels (if done) may show elevated soluble IL-1, IL-2R, IL-6, IL-8, and TNF-a[49,58]

Complete Blood Count with Differential: Lymphopenia with neutrophilia, anemia, thrombocytopenia

Complete Metabolic Panel: hyponatremia, elevated creatinine and/or BUN, elevated AST and/or ALT

Blood gas: metabolic acidosis

Cardiac/Perfusion: Elevated troponin, elevated BNP or pro-BNP, elevated lactate

Coagulation: elevated PT, INR, and D-dimer

SARS-CoV-2: Positive antibody testing

Echocardiogram: Impaired ejection fraction of the left ventricle, coronary artery dilations, or aneurysms

Electrocardiogram: Heart block (first or second degree) or non-specific ST wave changes

Chest radiograph: Pulmonary edema

[a]Patients must have elevated inflammatory markers to meet diagnostic criteria; other laboratory derangements may or may not be present. Serial evaluation is often indicated until abnormalities normalize.

---

individual with COVID-19, and occurrence of other symptoms. Careful physical examination should be performed with special attention to findings such as meningismus, mental status, conjunctivitis, dry, cracked lips, abdominal pain, extremity swelling, palmar or sole erythema, and rash.

Additional testing to rule out other infectious and noninfectious etiologies should be performed. Other infectious considerations include sepsis, rickettsial illness (particularly Rocky Mountain Spotted Fever), TSS, Staph Scalded Skin Syndrome, or severe adenovirus infection. Clinicians should consider obtaining a blood culture, urinalysis and culture, group A streptococcus testing, PCRs for other respiratory viral pathogens, and Rocky Mountain Fever Syndrome or Ehrlichia serologies (depending on geographic location and season). Hemophagocytic lymphohistiocytosis (HLH) or macrophage activation syndrome (MAS) should be considered in the appropriate clinical scenario.

SEVERE COVID-19 TREATMENT AND OUTCOMES
Treatment

Most children with moderate to severe COVID-19 will improve with supportive care alone. Data are lacking regarding optimal treatment strategies of children with COVID-19 as severe disease in children is very uncommon and children were not enrolled in prior published clinical trials.[50] The Pediatric Infectious Diseases Society suggests the use of a 5-day course of remdesivir in children with severe COVID-19.[51] Pharmacokinetic/pharmacodynamic clinical trials are ongoing to determine optimal dosing strategies (NCT04431453).[52] Dexamethasone has been widely used in children with severe disease, given results in adults from the RECOVERY trial, and while considered safe, efficacy data are lacking children.[53] Other immunomodulatory therapies such as tocilizumab, anakinra, and baricitinib have also been given to some children following some successful results in adults, but no data exist to support their use.

There is no evidence to support the use of azithromycin, hydroxychloroquine, iver-mectin, other antiviral therapies, or convalescent plasma in children.

Similar techniques of ICU management including optimal ventilation strategies, proning, and other optimal intensive care unit management of ARDS have also been used in children. Status asthmaticus is managed with standard asthma protocols.[54] Fluid management is essential. Adolescents are often anticoagulated, as are those who are obese or have another coexisting condition.

For treatment and outcomes of the overlapping phenotype between MIS-C and se-vere COVID-19, these children generally receive hybrid treatment strategies including steroids both for antiinflammatory effect and ARDS. IVIG and/or remdesivir may also be used.

Outcomes

An estimated 5% to 20% of cases require hospitalization, and about 2% of cases require admission to the intensive care unit versus the general pediatric floor. Of those admitted to the intensive care unit, the mortality rate was less than 2% even in a large national multicenter study.[5] Long-term pulmonary outcomes are unknown given that this is a novel disease.

MIS-C TREATMENT AND OUTCOMES
Treatment

Of the MIS-C cases in the United States, multicenter studies have shown that about two-thirds of patients diagnosed with MIS-C require admission to the intensive care unit.[8] Given the ongoing worldwide pandemic and the rarity of MIS-C, data regarding optimal treatment of MIS-C are sparse and largely from observational studies. Current treatment strategies from consensus recommendations focus on immunomodulation similar to the treatment of KD, typically with intravenous immunoglobulin (IVIG) and/or corticosteroids. Corticosteroids are usually initiated intravenously, then transitioned to an oral regimen with a physiologic taper until after hospital discharge.

A recent US-based study of very severe patients in the Overcoming COVID-19 US Network (47% were on vasopressors and 41% had impaired ejection fraction) showed improved outcomes when given IVIG plus steroids on the first day of treatment.[55] Addition of other immunomodulatory treatments after the initial treatment day was also significantly decreased. However, the Best Available Treatment Study (BATS), which was international, showed no difference in recovery from MIS-C when comparing groups given IVIG alone, corticosteroids alone, or IVIG and corticosteroids together.[56] The BATS study population used a broader definition for MIS-C, and their patients were markedly less ill than the US cohort. Therefore, in critically ill patients it is likely prudent to treat more aggressively initially to resolve the cardiovascular compli-cations more quickly. Other immunomodulatory therapies have been trialed such as anakinra, an IL-1 inhibitor, and tocilizumab, an IL-6 inhibitor, though data are lacking whether these are effective. Some institutions have used anakinra for refractory MIS-C that has not responded initially to steroids and/or IVIG. A recent single-center study reported quicker recovery in children given IVIG plus infliximab (a TNF-a inhibitor).[57]

In addition to immunomodulatory therapies, anticoagulation is typically adminis-tered to patients with laboratory markers consistent with a hypercoagulable state, given potential CAA and risk of thrombosis. While hospitalized in the ICU, low-molecular-weight heparin is usually initiated. In some centers, patients are also given low-dose aspirin, as is the standard of care in KD. Ultimate duration of optimal antico-agulation remains unclear. Most institutions continue anticoagulants until after discharge when a follow-up echocardiogram has been obtained and longer if the patient has a CAA.

Supportive care is always provided, including vasoactive support if needed and careful fluid management. Echocardiograms should be performed serially to follow decreased cardiac function. Antibiotics are usually administered until the blood and other cultures result negative, as sepsis must be ruled out.

Outcomes

The great majority of children with MIS-C have recovered. The mortality rate in the US in patients with MIS-C is 1% to 2%.[5,23] A recent UK case series showed that 6 to 12 months after diagnosis, most patients had a resolution of their hyperinflammatory state.[43] For cardiac outcomes. 4% to 17.5% percent of patients have had coronary aneurysms diagnosed while hospitalized, and at 90-day follow up, the majority of these coronary aneurysms have resolved.[5,39,42] Data are still being collected about long-term outcomes of these children, though data suggest that full recovery typically occurs after aggressive treatment on presentation. Studies are ongoing to determine the longer-term effects on the heart. Children who are diagnosed with MIS-C are often followed by a multidisciplinary team after discharge including rheumatology, cardiology, and in some cases, infectious disease specialists.

SUMMARY

Both severe acute COVID-19 and MIS-C can cause life-threatening illness in children and adolescents. Fortunately, the clinical outcomes for severe COVID-19 are markedly better in children than in adults, and mortality is uncommon. Optimal treatment strategies for severe, acute COVID-19 and MIS-C are difficult to study due to the low frequency of these conditions and there is a paucity of strong evidence in the pediatric population. Most institutions have applied the evidence gained from adult studies to children with acute COVID-19 critical illness. Consensus guidelines have been developed for the diagnosis and treatment of MIS-C, with treatment algorithms similar to what is used for KD.

CLINICS CARE POINTS

- Severe, acute COVID-19 is uncommon in children and adolescents but is most likely to present with pulmonary involvement as it does in adults.
- MIS-C is a novel clinical entity that is driven by systemic inflammation and most commonly affects the cardiovascular and mucocutaneous systems.
- Children with suspected MIS-C are at risk for thrombosis and neurologic complications.
- Immunomodulation, given promptly in children with MIS-C who are critically ill, will shorten the duration of cardiovascular dysfunction, but the optimal treatment of milder cases of MIS-C is unclear.

DISCLOSURE

AMB is funded by T32 GM75766-13/National Institutes of General Medical Science.

REFERENCES

1. Levin M. Childhood multisystem inflammatory syndrome — a new Challenge in the pandemic. NEJM 2020;383(4):393–5.

2. Shekerdemian LS, Mahmood NR, Wolfe KK, et al. Characteristics and outcomes of children with Coronavirus disease 2019 (COVID-19) infection admitted to US and Canadian pediatric intensive care Units. JAMA Pediatr 2020;2019:1–6.

3. Whitworth H, Sartain S, Kumar R, et al. Rate of thrombosis in children and adolescents hospitalized with COVID-19 or MIS-C. Blood 2021;138(2):190–8.

4. LaRovere KL, Riggs BJ, Poussaint TY, et al. Neurologic involvement in children and adolescents hospitalized in the United States for COVID-19 or multisystem inflammatory syndrome. JAMA Neurol 2021;78(5):536–47.

5. Feldstein LR, Tenforde MW, Friedman KG, et al. Characteristics and outcomes of US children and adolescents with multisystem inflammatory syndrome in children (MIS-C) compared with severe acute COVID-19. JAMA 2021;325(11):1074–87.

6. She J, Liu L, Liu W. COVID-19 epidemic: disease characteristics in children. J Med Virol 2020;92(7):747–54.

7. Swann Ov, Holden KA, Turtle L, et al. Clinical characteristics of children and young people admitted to hospital with covid-19 in United Kingdom: Prospective multicentre observational cohort study. BMJ 2020;370. https://doi.org/10.1136/BMJ.M3249.

8. Delahoy MJ, Ujamaa D, Whitaker M, et al. Hospitalizations associated with COVID-19 among children and adolescents — COVID-NET, 14 states, March 1, 2020–August 14, 2021. MMWR Morbidity Mortality Weekly Rep 2021;70(36):1255–60.

9. Kim L, Whitaker M, O'Halloran A, et al. Hospitalization rates and characteristics of children aged 18 Years hospitalized with laboratory-confirmed COVID-19 — COVID-NET, 14 states, March 1–July 25, 2020. MMWR Morbidity Mortality Weekly Rep 2020;69(32):1081–8.

10. Boehmer TK, Kompaniyets L, Lavery AM, et al. Association between COVID-19 and myocarditis using hospital-based Administrative data — United States, March 2020–January 2021. MMWR Morbidity Mortality Weekly Rep 2021;70(35):1228–32.

11. Dinnes J, Deeks JJ, Berhane S, et al. Rapid, point-of-care antigen and molecular-based tests for diagnosis of SARS-CoV-2 infection. Cochrane Database Syst Rev 2021;2021(3). https://doi.org/10.1002/14651858.CD013705.PUB2.

12. Kompaniyets L, Agathis NT, Nelson JM, et al. Underlying medical conditions associated with severe COVID-19 illness among children. JAMA Netw Open 2021;4(6):e2111182.

13. Govil-Dalela T, Sivaswamy L. Neurological effects of COVID-19 in children. Pediatr Clin North America 2021;68(5):1081.

14. Toubiana J, Poirault C, Corsia A, et al. Kawasaki-like multisystem inflammatory syndrome in children during the covid-19 pandemic in Paris, France: Prospective observational study. BMJ (Clinical research ed) 2020;369:m2094.

15. Verdoni L, Mazza A, Gervasoni A, et al. An Outbreak of severe Kawasaki-like disease at the Italian Epicentre of the SARS-CoV-2 epidemic: an observational cohort study. Lancet 2020;395(10239):1771–8.

16. Chiotos K, Bassiri H, Behrens EM, et al. Multisystem inflammatory syndrome in children during the Coronavirus 2019 pandemic: a case series. J Pediatr Infect Dis Soc 2020;9(3):393–8.

17. Riphagen S, Gomez X, Gonzalez-Martinez C, Wilkinson N, Theocharis P. Hyperinflammatory shock in children during COVID-19 pandemic. Lancet 2020;395(10237):1607.

18. Feldstein LR, Rose EB, Horwitz SM, et al. Multisystem inflammatory syndrome in U.S. Children and adolescents. NEJM 2020;1–13. https://doi.org/10.1056/NEJMoa2021680.

19. The Centers for Disease Control & Prevention. Multisystem inflammatory syndrome in children (MIS-C) associated with Coronavirus disease 2019 (COVID-19). Health Alert Network. 2020. https://emergency.cdc.gov/han/2020/han00432.asp. Accessed July 29, 2020.

20. World Health Organization. Multisystem inflammatory syndrome in children and adolescents temporally related to COVID-19. 2020. https://www.who.int/news-room/commentaries/detail/multisystem-inflammatory-syndrome-in-children-and-adolescents-with-covid-19. Accessed September 27, 2021.

21. Royal College of Paediatrics and Child Health. Guidance: Paediatric multisystem inflammatory syndrome temporally associated with COVID-19. 2020. https://www.rcpch.ac.uk/sites/default/files/2020-05/COVID-19-Paediatric-multisystem-%20inflammatory%20syndrome-20200501.pdf. Accessed September 26, 2021.

22. Godfred-Cato S. COVID-19–Associated multisystem inflammatory syndrome in children — United States, March–July 2020. MMWR Morbidity Mortality Weekly Rep 2020;69(32):1074–80.

23. The Centers for Disease Control & Prevention. CDC COVID data tracker. 2021. https://covid.cdc.gov/covid-data-tracker/#mis-national-surveillance. Accessed October 3, 2021.

24. Flood J, Shingleton J, Bennett E, et al. Paediatric multisystem inflammatory syndrome temporally associated with SARS-CoV-2 (PIMS-TS): Prospective, national surveillance, United Kingdom and Ireland, 2020. Lancet Reg Health – Europe 2021;3. https://doi.org/10.1016/J.LANEPE.2021.100075.

25. Lima-Setta F, Magalhães-Barbosa MC, Rodrigues-Santos G, et al. Multisystem inflammatory syndrome in children (MIS-C) during SARS-CoV-2 pandemic in Brazil: a multicenter, Prospective cohort study. Jornal de Pediatria 2021;97(3):354–61.

26. Antúnez-Montes OY, Escamilla MI, Figueroa-Uribe AF, et al. COVID-19 and multisystem inflammatory syndrome in Latin American children: a Multinational study. Pediatr Infect Dis J 2021;40(1). https://doi.org/10.1097/INF.0000000000002949.

27. García-Salido A, de Carlos Vicente JC, Belda Hofheinz S, et al. Severe manifestations of SARS-CoV-2 in children and adolescents: from COVID-19 Pneumonia to multisystem inflammatory syndrome: a multicentre study in pediatric intensive care Units in Spain. Crit Care 2020;24(1):666.

28. Balagurunathan M, Natarajan T, Karthikeyan J, Palanisamy V. Clinical Spectrum and Short-term outcomes of multisystem inflammatory syndrome in children in a South Indian hospital. Clin Exp Pediatr 2021. https://doi.org/10.3345/CEP.2021.00374.

29. van Heerden J, Nel J, Moodley P, et al. Multisystem inflammatory syndrome (MIS): a multicentre retrospective review of adults and adolescents in South Africa. Int J Infect Dis 2021;111:227–32.

30. Dufort EM, Koumans EH, Chow EJ, et al. Multisystem inflammatory syndrome in children in New York state. New Engl J Med 2020;383(4):347–58.

31. Payne A, Gilani Z, Godfred-Cato S, et al. Incidence of multisystem inflammatory syndrome in children among US persons infected with SARS-CoV-2. JAMA Netw Open 2021;4(6). https://doi.org/10.1001/JAMANETWORKOPEN.2021.16420.

32. Chou J, Platt CD, Habiballah S, et al. Mechanisms underlying genetic Susceptibility to multisystem inflammatory syndrome in children (MIS-C). J Allergy Clin Immunol 2021. https://doi.org/10.1016/J.JACI.2021.06.024.

33. Belay ED, Abrams J, Oster ME, et al. Trends in geographic and temporal Distribution of US children with multisystem inflammatory syndrome during the COVID-19 pandemic. JAMA Pediatr 2021;175(8):837–45.

34. Abrams JY, Oster ME, Godfred-Cato SE, et al. Factors linked to severe outcomes in multisystem inflammatory syndrome in children (MIS-C) in the USA: a retrospective surveillance study. Lancet Child Adolesc Health 2021;5(5):323.

35. Lee PY, Platt CD, Weeks S, et al. Immune dysregulation and multisystem inflammatory syndrome in children (MIS-C) in individuals with Haploinsufficiency of SOCS1. J Allergy Clin Immunol 2020;146(5):1194.

36. Morris S, Schwartz N, Patel P, et al. Case series of multisystem inflammatory syndrome in adults associated with SARS-CoV-2 infection — United Kingdom and United States, March–August 2020. MMWR Morbidity Mortality Weekly Rep 2020;69(40):1450–6.

37. Patel P, DeCuir J, Abrams J, Campbell AP, Godfred-Cato S, Belay ED. Clinical characteristics of multisystem inflammatory syndrome in adults: a Systematic review. JAMA Netw Open 2021;4(9):e2126456.

38. Vella LA, Giles JR, Baxter AE, et al. Deep immune Profiling of MIS-C demonstrates marked but transient immune activation Xompared to adult and pediatric COVID-19. Sci Immunol 2021;6(57). https://doi.org/10.1126/SCIIMMUNOL.ABF7570.

39. McMurray JC, May JW, Cunningham MW, Jones OY. Multisystem inflammatory syndrome in children (MIS-C), a post-viral myocarditis and systemic vasculitis—a critical review of its pathogenesis and treatment. Front Pediatr 2020;8:626182. https://doi.org/10.3389/FPED.2020.626182.

40. Rivas MN, Porritt RA, Cheng MH, Bahar I, Arditi M. COVID-19–associated multisystem inflammatory syndrome in children (MIS-C): a novel disease that mimics Toxic shock syndrome—the superantigen Hypothesis. J Allergy Clin Immunol 2021;147(1):57–9.

41. Niaz T, Hope K, Fremed M, et al. Role of a pediatric cardiologist in the COVID-19 pandemic. Pediatr Cardiol 2021;42(1):19–35.

42. Matsubara D, Kauffman H, Wang Y, et al. Echocardiographic findings in pediatric multisystem inflammatory syndrome associated with COVID-19 in the United States. J Am Coll Cardiol 2020;76(17):1947–61.

43. Farooqi KM, Chan A, Weller RJ, et al. Longitudinal outcomes for multisystem inflammatory syndrome in children. Pediatrics 2021;148(2). e2021051155.

44. Chen T-H, Kao W-T, Tseng Y-H. Gastrointestinal involvements in children with COVID-related multisystem inflammatory syndrome. Gastroenterology 2021;160(5):1887.

45. Assa A, Benninga MA, Borrelli O, et al. Gastrointestinal Perspective of Coronavirus disease 2019 in children-an Updated review. J Pediatr Gastroenterol Nutr 2021;73(3):299–305.

46. Blatz AM, Oboite M, Chiotos K, et al. Cutaneous findings in SARS-CoV-2-associated multisystem inflammatory disease in children. Open Forum Infect Dis 2021;8(3). https://doi.org/10.1093/OFID/OFAB074.

47. Naka F, Melnick L, Gorelik M, Morel KD. A Dermatologic Perspective on multisystem inflammatory syndrome in children. Clin Dermatol 2021;39(1):163.

48. Young TK, Shaw KS, Shah JK, et al. Mucocutaneous manifestations of multisystem inflammatory syndrome in children during the COVID-19 pandemic. JAMA Dermatol 2021;157(2):207–12.

49. DeBiasi R, Harahsheh A, Srinivasalu H, et al. Multisystem inflammatory syndrome of children: Subphenotypes, risk factors, Biomarkers, cytokine Profiles, and viral Sequencing. J Pediatr 2021;237:125–35.e18.

50. Hwang TJ, Randolph AG, Bourgeois FT. Inclusion of children in clinical trials of treatments for Coronavirus disease 2019 (COVID-19). JAMA Pediatr 2020; 174(9):825–6.

51. Chiotos K, Hayes M, Kimberlin DW, et al. Multicenter interim guidance on use of antivirals for children with COVID-19/SARS-CoV-2. J Pediatr Infect Dis Soc 2021; 10(1):34–48.

52. ClinicalTrials.gov. Study to evaluate the safety, Tolerability, Pharmacokinetics, and efficacy of remdesivir (GS-5734™) in Participants from Birth to < 18 Years of age with Coronavirus disease 2019 (COVID-19) (CARAVAN). 2020. https://www.clinicaltrials.gov/ct2/show/NCT04431453. Accessed September 27, 2021.

53. The RECOVERY Collaborative Group. Dexamethasone in hospitalized patients with covid-19. NEJM 2020;384(8):693–704.

54. Abrams EM, Sinha I, Fernandes RM, Hawcutt DB. Pediatric asthma and COVID-19: the Known, the unknown, and the controversial. Pediatr Pulmonology 2020; 55(12):3573–8.

55. Son MBF, Murray N, Friedman K, et al. Multisystem inflammatory syndrome in children - initial Therapy and outcomes. NEJM 2021;385(1):23–34.

56. McArdle AJ, Vito O, Patel H, et al. Treatment of multisystem inflammatory syndrome in children. NEJM 2021;385(1):11–22.

57. Cole LD, Osborne CM, Silveira LJ, et al. IVIG compared to IVIG plus infliximab in multisystem inflammatory syndrome in children. *Pediatr* Published Online September 2021;21. https://doi.org/10.1542/PEDS.2021-052702. e2021052702.

58. Diorio C, Henrickson SE, Vella LA, et al. Multisystem inflammatory syndrome in children and COVID-19 are distinct presentations of SARS–CoV-2. J Clin Invest 2020;130(11). https://doi.org/10.1172/JCI140970.

Review of Anti-inflammatory and Antiviral Therapeutics for Hospitalized Patients Infected with Severe Acute Respiratory Syndrome Coronavirus 2

Jen-Ting Chen, MD, MS[a],*, Marlies Ostermann, MD, PhD[b]

KEYWORDS

- Anti-inflammatory • Cytokines • Interleukins • COVID-19 • SARS-CoV-2 • Antiviral
- Glucocorticoids • Antibody

KEY POINTS

- Severe acute respiratory syndrome coronavirus 2 (SARS-CoV-2) infection can lead to dysregulated cytokine production causing imbalance in host immunity.
- Glucocorticoids, such as dexamethasone, decrease mortality in hospitalized patients with SARS-CoV-2 requiring oxygen.
- Early use of interleukin-6 antagonists is beneficial for hypoxemic patients with COVID-19.
- Janus kinase inhibition is effective in preventing SARS-CoV-2 progression and has the potential to decrease mortality in patients requiring low-flow oxygen but not in those with severe symptoms.
- Antiviral therapy with remdesivir, intravenous immunoglobulin, or convalescent plasma is not beneficial in hospitalized symptomatic patients.

INTRODUCTION

Inflammation in Sepsis and Acute Respiratory Distress Syndrome

Sepsis is defined as a dysregulated host response to infection with an imbalance of proinflammatory and anti-inflammatory cytokines.[1] As the first line of defense to

[a] Division Critical Care Medicine, Department of Medicine, Montefiore Medical Center, Albert Einstein College of Medicine, 111 East 210th Street, Bronx, NY 10467, USA; [b] Department of Critical Care, King's College London, Guy's & St Thomas' NHS Foundation Hospital, Westminster Bridge Road, London SE1 7EH, United Kingdom
* Corresponding author.
E-mail address: jeche@montefiore.org
Twitter: @tchen383 (J.-T.C.)

Crit Care Clin 38 (2022) 587–600
https://doi.org/10.1016/j.ccc.2022.02.002
0749-0704/22/© 2022 Elsevier Inc. All rights reserved.

criticalcare.theclinics.com

infection, the innate immune system is activated and produces proinflammatory cytokines leading to indiscriminate destruction of foreign or infected cells. Proinflammatory mediators then further trigger downstream physiologic processes leading to activation of coagulation pathways, endothelial dilatation and increased permeability, complement activation, recruitment of adaptive immunity, and ultimately, production of anti-inflammatory cytokines to balance the proinflammatory state.[2] When left unchecked, hyperinflammation may occur, resulting in tissue damage, acute respiratory distress syndrome (ARDS), vasodilatory shock, disseminated intravascular coagulopathy, intravascular formation of microthrombi, and death. This unchecked hyperinflammatory state is sometimes referred to as "cytokine storm."[3]

During the severe acute respiratory syndrome coronavirus 2 (SARS-CoV-2) pandemic in 2020, some hospitalized patients with severe SARS-CoV-2 infection were reported to have lymphopenia and thrombocytopenia, as well as elevated acute phase reactants, such as ferritin and C-reactive protein (CRP), and raised liver enzymes and D-dimer.[4] Not surprisingly, the derangement of these biomarkers was directly associated with worse outcomes.[5] The inflammatory profile of patients with moderate to severe SARS-CoV-2 infection is similar to that of patients with ARDS and sepsis.[5–7] In a prospective study, Wilson and colleagues[6] compared the cytokine profiles of patients with coronavirus disease 2019 (COVID-19) with historical patients suffering from ARDS or sepsis. They found no difference in 6 major cytokines (interleukins [IL]-1β, IL-1RA, IL-6, IL-8, IL-18, and tumor necrosis factor [TNF]-α).

Immune Response in Severe Acute Respiratory Syndrome Coronavirus 2 Infection

Elevated cytokine concentrations are associated with increased severity of SARS-CoV-2 infections.[8] The pathogenesis of SARS-CoV-2 infection includes various phases (**Fig. 1**). In the early phase, the virus enters the cells after binding of the spike unit to the angiotensin-converting enzyme 2 receptor.[9] The host cell protease facilitates viral fusion and cell entry following which viral RNA processing occurs. The viral N-protein inhibits interferon production, which decreases recruitment of innate immunity cells and viral clearance.[9–11] As viral replication continues, host cell death ensues, resulting in the release of excessive intracellular material, including cytokines and chemokines. Symptomatically, the host experiences hypoxemia and can develop ARDS and additional organs dysfunction. A myriad of cytokines may be involved in this process.[12] Clinical trials have demonstrated improved outcomes in patients with severe or critical COVID-19 with immunomodulatory therapies. In this article, the authors review the current level of evidence.

IMMUNE MODULATION IN SEVERE ACUTE RESPIRATORY SYNDROME CORONAVIRUS 2 INFECTIONS
Glucocorticoids

Glucocorticoids are fat-soluble hormones that bind to transmembrane receptors as well as intracellular receptors. In the setting of stress, glucocorticoids are released by the adrenal glands and bind to the glucocorticoid receptor, a transcription factor in target cells. Glucocorticoid receptor binding has strong anti-inflammatory downstream effects ranging from transcriptional action, protein modification, and direct cell type–specific directives (**Table 1**).[13] A variety of glucocorticoids, including dexamethasone, prednisone, hydrocortisone, and methylprednisolone, have been trialed; the largest study, conducted by the RECOVERY collaborative group, examined dexamethasone.[14–17] Therapy with dexamethasone has become standard of care for patients with SARS-CoV-2 requiring oxygen therapy.

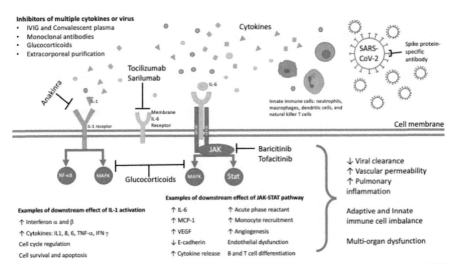

Fig. 1. Potential targets for anti-inflammation and antiviral in SARS-CoV-2 infection.[12,33,59] (*Adapted from* Ni, Y., Alu, A., Lei, H. et al. Immunological perspectives on the pathogenesis, diagnosis, prevention and treatment of COVID-19. Mol Biomed 2, 1 (2021). https://doi.org/10.1186/s43556-020-00015-y; under CC BY 4.0 http://creativecommons.org/licenses/by/4.0/.)

Timing of steroids

Uncontrolled inflammation can result in progression from severe to critical SARS-CoV-2 infection. Careful selection of the right cohort of patients to receive glucocorticoids for pan-immune suppression is key, as premature immune modulation may impede viral clearance. Historically, the use of steroids in critically ill patients infected with influenza, SARS-CoV-1, or Middle East respiratory syndrome coronavirus has not demonstrated any benefit in patient-centered outcomes, but is associated with delayed viral clearance.[18–20] Indeed, the early use of systemic steroids in patients with SARS-CoV-2 with mild symptoms is likely to be harmful. Sahu and colleagues[21] conducted a systematic review of the use of systemic steroids using data of 2214 patients included in 3 randomized controlled trials (RCTs) and 4 propensity score matched studies. They demonstrated that in patients without oxygen requirement, steroid therapy was associated with an increased risk of disease progression. The mean duration to viral clearance was also longer in the group receiving glucocorticoids compared with the control arm (18.9 days vs 16.5 days; odds ratio [OR] 0.20, 95% confidence interval [CI] 0.04–0.36).[21]

However, SARS-CoV-2 inflammation in moderate to severe disease behaves differently. The RECOVERY trial,[14] the largest steroid trial in SARS-CoV-2 to date, was an open-label, RCT and included 6525 patients of whom 2104 patients were assigned to receive dexamethasone and 4321 were assigned to receive usual care. At the time of randomization, 24% of patients were not on oxygen; the remainder were either on noninvasive oxygen therapy (61%) or on invasive mechanical ventilation (16%). The study demonstrated a reduction in 28-day mortality (OR, 0.83; 95% CI, 0.75–0.93) in patients receiving steroids. However, in those who did not require oxygen therapy at time of randomization, there was no significant benefit (OR, 1.19; 95% CI, 0.92, 1.55), and a trend toward harm. A meta-analysis of 7 RCTs by the World Health Organization (WHO) Rapid Evidence Appraisal for COVID-19 Therapeutics (REACT) Working Group consistently demonstrated that patients with respiratory symptoms

Table 1
Glucocorticoid mechanisms of action in severe acute respiratory syndrome coronavirus 2

Effects of Glucocorticoids	Action
Genomic actions	• Direct and indirect binding through other transcription factors • Decrease of IL-2 expression through AP1, NFAT, and NFKB • Shift from TH1 cellular immunity to TH2 humoral immunity through decrease of IL-2, IFN-γ, and STAT4 • Chromatin structure alteration by interaction of histone acetyltransferase activity
Nongenomic actions	• Direct negative interaction with PI3K, JNK, 14-3-3 proteins in T-cell receptor signaling complex • Enters thymocyte mitochondria and induces apoptosis • Recruitment of multiprotein chaperone complex for signaling pathways
Cell type–specific actions	• Monocyte and macrophage survival and function: improves phagocytic activity and stimulates clearance of harmful elements • Dendritic cells: Maturation, survival, and migration toward lymph nodes. Reduces ability of DC cells to stimulate T cells by upregulation of costimulatory IL-6, IL-12, and TNF-alpha, and tolerance-inducing transcription factors • Neutrophils: Leukocyte extravasation and favoring their egress from bone marrow and modulating their migration to perivascular space • T cells: Decreases number by migration back to bone marrow or lymphoid tissues with induction of chemokines. Favors T-cell apoptosis. Limits naïve T-cell differentiation
Hemodynamic effects	• Potentiation of vasoconstrictor hormones • Retention of fluid

Abbreviations: AP1, activator protein 1; DC, dendritic cell; NFAT, nuclear factor of activated T cells; NFKB, nuclear factor-κB; PI3K, Phosphoinositide 3-kinase; TH, T helper.

Adapted from Liberman AC, Budziński ML, Sokn C, Gobbini RP, Steininger A and Arzt E (2018) Regulatory and Mechanistic Actions of Glucocorticoids on T and Inflammatory Cells. Front. Endocrinol. 9:235. https://doi.org/10.3389/fendo.2018.00235; under CC BY 4.0 https://creativecommons.org/licenses/by/4.0/.

requiring oxygen benefited from systemic glucocorticoid therapy with the largest benefit seen in those on mechanical ventilation.[17] The beneficial role of steroids on systemic inflammation is further supported by a decrease in mortality in patients with a prolonged course of illness (>7 days of symptoms).[17]

Currently, the evidence for the use of systemic glucocorticoids for persistent diffuse lung parenchymal disease is limited. In an observational cohort study, 4.8% of survivors of severe SARS-CoV-2 infections had residual symptoms and persistent radiographic evidence of interstitial lung disease with a predominant organizing pneumonia pattern 4 weeks after initial hospital admission.[22] It is recommended to involve multidisciplinary medical teams to determine the best course of action in this patient population.[22,23]

Glucocorticoid selection

Hydrocortisone is the equivalent of cortisol when used as a drug; other formulations are compared with hydrocortisone,[13] in terms of potency and duration of action. Dexamethasone is the most potent anti-inflammatory and longest-acting corticosteroid followed by methylprednisolone, prednisone, and hydrocortisone (least potent). They have all been used to treat oxygen-requiring patients with SARS-CoV-2 infection.

Dexamethasone is known to suppress IL-1 signaling pathways, specifically c-Jun N-terminal kinase (JNK)-p38, leading to suppression of macrophage release of downstream cytokines, such as IL-6, IL-8, and TNF.[24] Similarly, hydrocortisone use in patients with severe sepsis has been shown to significantly decrease IL-1β, interferon-γ (IFN-γ), TNF-α, and IL-6 levels.[25] Methylprednisolone has been reported to have some benefit in acute lung injury.[26]

Dexamethasone, hydrocortisone, and methylprednisolone have been used in ARDS clinical trials. In the DEXA-ARDS study, Villar and colleagues[27] investigated the role of dexamethasone (20 mg for 5 days followed by 10 mg for 5 more days). Hospital mortality was reduced by 12.5% (95% CI, −22.9 to −1.7) with an increase in ventilator-free days of 4.8 (95% CI, 2.57–7.03) in those treated with dexamethasone.

The COVID-19 Dexamethasone RCT has been completed in Brazil.[28] It included mechanically ventilated patients with moderate to severe ARDS who were randomized to receive 20 mg of dexamethasone for 5 days followed by 10 mg of dexamethasone for 5 additional days. There was not a significant difference in all-cause mortality between the 2 groups, in contrast to the original DEXA-ARDS results.[27,28] Furthermore, both the CAPE-COVID (community-acquired pneumonia-COVID) trial and the randomized, embedded, multifactorial adaptive platform trial for community-acquired pneumonia (REMAP-CAP) trial randomized patients to 200 mg of daily hydrocortisone (equivalent of dexamethasone 7 mg) or placebo.[15] There was no significant mortality benefit or difference in organ support-free days.[15,29] Methylprednisone infusion also did not lead to significant mortality benefits.[16] None of the studies showed differences in serious adverse events between the glucocorticoid and placebo arms.

The RECOVERY trial compared Dexamethasone 6 mg daily for 10 days versus standard care and demonstrated a significantly lower mortality.[14] Although there was no significant difference between dexamethasone 6 mg per day versus 12 mg per day in clinical outcomes, the mortality at 28 and 90 days trended toward benefit in the higher dose group in the COVID STEROID 2 Trial.[30] Smaller clinical trials examining the use of other formulations and different dosages of hydrocortisone and methylprednisolone were examined in a meta-analysis by the WHO-REACT working group.[17] Significant benefit was seen in the dexamethasone subgroup and not in either hydrocortisone or methylprednisolone subgroups groups.

In conclusion, current evidence supports the use of dexamethasone 6 mg daily for 10 days in hospitalized patients with SARS-CoV-2 requiring oxygen therapy (**Table 2**). Steroids should be avoided in asymptomatic or mild disease. Increasing the dose to 12 mg can be considered. The actions of dexamethasone are likely to be more systemic rather than intrapulmonary.

Interleukin-6 Antagonists

IL-6 is a key cytokine in the pathogenesis of severe to critical SARS-CoV-2 infection. Cellular stress induces IL-6 secretion.[12] IL-6 receptors are soluble and transmembrane structures.[31] After binding with IL-6, the IL-6 receptor complex binds with another molecule gp130 in either membrane form or soluble form in blood. The membrane-bound gp130-IL-6/IL-6 receptor complex is associated with Janus kinase (JAK), a tyrosine kinase.[32] The binding of soluble gp130 to the IL-6 receptor complex has an inhibitory effect on IL-6 downstream activities (see **Fig. 1**). IL-6–mediated clinical signs include patients' fever, weight loss, flulike symptoms, and an elevation in acute phase reactants like CRP.[32] In addition, angiogenesis is triggered, and neutrophils are recruited to the site of inflammation. IL-6 also promotes B- and T-cell differentiation and is involved in the differentiation of naïve T cell to CD4+ T-helper cells. Inflammation with elevated IL-6 levels can be seen in severe to critical SARS-CoV-2

Table 2
Anti-inflammatory therapeutics with evidence-based data in support of use

Therapeutics	Dose	Timing	Benefit
Glucocorticoids: Dexamethasone	6 mg daily for 10 days, oral or intravenous	Hospitalized patients requiring oxygen	Decreased mortality
IL-6 antagonists: Tocilizumab	400 mg or 8 mg/kg (maximum 800 mg) single dose Use with systemic glucocorticoids	Hospitalized patients requiring oxygen or noninvasive ventilatory support Not in patients treated with mechanical ventilation or ECMO More effective in patients with CRP ≥75 mg/L	Decreased mortality
JAK inhibitors: Baricitinib	4 mg daily for up to 14 days, orally. Use with systemic glucocorticoids	Hospitalized patients requiring oxygen	Faster time to symptom resolution Potential decrease mortality

Abbreviation: ECMO, extracorporeal membrane oxygenation.

infection,[25,33] and excessive IL-6 levels may lead to an imbalance in innate and adaptive immunity.[34] Therefore, IL-6 antagonism has a role in the management of severe critical COVID-19.

Multiple studies have examined the efficacy of using a fixed-single dose of tocilizumab 400 mg or weight-based dose at 8 mg/kg, or sarilumab at 400 mg intravenously in hospitalized patients with SARS-CoV-2 with variable results.[35–42] A potential explanation for the different findings may be administration of the drug at different stages of the disease process and severity of illness. The largest study was the RECOVERY trial, which compared tocilizumab with placebo in 4116 patients; most participants concurrently received dexamethasone.[38] Study drug was initiated at a median of 2 days from hospital admission. A substantial proportion of patients did not require ventilatory support (45%); 41% received noninvasive ventilation (NIV), and a small group required mechanical ventilation. There was a 15% reduction in 28-day mortality (OR, 0.58; 95% CI, 0.76–0.74). A subgroup analysis revealed that there was no benefit in those on ventilatory support, or in those not receiving concomitant corticosteroids. The REMAP-CAP group enrolled 865 patients, with mostly patients on high-flow nasal cannula (29%) or NIV (42%); 29% of patients were already on invasive mechanical ventilation.[37] Patients were randomized within 24 hours of initiation of respiratory support. The study was stopped early after an interim analysis showed significantly more days alive without need for organ support in patients treated with tocilizumab (OR, 1.64; 95% CI, 1.24–2.14) or sarilumab (OR, 1.76; 95% CI, 1.17–2.91) compared with placebo. Patients in the intervention arm were more likely to survive to hospital discharge (pooled OR, 1.64; 95% CI, 1.15–2.35).[37] Subgroup analysis showed that in patients on mechanical ventilation, treatment with an IL-6 antagonist did not improve outcomes (adjusted OR, 1.27; 95% CI, 0.84–1.94). Other smaller clinical studies showed mixed results, most likely because of the inclusion of patients with variable severity of disease,[36,39–41,43] and lack of concomitant steroid use. Three of these trials included moderate patients on low-flow nasal canula,[36,39,40] whereas others included patients who were already on mechanical ventilation in critical disease.[41,43,44] The heterogeneity of disease severity within the studies might have impacted the outcome of the analysis.

A meta-analysis by the WHO REACT group including 27 studies comparing IL-6 antagonists with usual care or placebo showed an overall all-cause mortality reduction of 14% (OR, 0.86; 95% CI, 0.79–0.95).[35] In a subgroup analysis, the benefit of IL-6 antagonism was only seen with concomitant use of corticosteroid use. In addition, the protection from IL-6 antagonism was more pronounced in patients with CRP $\geq$ 75. Indeed, a follow-up report of the CORIMUNO-TOCU-1 study showed that a CRP cutoff of 150 mg/L was associated with reduced 90-day mortality (OR, 0.18; 95% CI, 0.04–0.89).[45] Furthermore, patients with critical disease requiring mechanical ventilation or extracorporeal membrane oxygenation were least likely to benefit in contrast to patients treated with supplemental oxygen or NIV.[35]

In conclusion, early use of IL-6 antagonists is beneficial for hypoxemic patients with COVID-19 requiring oxygen (see **Table 2**). The use of IL-6 receptor inhibitor therapy in patients on mechanical ventilation is likely too late and unlikely to improve outcomes. IL-6 antagonists should be used in conjunction with corticosteroids. CRP levels may identify individuals with more potential to benefit.

Janus Kinase Inhibitors

The JAK-signal transducer and activator of transcription (JAK-STAT) signaling pathway mediates extracellular interleukins and interferons signal, through membrane receptor activation, and leads to T-cell proliferation and maturation.[46] Cytokine receptor binding phosphorylates JAK and allows docking for cytoplasmic STATs (see **Fig. 1**).[12] JAK phosphorylates STAT protein, allowing STAT to move into the nucleus. STAT regulates inflammatory and immune response, viral clearance, cell proliferation and survival, endothelial integrity, and coagulation pathways.[47] IL-6 receptor downstream activity is mediated by JAK-STAT pathway; specifically, IL-6 receptor activation of STAT3 is associated with lung fibrosis and injury, thrombosis, and delayed viral clearing by blocking IFN response of STAT-1. The rationale for baricitinib was based not only on its anti-inflammatory property to inhibit JAK but also on the ability to inhibit other kinases associated with viral endocytosis.[48] In addition, the JAK-STAT pathway mediates angiotensin II function in the cardiovascular system.[31] An observational study in patients with SARS-CoV-2 showed that baricitinib significantly reduced CRP and increased T-lymphocyte count with an increase of the $CD4^+$ to $CD8^+$ cell ratio.[49] Reduction in STAT3 activity improves NK cell-mediated surveillance against pathogens and blocks the release of inflammatory cytokines.

RCTs investigating JAK antagonists are limited. Two international studies used oral baricitinib at 4 mg per day for 14 days with dose adjustment for impaired renal function.[50,51] The first study using a JAK-inhibitor was the Adaptive COVID-19 Treatment Trial 2 study, which included 1033 patients of whom 68.3% had moderate disease (National Institute of Allergy and Infectious Disease Ordinal Scale [NIAID-OS] 4 [no oxygen] and 5 [low-flow supplemental oxygen] and 31.6% had severe symptoms [NIAID-OS 6 using NIV or high flow oxygen]).[51] Patients were randomized to a combination of remdesivir with baricitinib or remdesivir alone. In this study, patients receiving glucocorticoid treatment were excluded. Patients treated with the combination of remdesivir and baricitinib were more likely to recover to no or mild symptoms (NIAID-OS 1–3) 1 day faster (rate ratio [RR], 0.16; 95% CI, 0.10–1.32). There was no survival benefit with combination therapy of remdesivir and baricitinib. The exclusion of glucocorticoid treatment is an important limitation of this study.

The COV-BARRIER study, another trial examining the role of baricitinib, included participants treated with dexamethasone at a dose of 20 mg/d or less. Most patients (63.4%) had moderate disease (NIAID-OS 5), and 24.4% had NIAID-OS 6.[50] There was no difference in progression on the ordinal scale or death between the baricitinib and placebo arm. However, all-cause 28-day mortality was lower in the baricitinib group (hazard ratio, 0.57; 95% CI, 0.41–0.78). This protective effect persisted to 60 days. A subgroup analysis investigating the impact of different oxygen requirements at the time of randomization showed that patients who required NIV or high-flow oxygen had significantly lower 28-day mortality, regardless of concomitant steroid use.

The STOP-COVID group tested the efficacy of another JAK 1, 2, and 3 inhibitor, tofacitinib, in 289 hospitalized patients with mild to moderate disease.[52] Patients were randomized to receive oral tofacitinib 10 mg twice a day for 14 days versus placebo. At day 28, the composite outcome of death or respiratory failure (NIAID-OS 6 or more) was lower in the tofacitinib versus placebo arm (18.1% vs 29.0%; RR, 0.63; 95% CI, 0.41–0.97). A meta-analysis of observational studies and clinical trials using the JAK inhibitors, baricitinib or ruxolitinib, showed lower mortality in the treatment group (RR, 0.42; 95% CI, 0.30–0.56).[53]

In summary, JAK inhibition is effective in preventing SARS-CoV-2 progression and has the potential to decrease mortality in patients requiring low-flow oxygen but not in those with severe symptoms. JAK inhibitors should be used concomitantly with glucocorticoids (see **Table 2**).

Anakinra

IL-1β is transcribed by monocytes, macrophages, and dendritic cells following Toll-like receptor activation by pathogens.[54] IL-1 binding triggers protein complexes at the intracellular membrane with 2 further downstream pathways: activation pathway for cellular survival and inhibitory pathway for B-cell maturation.[55,56]

The use of anakinra in mild to moderate SARS-CoV-2 infection was not supported by a recent RCT.[57] One hundred sixteen patients were randomized to receive anakinra versus usual care. Only a small proportion of the patients received glucocorticoids (14%). There was no difference in terms of symptom progression at day 4 and day 14 in the primary outcomes and the overall survival.

ANTIVIRAL THERAPY FOR HOSPITALIZED SEVERE ACUTE RESPIRATORY SYNDROME CORONAVIRUS 2 *INFECTION*
Antiviral Drugs

In the early phase of the COVID-19 pandemic, multiple antiviral drugs were repurposed as potential to treat SARS-CoV-2 infection, including lopinavir-ritonavir and remdesivir.[58,59] The viral protease inhibitor combination, lopinavir-ritonavir, is not effective in SARS-CoV-2 infection.[58,60,61] Remdesivir is an inhibitor of viral RNA-dependent RNA polymerase. In a large RCT including 1062 patients, remdesivir decreased time to recovery by 5 days, and this overall effect was mostly driven by patients receiving oxygen.[59] In patients with severe to critical infection at time of enrollment, remdesivir did not shorten time to recovery. Ultimately, the meta-analysis by the WHO Solidarity group did not show a mortality benefit with the use of remdesivir regardless of subgroups by age or by severity of infection.[60] Furthermore, the WHO living guideline suggests against the use of remdesivir in hospitalized patients with SARS-CoV-2 infection.[62]

New antiviral drugs against SARS-CoV-2 are rapidly emerging as this review is being prepared. Molnupiravir, an oral prodrug of ribonucleoside analogue against RNA viruses, has good tolerability and potential in decrease viral load in early SARS-CoV-2 infection.[63,64] Further phase 3 studies are necessary to determine the efficacy.

Hyperimmune Immunoglobulin and Convalescent Plasma

In viral infection, intravenous immunoglobulin (IVIG) has been proposed to provide passive immunity to mediate antibody-dependent cellular cytotoxicity and acts as decoy receptor to prevent viral binding and entry.[65] However, no large RCT for efficacy has been published to date. In a meta-analysis of 7 observational studies, use of IVIG in critically patients with SARS-CoV-2 (n = 122) was associated with decreased mortality (RR, 0.57; 95% CI, 0.42–0.79).[66] However, no mortality reduction was seen in severe patients (n = 201; RR, 0.76; 95% CI, 0.51–1.14) or moderately ill (n = 92; RR, 1.39; 95% CI, 0.23–8.29) patients.[66] Trends in hospital or intensive care unit length of stay were inconsistent among the studies, as was the dosing of IVIG.[66]

Similar to the concept of using immunoglobulin binding, convalescent plasma from a previously SARS-CoV-2–infected individual was initially thought to potentially confer passive immunity in currently infected individuals. In a multicenter, double-blinded RCT of 334 patients with moderate SARS-CoV-2 symptoms, convalescent plasma infusion failed to improve clinical status at 30 days.[67] The RECOVERY study group tested the efficacy of convalescent plasma in 11,558 patients with most of them requiring oxygen in the hospital (87%).[68] There was no mortality or other clinical benefit in the treatment group. A large meta-analysis found no efficacy associated with the use of convalescent plasma and pointed out the high risk of bias in the included studies.[69]

Neutralizing Monoclonal Antibody

Two combinations of neutralizing antibodies: casirivimab with imdevimab (Regen-COV) and bamlanivimab with etesevimab, targeting SARS-CoV-2 surface spike protein decrease viral load compared with placebo in patients with mild to moderate symptoms.[70,71] Used in the ambulatory settings, these monoclonal antibody cocktails prevent hospitalization.[71,72] However, hospitalized patients treated with anti–SARS-CoV-2 antibodies did not have different symptom progression compared with standard of care.[73] The RECOVERY study examined the use of casirivimab with imdevimab in hospitalized patients only and found mortality benefit in a subgroup of patients who were seronegative of SARS-CoV-2 at time of randomization.[74]

Plasma Exchange and Absorption

Limited data are available for the use of plasma exchange in patients with severe to critical SARS-CoV-2 infection. An open-label study randomized patients to therapeutic plasma exchange and usual care. There was no significant mortality benefit despite sustained decrease in IL-6 levels.[75] Currently, there is no clinical evidence to support the use of these methods.[76–78]

SUMMARY

SARS-CoV-2 infection leads to dysregulation of immune pathways. Therapies focusing on suppressing cytokine activity demonstrate some success. Current evidence supports the use of dexamethasone in hospitalized patients requiring oxygen.

Early use of IL-6 inhibitors is also beneficial in hypoxemic patients. CRP level can serve to identify patients who may benefit from IL-6 inhibitors. JAK inhibition in combination with glucocorticoids is emerging as a potential therapeutic option for patients with moderate to severe symptoms. Direct antiviral therapy is not effective in hospitalized patients with severe symptoms. Data on anakinra, hyperimmune immunoglobulin/convalescent plasma, or plasma purification are limited and inconclusive.

CLINICS CARE POINTS

- Severe and critical syndrome from Severe acute respiratory syndrome coronavirus 2 (SARS-CoV-2) is mainly driven by dysregulation of host inflammatory response.
- Anti-inflammatory therapy using dexamethasone 6 mg daily for 10 days for SARS-CoV-2 infected patients requiring supplemental oxygen decreases mortality in this population.
- Biologics such as interleukin-6 antagonists in early severe syndrome and Janus kinase inhibition in low flow oxygen-requiring patients are also effective in improving the outcomes of this population.

DISCLOSURE

J.-T. Chen Served on Gilead Medical Affairs Sentinel Panel 2020 to 2021. M. Ostermann received research funding from BioMerieux.

REFERENCES

1. Angus DC, van der Poll T. Severe sepsis and septic shock. N Engl J Med 2013; 369(9):840–51.
2. Bosmann M, Ward PA. The inflammatory response in sepsis. Trends Immunol 2013;34(3):129–36.
3. Fajgenbaum DC, June CH. Cytokine storm. N Engl J Med 2020;383(23):2255–73.
4. Huang C, Wang Y, Li X, et al. Clinical features of patients infected with 2019 novel coronavirus in Wuhan, China. Lancet 2020;395(10223):497–506.
5. Zafer MM, El-Mahallawy HA, Ashour HM. Severe COVID-19 and sepsis: immune pathogenesis and laboratory markers. Microorganisms 2021;9(1). https://doi.org/10.3390/microorganisms9010159.
6. Wilson JG, Simpson LJ, Ferreira AM, et al. Cytokine profile in plasma of severe COVID-19 does not differ from ARDS and sepsis. JCI Insight 2020;(17):5. https://doi.org/10.1172/jci.insight.140289.
7. Hue S, Beldi-Ferchiou A, Bendib I, et al. Uncontrolled innate and impaired adaptive immune responses in patients with COVID-19 acute respiratory distress syndrome. Am J Respir Crit Care Med 2020;202(11):1509–19.
8. Petrey AC, Qeadan F, Middleton EA, Pinchuk IV, Campbell RA, Beswick EJ. Cytokine release syndrome in COVID-19: innate immune, vascular, and platelet pathogenic factors differ in severity of disease and sex. J Leukoc Biol 2021;109(1): 55–66.
9. Tsang HF, Chan LWC, Cho WCS, et al. An update on COVID-19 pandemic: the epidemiology, pathogenesis, prevention and treatment strategies. Expert Rev Anti Infect Ther 2021;19(7):877–88.
10. Mason RJ. Pathogenesis of COVID-19 from a cell biology perspective. Eur Respir J 2020;55(4). https://doi.org/10.1183/13993003.00607-2020.

11. Li G, Fan Y, Lai Y, et al. Coronavirus infections and immune responses. J Med Virol 2020;92(4):424–32.
12. Ni Y, Alu A, Lei H, Wang Y, Wu M, Wei X. Immunological perspectives on the pathogenesis, diagnosis, prevention and treatment of COVID-19. Mol Biomed 2021; 2(1). https://doi.org/10.1186/s43556-020-00015-y.
13. Liberman AC, Budzinski ML, Sokn C, Gobbini RP, Steininger A, Arzt E. Regulatory and mechanistic actions of glucocorticoids on T and inflammatory cells. Front Endocrinol (Lausanne) 2018;9:235. https://doi.org/10.3389/fendo.2018.00235.
14. Group RC, Horby P, Lim WS, et al. Dexamethasone in hospitalized patients with Covid-19. N Engl J Med 2021;384(8):693–704.
15. Angus DC, Derde L, Al-Beidh F, et al. Effect of hydrocortisone on mortality and organ support in patients with severe COVID-19: the REMAP-CAP COVID-19 corticosteroid domain randomized clinical trial. JAMA 2020;324(13):1317–29.
16. Jeronimo CMP, Val FFA, Sampaio VS, for the Metcovid Team. Methylprednisolone as adjunctive therapy for patients hospitalized with coronavirus disease 2019 (COVID-19; Metcovid): a randomized, double-blind, phase IIb, placebo-controlled trial. Clin Infect Dis 2021;72(9):e373–81.
17. Group WHOREAfC TW, Sterne JAC, Murthy S, et al. Association between administration of systemic corticosteroids and mortality among critically ill patients with COVID-19: a meta-analysis. JAMA 2020;324(13):1330–41.
18. Arabi YM, Mandourah Y, Al-Hameed F, et al. Corticosteroid therapy for critically ill patients with Middle East respiratory syndrome. Am J Respir Crit Care Med 2018; 197(6):757–67.
19. Lee N, Allen Chan KC, Hui DS, et al. Effects of early corticosteroid treatment on plasma SARS-associated coronavirus RNA concentrations in adult patients. J Clin Virol 2004;31(4):304–9.
20. Cao Y, Wei J, Zou L, et al. Ruxolitinib in treatment of severe coronavirus disease 2019 (COVID-19): a multicenter, single-blind, randomized controlled trial. J Allergy Clin Immunol 2020;146(1):137–146 e3.
21. Sahu AK, Mathew R, Bhat R, et al. Steroids use in non-oxygen requiring COVID-19 patients: a systematic review and meta-analysis. QJM 2021. https://doi.org/10. 1093/qjmed/hcab212.
22. Myall KJ, Mukherjee B, Castanheira AM, et al. Persistent post-COVID-19 interstitial lung disease. An observational study of corticosteroid treatment. Ann Am Thorac Soc 2021;18(5):799–806.
23. Bieksiene K, Zaveckiene J, Malakauskas K, Vaguliene N, Zemaitis M, Miliauskas S. Post COVID-19 organizing pneumonia: the right time to interfere. Medicina (Kaunas) 2021;57(3). https://doi.org/10.3390/medicina57030283.
24. Liu Y, Shepherd EG, Nelin LD. MAPK phosphatases–regulating the immune response. Nat Rev Immunol 2007;7(3):202–12.
25. Zhou Y, Fu X, Liu X, et al. Use of corticosteroids in influenza-associated acute respiratory distress syndrome and severe pneumonia: a systemic review and meta-analysis. Scientific Rep 2020;10(1):3044.
26. Villar J, Confalonieri M, Pastores SM, et al. Rationale for prolonged corticosteroid treatment in the acute respiratory distress syndrome caused by coronavirus disease 2019. Crit Care Explor 2020;2(4):e0111. https://doi.org/10.1097/CCE. 0000000000000111.
27. Villar J, Ferrando C, Martínez D, et al. Dexamethasone treatment for the acute respiratory distress syndrome: a multicentre, randomised controlled trial. Lancet Respir Med 2020;8(3):267–76.

28. Tomazini BM, Maia IS, Cavalcanti AB, et al. Effect of dexamethasone on days alive and ventilator-free in patients with moderate or severe acute respiratory distress syndrome and COVID-19: the CoDEX randomized clinical trial. JAMA 2020;324(13):1307–16.

29. Dequin PF, Heming N, Meziani F, et al. Effect of hydrocortisone on 21-day mortality or respiratory support among critically ill patients with COVID-19: a randomized clinical trial. JAMA 2020;324(13):1298–306.

30. Group CST, Munch MW, Myatra SN, et al. Effect of 12 mg vs 6 mg of dexamethasone on the number of days alive without life support in adults with COVID-19 and severe hypoxemia: the COVID STEROID 2 randomized trial. JAMA 2021; 326(18):1807–17.

31. Yarmohammadi A, Yarmohammadi M, Fakhri S, Khan H. Targeting pivotal inflammatory pathways in COVID-19: a mechanistic review. Eur J Pharmacol 2021;890: 173620.

32. Mihara M, Hashizume M, Yoshida H, Suzuki M, Shiina M. IL-6/IL-6 receptor system and its role in physiological and pathological conditions. Clin Sci (Lond) 2012;122(4):143–59.

33. Wang J, Jiang M, Chen X, Montaner LJ. Cytokine storm and leukocyte changes in mild versus severe SARS-CoV-2 infection: review of 3939 COVID-19 patients in China and emerging pathogenesis and therapy concepts. J Leukoc Biol 2020; 108(1):17–41.

34. Carsetti R, Zaffina S, Piano Mortari E, et al. Different innate and adaptive immune responses to SARS-CoV-2 infection of asymptomatic, mild, and severe cases. Front Immunol 2020;11:610300.

35. Group WHOREAfC-TW, Shankar-Hari M, Vale CL, et al. Association between administration of IL-6 antagonists and mortality among patients hospitalized for COVID-19: a meta-analysis. JAMA 2021;326(6):499–518.

36. Hermine O, Mariette X, Tharaux PL, et al. Effect of tocilizumab vs usual care in adults hospitalized with COVID-19 and moderate or severe pneumonia: a randomized clinical trial. JAMA Intern Med 2021;181(1):32–40.

37. Investigators R-C, Gordon AC, Mouncey PR, et al. Interleukin-6 receptor antagonists in critically ill patients with covid-19. N Engl J Med 2021;384(16):1491–502.

38. Group RC. Tocilizumab in patients admitted to hospital with Covid-19 recovery: a randomised, controlled, open-label, platform trial. Lancet 2021;397:1637–45.

39. Salama C, Han J, Yau L, et al. Tocilizumab in patients hospitalized with Covid-19 pneumonia. N Engl J Med 2021;384(1):20–30.

40. Stone JH, Frigault MJ, Serling-Boyd NJ, et al. Efficacy of tocilizumab in patients hospitalized with Covid-19. N Engl J Med 2020;383(24):2333–44.

41. Rosas IO, Brau N, Waters M, et al. Tocilizumab in hospitalized patients with severe Covid-19 pneumonia. N Engl J Med 2021;384(16):1503–16.

42. Paccaly AJ, Kovalenko P, Parrino J, et al. Pharmacokinetics and pharmacodynamics of subcutaneous sarilumab and intravenous tocilizumab following single-dose administration in patients with active rheumatoid arthritis on stable methotrexate. J Clin Pharmacol 2021;61(1):90–104.

43. Salvarani C, Dolci G, Massari M, et al. Effect of tocilizumab vs standard care on clinical worsening in patients hospitalized with COVID-19 pneumonia: a randomized clinical trial. JAMA Intern Med 2021;181(1):24–31.

44. Veiga VC, Prats J, Farias DLC, et al. Effect of tocilizumab on clinical outcomes at 15 days in patients with severe or critical coronavirus disease 2019: randomised controlled trial. BMJ 2021;372:n84. https://doi.org/10.1136/bmj.n84.

45. Xavier Mariette M, Olivier Hermine M, Pierre-Louis Tharaux M, et al. Effectiveness of tocilizumab in patients hospitalized with COVID-19: a follow-up of the CORIMUNO-TOCI-1 randomized clinical trial. JAMA Intern Med 2021;181(9): 1241–2.

46. Seif F, Khoshmirsafa M, Aazami H, Mohsenzadegan M, Sedighi G, Bahar M. The role of JAK-STAT signaling pathway and its regulators in the fate of T helper cells. Cell Commun Signal 2017;15(1):23.

47. Jafarzadeh A, Nemati M, Jafarzadeh S. Contribution of STAT3 to the pathogenesis of COVID-19. Microb Pathog 2021;154:104836. https://doi.org/10.1016/j.micpath.2021.104836.

48. Richardson P, Griffin I, Tucker C, et al. Baricitinib as potential treatment for 2019-nCoV acute respiratory disease. Lancet 2020;395(10223):e30–1.

49. Bronte V, Ugel S, Tinazzi E, et al. Baricitinib restrains the immune dysregulation in patients with severe COVID-19. J Clin Invest 2020;130(12):6409–16.

50. Marconi VC, Ramanan AV, de Bono S, et al. Efficacy and safety of baricitinib for the treatment of hospitalised adults with COVID-19 (COV-BARRIER): a randomised, double-blind, parallel-group, placebo-controlled phase 3 trial. Lancet Respir Med 2021. https://doi.org/10.1016/s2213-2600(21)00331-3.

51. Kalil AC, Patterson TF, Mehta AK, et al. Baricitinib plus remdesivir for hospitalized adults with Covid-19. N Engl J Med 2021;384(9):795–807.

52. Guimaraes PO, Quirk D, Furtado RH, et al. Tofacitinib in patients hospitalized with Covid-19 pneumonia. N Engl J Med 2021;385(5):406–15.

53. Chen CX, Wang JJ, Li H, Yuan LT, Gale RP, Liang Y. JAK-inhibitors for coronavirus disease-2019 (COVID-19): a meta-analysis. Leukemia 2021;35(9):2616–20.

54. Dayer JM, Oliviero F, Punzi L. A brief history of IL-1 and IL-1 Ra in rheumatology. Front Pharmacol 2017;8:293. https://doi.org/10.3389/fphar.2017.00293.

55. Acuner Ozbabacan SE, Gursoy A, Nussinov R, Keskin O. The structural pathway of interleukin 1 (IL-1) initiated signaling reveals mechanisms of oncogenic mutations and SNPs in inflammation and cancer. Plos Comput Biol 2014;10(2): e1003470. https://doi.org/10.1371/journal.pcbi.1003470.

56. Chang L, Karin M. Mammalian MAP kinase signalling cascades. Nature 2001; 410(6824):37–40.

57. Tharaux P-L, Pialoux G, Pavot A, et al. Effect of anakinra versus usual care in adults in hospital with COVID-19 and mild-to-moderate pneumonia (CORIMUNO-ANA-1): a randomised controlled trial. Lancet Respir Med 2021;9(3): 295–304.

58. Horby PW, Mafham M, Bell JL, et al. Lopinavir–ritonavir in patients admitted to hospital with COVID-19 (RECOVERY): a randomised, controlled, open-label, platform trial. Lancet 2020;396(10259):1345–52.

59. Beigel JH, Tomashek KM, Dodd LE, et al. Remdesivir for the treatment of Covid-19 - final report. N Engl J Med 2020;383(19):1813–26.

60. Consortium WHOST, Pan H, Peto R, et al. Repurposed antiviral drugs for Covid-19 - interim WHO solidarity trial results. N Engl J Med 2021;384(6):497–511.

61. Cao B, Wang Y, Wen D, et al. A trial of lopinavir-ritonavir in adults hospitalized with severe Covid-19. N Engl J Med 2020;382(19):1787–99.

62. Rochwerg B, Agarwal A, Siemieniuk RA, et al. A living WHO guideline on drugs for Covid-19. Bmj 2020;370:m3379. https://doi.org/10.1136/bmj.m3379.

63. Painter WP, Holman W, Bush JA, et al. Human safety, tolerability, and pharmacokinetics of molnupiravir, a novel broad-spectrum oral antiviral agent with activity against SARS-CoV-2. Antimicrob Agents Chemother 2021. https://doi.org/10.1128/AAC.02428-20.

64. Fischer W, Eron JJ, Holman W, et al. Molnupiravir, an oral antiviral treatment for COVID-19. medRxiv 2021. https://doi.org/10.1101/2021.06.17.21258639.
65. Moradimajd P, Samaee H, Sedigh-Maroufi S, Kourosh-Aami M, Mohsenzadagan M. Administration of intravenous immunoglobulin in the treatment of COVID-19: a review of available evidence. J Med Virol 2021;93(5): 2675–82.
66. Xiang HR, Cheng X, Li Y, Luo WW, Zhang QZ, Peng WX. Efficacy of IVIG (intravenous immunoglobulin) for corona virus disease 2019 (COVID-19): a meta-analysis. Int Immunopharmacol 2021;96:107732. https://doi.org/10.1016/j.intimp.2021.107732.
67. Simonovich VA, Burgos Pratx LD, Scibona P, et al. A randomized trial of convalescent plasma in Covid-19 severe pneumonia. N Engl J Med 2021;384(7): 619–29.
68. Abani O, Abbas A, Abbas F, et al. Convalescent plasma in patients admitted to hospital with COVID-19 (RECOVERY): a randomised controlled, open-label, platform trial. Lancet 2021;397(10289):2049–59.
69. Piechotta V, Chai KL, Valk SJ, et al. Convalescent plasma or hyperimmune immunoglobulin for people with COVID-19: a living systematic review. Cochrane Database Syst Rev 2020;7:CD013600. https://doi.org/10.1002/14651858.CD013600.pub2.
70. Dougan M, Nirula A, Azizad M, et al. Bamlanivimab plus etesevimab in mild or moderate Covid-19. N Engl J Med 2021. https://doi.org/10.1056/NEJMoa2102685.
71. Weinreich DM, Sivapalasingam S, Norton T, et al. REGN-COV2, a neutralizing antibody cocktail, in outpatients with Covid-19. N Engl J Med 2021;384(3): 238–51.
72. Gottlieb RL, Nirula A, Chen P, et al. Effect of bamlanivimab as monotherapy or in combination with etesevimab on viral load in patients with mild to moderate COVID-19: a randomized clinical trial. JAMA 2021;325(7):632–44.
73. Group A-TL-CS, Lundgren JD, Grund B, et al. A neutralizing monoclonal antibody for hospitalized patients with Covid-19. N Engl J Med 2021;384(10):905–14.
74. Abani O, Abbas A, Abbas F, et al. Casirivimab and imdevimab in patients admitted to hospital with COVID-19 (RECOVERY): a randomised, controlled, open-label, platform trial. The Lancet 2022;399(10325):665–76.
75. Faqihi F, Alharthy A, Abdulaziz S, et al. Therapeutic plasma exchange in patients with life-threatening COVID-19: a randomised controlled clinical trial. Int J Antimicrob Agents 2021;57(5):106334.
76. Clark EG, Hiremath S, McIntyre L, Wald R, Hundemer GL, Joannidis M. Haemoperfusion should only be used for COVID-19 in the context of randomized trials. Nat Rev Nephrol 2020;16(12):697–9.
77. Ronco C, Bagshaw SM, Bellomo R, et al. Extracorporeal blood purification and organ support in the critically ill patient during COVID-19 pandemic: expert review and recommendation. Blood Purif 2021;50(1):17–27.
78. Rizvi S, Danic M, Silver M, LaBond V. Cytosorb filter: an adjunct for survival in the COVID-19 patient in cytokine storm? a case report. Heart Lung 2021;50(1):44–50.

High-Flow Nasal Oxygen and Noninvasive Ventilation for COVID-19

Hasan M. Al-Dorzi, MD[a], John Kress, MD[b],
Yaseen M. Arabi, MD, FCCP, FCCM[a,*]

KEYWORDS

- COVID-19 • Noninvasive ventilation • HFNO
- Acute hypoxemic respiratory failure (AHRF)

KEY POINTS

- Invasive mechanical ventilation has been associated with high mortality in patients with acute hypoxemic respiratory failure due to COVID-19.
- Hence, High flow nasal oxygen and noninvaive ventilation were increasing used as first-line respiratory support in most affceted patients.
- Based on observational studies, the use of high flow nasal oxygen and noninvasive ventilation have been associated with a reduction in the need for invasive mechanical ventilation and possibly mortality.
- Results from ongoing randomized controlled trials are awaited.

INTRODUCTION

The novel severe acute respiratory syndrome coronavirus 2 (SARS-CoV-2) has led to more than 347 million cases of coronavirus disease 2019 (COVID-19) and approximately 5.7 million fatalities by January 22, 2022.[1] COVID-19 is a systemic disease, with a wide spectrum of disease severity ranging from asymptomatic to life-threatening. The main reason for hospitalization and admission to an intensive care unit (ICU) is the development of acute hypoxemic respiratory failure (AHRF),[2] which is frequently severe.[3,4] The International Severe Acute Respiratory and Emerging Infection Consortium (ISARIC) database suggests that 15% of hospitalized patients with COVID-19 are admitted to an ICU or a high dependency unit at some point during their illness.[5]

[a] College of Medicine, King Saud bin Abdulaziz University for Health Sciences, King Abdullah International Medical Research Center and Intensive Care Department, King Abdulaziz Medical City, Ministry of National Guard Health Affairs, ICU2, Mail Code 1425, PO Box 22490, Riyadh 11426, Saudi Arabia; [b] Section of Pulmonary and Critical Care, Medical ICU, University of Chicago, 5841 South Maryland Avenue, MC 6026, Chicago, IL 60637, USA
* Corresponding author.
E-mail address: arabi@ngha.med.sa

Crit Care Clin 38 (2022) 601–621
https://doi.org/10.1016/j.ccc.2022.01.006
0749-0704/22/© 2022 Elsevier Inc. All rights reserved.

criticalcare.theclinics.com

Abbreviations	
COVID-19	Coronasvirus Disease 2019
AHRF	acute hypoxemic respiratory failure
SARS-CoV-2	acute respiratory syndrome coronavirus 2
HFNO	high-flow nasal oxygen
NIV	noninvasive ventilation
ARDS	acute respiratory distress syndrome
CPAP	continuous positive airway pressure
ICU	intensive care unit
RCT	randomized controlled trial
HR	hazard ratio
CI	confidence interval
ISARIC	International Severe Acute Respiratory and Emerging Infection Consortium
HCW	health care worker

Respiratory support options for patients with AHRF in COVID-19 pneumonia include conventional oxygen therapy, high-flow nasal oxygen (HFNO), and noninvasive positive pressure ventilation (NIV) in addition to invasive mechanical ventilation.[6–8] The ISARIC database showed that HFNO was used in 20.3%, NIV was used in 9.8%, and invasive mechanical ventilation was used in 9.3% of hospitalized patients.[5] Early in the pandemic, invasive mechanical ventilation was the preferred modality for treating severe cases, partly because of the concerns over aerosolization associated with other forms of oxygen therapy, especially with reports of intrahospital transmission among health care workers (HCWs).[9] Early clinical practice guidelines on the use of NIV and HFNO in COVID-19 were cautious. For example, the World Health Organization interim guidelines published in May 2020 stated that a trial of HFNO and NIV may be used in selected patients with COVID-19 and mild acute respiratory distress syndrome (ARDS).[10] As high mortality was observed in intubated patients (**Table 1**), NIV and HFNO were increasingly used,[11] which paved the way for conducting clinical studies.

In this review, the authors focus on the published evidence of the safety and effectiveness of HFNO and NIV for the management of patients with AHRF owing to COVID-19.

MECHANISMS OF ACTION OF HIGH-FLOW NASAL OXYGEN AND NONINVASIVE VENTILATION IN ACUTE HYPOXEMIC RESPIRATORY FAILURE

HFNO achieves its main beneficial effects through the provision of high flow of gases. It uses humidification and heat to allow the delivery of up to 100% oxygen at high-flow rates (usually 40–60 L/min) that can be tolerated by patients for extended time periods. The main mechanisms of action are the following: (1) washout of nasopharyngeal dead space, thus reducing the overall dead space, improving the elimination of carbon dioxide and enhancing oxygenation; (2) attenuation of the inspiratory resistance of the nasopharynx, and thus reducing the related work of breathing; (3) improving conductance and pulmonary compliance by the adequately warmed and humidified gas compared with dry, cooler gas; (4) reducing the metabolic work associated with gas conditioning; and (5) the application of positive distending pressure for lung recruitment.[12] HFNO generates a very low positive end-expiratory pressure (PEEP) effect (3 cm H_2O on average), although it is higher with increasing flow.[13] The utilization of delivered oxygen is higher with HFNO compared with NIV at the same set fraction of inspired oxygen (Fio_2), hence increasing the risk of depletion of hospital oxygen supply.

Table 1
Studies that reported the use of high-flow nasal oxygen and/or noninvasive positive pressure ventilation for patients with COVID-19

Study	Study Type	Patients/Setting/Country	Respiratory Support	Outcomes
Chen et al,[61] 2020	Retrospective observational (single-center)	145 patients with COVID-19 (43 severely ill) (China)	HFNO: 6 patients IMV: 1 patient	Not reported
Lagi et al,[62] 2020	Retrospective observational (single-center)	84 patients with COVID-19 admitted to the Infectious and Tropical Disease Unit in February–March 2020; nurse and physician coverage intensified with time (Italy)	HFNO: 9 patients IMV: 1 patient	1/9 (11.1%) patients treated with HFNO required ICU admission and intubation[a]
Calligaro et al,[63] 2020	Prospective observational (multicenter)	293 consecutive patients with COVID-19 and AHRF in April–June 2020 (South Africa)	HFNO: 293 patients	HFNO success: 134/293 (47%) HFNO failure: 156/293 (53%) with 111 received IMV and 45 died without intubation 84/111 (75.7%) who received IMV died[a]
Zhou et al,[64] 2020	Retrospective observational (multicenter)	191 patients with COVID-19 admitted to 2 hospitals in December 2019–January 2020; 50 were admitted to ICU (Wuhan, China)	HFNO: 41 patients NIV: 26 patients IMV: 32 patients	33/41 (80.5%) patients treated with HFNO died 24/26 (92.3%) patients treated with NIV died 31/32 (96.9%) patients treated with IMV died
Yang et al,[65] 2020	Retrospective observational (single-center)	52 critically ill patients with COVID-19 December 2019–January 2020 (Wuhan, China)	HFNO: 33 patients NIV: 29 patients IMV: 22 patients	16/33 (48.5%) patients treated with HFNO died 23/29 (79.3%) patients treated with NIV died 19/22 (86.4%) patients treated with IMV died

(continued on next page)

Table 1
(continued)

Study	Study Type	Patients/Setting/Country	Respiratory Support	Outcomes
Grasselli et al,[2] 2020	Retrospective observational (multicenter)	1591 patients admitted to the ICU in February–March 2020 (Italy)	NIV: 137 (11%) patients IMV: 1150 (88%) patients	No outcome reported for patients who were treated with NIV or IMV[a]
Avdeev et al,[66] 2021	Retrospective observational (multicenter)	61 patients receiving NIV for AHRF in wards in April–June 2020 (Russia)	NIV: 61 patients	44/61 (72.1%) patients had NIV success 17/61 (27.9%) patients treated with NIV required intubation Mortality was 24.6%
Forrest et al,[45] 2021	Retrospective observational (multicenter)	688 adult patients with confirmed COVID-19 and hypoxia in March–April 2020 (New York City, USA)	NIV: 534 patients IMV: 154 patients	171/534 (32.0%) patients treated with NIV died 128/154 (83.1%) patients treated with IMV died Across all subgroups and propensity-matched analysis, IMV was associated with a greater risk of death than NIV
Bellani et al,[67] 2021	Prospective, single-day observational study (multicenter)	8753 patients with COVID-19 present in the participating hospitals on the study day in March 2020 (Italy)	909 (10%) patients received NIV outside the ICU (85%) with CPAP; delivered by helmet in 617 (68%) patients	300/909 (37.6%) patients had NIV failure 498/909 (62.4%) patients were discharged alive without intubation C-reactive protein, PF ratio, and platelet counts were independently associated with increased risk of NIV failure

Study	Design	Population	Groups	Results
Franco et al,[36] 2020	Retrospective observational (multicenter)	670 consecutive patients with confirmed COVID-19 in pulmonology units in 9 hospitals in March–May 2020 (Italy)	HFNO: 163 patients; CPAP/NIV: 507 patients	Intubation: 47 (28.8%) patients on HFNO, 82 (24.8%) patients on CPAP, and 49 (27.7%) patients on NIV; Mortality: 16%, 30%, and 30% for HFNO, CPAP and NIV, respectively
Karagiannidis et al,[11] 2021	Retrospective observational (multicenter)	Nationwide cohort of 7490 patients with COVID-19 hospitalized in 2 periods (February–May and October–November 2020) with hospital setting not specified (Germany)	NIV only: 1614 (21.5%) patients; NIV followed by intubation: 1247 (16.6%) patients; IMV: 3851 (51.4%) patients	1247/2861 (43.6%) patients had NIV failure; 624/1614 (38.7%) patients treated with NIV only died; 818/1247 (65.6%) patients with NIV failure died; 2003/3851 (52.0%) patients treated with IMV died
Faraone et al,[37] 2021	Retrospective observational (single-center)	50 consecutive patients with COVID-19 admitted to the general wards in March–May 2020 (Italy)	NIV: 50 patients	25 (50%) patients had do-not-intubate order; 22 patients were weaned from NIV and did not require intubation (6/25 patients with treatment limitation and 16/25 without treatment limitation); 9 (36%) patients had NIV failure and needed IMV
Menga et al,[68] 2021	Prospective observational (single-center)	85 consecutive patients with COVID-19 admitted to the ICU in March–April 20 (Italy)	Helmet NIV: 42 patients; Face-mask NIV: 19 patients; HFNO: 24 patients	Helmet NIV failure: 27/42 (64.3%); Face-mask NIV failure: 10/19 (52.6%); HFNO failure: 15/24 (62.5%); 21/52 (40.4%) of patient with NIV/HFNO failure died; Higher illness severity predicted NIV/HFNO failure

(continued on next page)

Table 1
(continued)

Study	Study Type	Patients/Setting/Country	Respiratory Support	Outcomes
Burns et al,[69] 2020	Retrospective observational (single-center)	28 patients with COVID-19 admitted to the ward in March–April 2020 (United Kingdom)	NIV: 28 patients	14/28 (50%) patients treated with NIV died
Xie et al,[70] 2020	Retrospective observational (multicenter)	733 patients with COVID-19 admitted to the ICU in January-February 2020 (China)	HFNO: 320 patients NIV: 164 patients IMV: 100	144/320 (%) patients treated with HFNO died 107/164 (%) patients treated with NIV died 75/100 (75%) patients treated with IMV died
Garcia et al,[71] 2020	Prospective observational (multicenter)	639 patients with COVID-19 admitted to the ICU after April 2020 (Europe)	HFNO: 25 patients NIV: 27 patients IMV: 317 patients	4/25 (16.0%) patients treated with HFNO died in the ICU[a] 9/27 (33.3%) patients treated with NIV died in the ICU[a] 58/317 (18.3%) patients treated with IMV died in the ICU[a]
Elhadi et al,[72] 2021	Prospective observational (multicenter)	465 consecutive COVID-19 critically ill patients May-December 2020 (Libya)	HFNO:20 patients NIV/CPAP: 20 patients	15/20 (75%) patients treated with HFNO died 18/20 (90%) patients treated with NIV died
Rahim et al,[73] 2020	Cross-sectional (single)	204 patients admitted to the ICU April–August 2020 (Pakistan)	NIV: 126 patients IMV: 78 patients	84/126 (66.7%) patients treated with NIV died 73/78 (93.6%) patients treated with IMV died
Carpagnano et al,[74] 2021	Retrospective (single-center)	78 consecutive patients with COVID-19 and moderate to severe ARDS hospitalized in an intermediate respiratory ICU, in March–April 2020 (Italy)	HFNO: 7 patients NIV: 61 patients	2/7 (28.6%) patients treated with HFNO died 25/61 (41.0%) patients treated with NIV died

Study	Design	Population	Groups	Outcomes
Rodríguez et al,[75] 2021	Prospective observational (multicenter)	1362 critically ill patients with confirmed COVID-19 disease and acute respiratory failure in February–May 2020 (Spain)	HFNO: 375 patients NIV: 140 patients IMV: 1172 patients	80/375 (21.3%) patients treated with HFNO died in ICU 42/140 (30.0%) patients treated with NIV died in ICU 458/1172 (39.1%) patients treated with IMV died in ICU
Roomi et al,[76] 2021	Retrospective observational (multicenter)	1204 patients with COVID-19 admitted to the ICU in March–August 2020 (Philadelphia area, USA)	HFNO: 573 patients NIV: 399 patients IMV: 713 patients	203/573 (35.4%) patients treated with HFNO died 187/399 (46.9%) patients treated with NIV died 373/713 (52.3%) patients treated with IMV died
Grosgurin et al,[77] 2021	Retrospective observational (single-center)	157 patients with COVID-19 admitted to the intermediate care unit in March–April 2020 (Switzerland)	HFNO alternating with NIV was provided to 85 patients with worsening respiratory failure	33/85 (39%) required ICU admission and IMV 52 (61%) were discharged to the ward without ICU admission
Grieco et al,[47] 2021	Randomized controlled trial (multicenter)	109 patients with COVID-19 and moderate-severe AHRF (PF ratio < 200) admitted to 4 ICUs (Italy)	Helmet-NIV group: helmet applied continuously for the first 48 h (PEEP: 10–12 cmH_2O; pressure support: 10–12 cmH_2O) followed by HFNO: 54 HFNO group at 60 L/min: 55	No difference in the duration of respiratory support at 28 d (primary outcome): mean difference 2 d, 95% CI, −2 to 6, $P = .26$) Intubation rate: 16/54 (30%) vs 28/55 (51%); $P = .03$ in favor of the Helmet NIV group Ventilator-free days within 28 d (median of 28 vs 25 d; mean difference; $P = .04$) 13/54 (24%) patients in the helmet-NIV group and 14/55 (25%) patients in HFNO group died in the hospital ($P = 1.0$)

(continued on next page)

Table 1
(*continued*)

Study	Study Type	Patients/Setting/Country	Respiratory Support	Outcomes
Perkins et al,[48] 2021	Randomized controlled trial (multicenter)	1272 hospitalized patients with acute respiratory failure due to COVID-19 (United Kingdom)	CPAP: 380 patients HFNO: 417 patients Conventional oxygen therapy: 475 patients	The primary outcome (composite of tracheal intubation or mortality within 30 d) was lower in the CPAP group (36.3%) compared with conventional oxygen therapy (44.4%; $P = .03$), but similar in the HFNO and conventional oxygen therapy groups ($P = .85$). The difference in between CPAP and HFNO was due to tracheal intubation Safety events were most common in the CPAP group (CPAP 34.2%; HFNO 20.6%; conventional oxygen therapy 13.9%, $P<.001$)

Abbreviation: IMV, invasive mechanical ventilation.
[a] Outcome data incomplete at the time of publication.

NIV is primarily a pressure-targeted modality delivered as continuous (CPAP) or biphasic positive airway pressure (mainly as pressure support ventilation). It improves arterial oxygenation by increasing functional residual capacity, shifting the tidal volume to a more compliant part of the pressure-volume curve, thus reducing both the work of breathing and the tidal opening and closure of the airways.[14] The face-mask and helmet interfaces are commonly used to deliver NIV. The helmet has the advantage of less air leaks and better tolerability in many patients, thus facilitating prolonged NIV treatments at higher PEEP.[15]

The main settings, strengths, and risks of HFNO, face-mask NIV, and helmet NIV are presented in **Fig. 1**.

SAFETY OF NONINVASIVE VENTILATION AND HIGH-FLOW NASAL OXYGEN IN PATIENTS WITH COVID-19

Both NIV and HFNO can avoid the complications associated with invasive mechanical ventilation, most importantly, ventilator-induced lung injury, cardiovascular decompensation, and infectious complications.[16,17] However, the concerns associated with NIV and HFNO use in patients with COVID-19 include patient self-inflicted lung

	High-flow nasal oxygen	Mask NIV/CPAP	Helmet NIV/CPAP
Picture			
Main settings	FiO$_2$: 0.21-1.0 start high and titrate to achieve SpO2 92-96% (usual target for most patients) Flow: 40-60 L/min Temperature: 31-37° C	FiO$_2$: 0.21-1.0; start high and titrate to achieve SpO2 92-96% (usual target for most patients) PSV/ PEEP: 8-10/5-8 cmH2O or CPAP 8-10 cmH2O	FiO$_2$: 0.21-1.0; start high and titrate to achieve SpO2 92-96% (usual target for most patients) PSV/PEEP 10-12/ 10-12 cmH2O or CPAP10-12 cmH2O Flow:≥60 L/min
Advantages/ strengths			
Easy to apply	+++	++	+
Easy to monitor	+++	++	+
Ability to drink and eat	+++	0	+
Ability to communicate	+++	+	++
Risks			
Mucosal irritation/ dryness	+	++	+
Claustrophobia	0	++	+++
Skin Injury	0/+	+++	+
pneumothorax	0	++	++
Minimizing the associated risks	Caution in patients with hemodynamic instability, decreased level of consciousness Monitoring mental status, respiratory rate, PF ratio, ROX index	Caution in patients with hemodynamic instability, decreased level of consciousness, agitation Monitoring mental status, work of breathing, respiratory rate, PF ratio, ROX index, HACOR scale, pressure-induced skin injury (nose bridge, face)	Caution in patients with hypercapnia, hemodynamic instability, decreased level of consciousness, agitation Monitoring mental status, work of breathing, respiratory rate, PF ratio, ROX index, pressure-induced skin injury (axilla)

Fig. 1. Settings, strengths, risks, and monitoring of HFNO and NIV/CPAP via face mask and helmet in patients with COVID-19 and AHRF. PF ratio, the ratio of arterial oxygen partial pressure to fractional inspired oxygen; PSV, pressure support ventilation.

injury, delayed intubation in the case of treatment failure, and virus nosocomial transmission.[18]

Patient Self-Inflicted Lung Injury

In patients with AHRF, hypoxemia and dysregulated inspiratory effort may induce spontaneous vigorous inspiratory efforts. The resulting high transpulmonary pressures along with altered respiratory mechanics and inhomogeneous lung inflation may induce further injury to the lung, which is described as patient self-inflicted lung injury.[15,19,20] HFNO and NIV may mitigate partially, but not fully, these pathophysiologic abnormalities. Patient self-inflicted lung injury is difficult to quantify or even detect, and related studies that compare noninvasive respiratory support versus invasive mechanical ventilation are lacking. From a mechanistic point of view, NIV has theoretic advantages over HFNO for the management of patients with COVID-19 and AHRF.[21] The ability of NIV to deliver higher PEEP compared with HFNO may render spontaneous breathing less injurious.[22]

Delayed Intubation

One of the concerns with the use of HFNO or NIV is delayed intubation that may worsen outcomes. Related studies showed mixed results and are based mainly on observational data. In a propensity score-matched retrospective study of 175 patients with non-COVID-19 respiratory failure who required intubation after HFNO failure (2013–2014), patients with early HFNO failure (intubated < 48 hours after initiation; n = 130) had significantly lower mortality compared with those failing greater than 48 hours after initiation (n = 45; 39.2% vs 66.7%, $P = .001$).[23] In a multicenter retrospective study, 164 out of 272 patients with COVID-19 managed with HFNO inside (n = 161) and outside (n = 111) the ICU were successfully weaned from HFNO.[24] HFNO failure occurred in 108 (39.7%) patients: 61 had early failures (< 48 hours) and 47 late failures.[24] Mortality after HFNO failure was high (45.4%) with no significant difference in hospital mortality (39.3% vs 53.2%; $P = .18$) or any of the secondary end points between early and late HFNO failure groups. The trend in mortality difference, although not statistically significant, raises the question of whether a larger trial might show a difference. Much larger trials will be needed to answer this question.[24]

Nosocomial Transmission

The viral dispersion with HFNO has been evaluated in simulation and clinical studies. A study measured smoke dispersion distance from a manikin model with HFNO at 60 L/min and demonstrated that smoke dispersion distance was limited, suggesting that dispersion was similar to the one observed with simple oxygen mask.[25,26] Wearing a surgical mask on top of HFNO further reduces the aerosol transmission during coughing or sneezing.[27] An experiment in healthy volunteers showed that cough-generated droplets spread to a mean (standard deviation) distance of 2.48 ± 1.03 m at baseline and 2.91 ± 1.09 m with HFNO (maximum cough distance of 4.50 m).[28] Face-mask NIV delivered through devices with single-limb circuits has been associated with more viral dispersion than HFNO.[29,30] Using a human-patient simulator on face-mask NIV, the exhaled air dispersion distance was shown to increase with higher inspiratory positive airway pressures and was within a 1-m region.[30] It has been suggested that NIV delivered through devices that use double-tube circuits (which includes selected NIV machines and ICU ventilators) is associated with less aerosol generation compared with single-tube circuits (only inspiratory tube).[31] Helmet NIV is associated with less viral dispersion than HFNO and face-mask NIV.[29] On the other hand, a study found that HFNO and NIV did not increase aerosol generation from the respiratory tract in healthy participants with no active pulmonary disease measured in a negative-pressure room.[32]

Clinical studies that link HFNO or NIV with nosocomial transmission of viruses are limited by their size and methodology.[33] These studies suggest that transmission to HCWs is uncommon with the use of infection control precautions, but it does exist. One study evaluated 73 HCWs exposed to patients with confirmed COVID-19 (n = 28) treated with HFNO for a median of 48 hours per person.[34] All HCWs wore appropriate personal protective equipment and underwent weekly COVID-19 polymerase chain reaction testing, and all HCWs had negative tests in the 14 days following exposure.[34] A study in 27 patients with confirmed COVID-19 treated with HFNO outside the ICU found that 1 nurse became infected among 44 exposed HCWs.[35] The HCWs applied airborne precautions, and the patients wore a surgical mask when an HCW entered the room.[35] In a cohort of 670 patients with confirmed COVID-19, closely monitored and treated in respiratory units outside the ICU with either HFNO (N = 163, 24.3%) or CPAP/NIV (n = 507, 75.7%; using helmet or face-mask interfaces), 42 (11.1%) HCWs tested positive for infection, despite appropriate protective equipment.[36] Only 3 HCWs required hospitalization.[36] In another study in which 50 patients with COVID-19 received NIV, HCWs caring for them underwent nasopharyngeal swabs for SARS-CoV-2 in case of COVID-19 symptoms and had periodic SARS-CoV-2 screening serology, and 2/124 (1.6%) HCWs were diagnosed with COVID-19.[37]

As the potential of nosocomial transmission of SARS-CoV-2 exists, it is prudent that HFNO and NIV are used with proper infection control precautions, that is, in single rooms or negative pressure airborne isolation rooms when possible.[28] Careful fitting of the interfaces on supported patients is recommended.[38] The risk of transmission may be decreased by using NIV devices that use double-tube circuits without exhalation ports.[31] The use of viral filters at exhalation ports may further reduce nosocomial transmission. HCWs caring for patients with COVID-19 using NIV or HFNO should be wearing full airborne personal protective equipment.[28]

Other Safety Concerns

The prolonged use of NIV and to a lesser extent HFNO in patients with COVID-19 is associated with the risk of pressure injury, especially in the nasal area, and with an increased risk of pulmonary barotrauma.[39] Helmet-NIV eliminates the risk of pressure injury associated with face-mask interfaces, but may uncommonly be associated with other pressure injuries around the neck seal and underneath the axillary straps.

EFFECTIVENESS OF HIGH-FLOW NASAL OXYGEN AND NONINVASIVE VENTILATION IN PATIENTS WITH ACUTE HYPOXEMIC RESPIRATORY FAILURE
Evidence from Randomized Controlled Trials in Non-COVID-19 Population

A meta-analysis of 9 randomized controlled trials (RCTs; n = 2093 patients) found no difference in mortality in patients with AHRF treated with HFNO (relative risk, 0.94; 95% confidence interval [CI], 0.67–1.31, moderate certainty) compared with conventional oxygen therapy, but a decreased risk of intubation (relative risk, 0.85; 95% CI, 0.74–0.99).[40] A meta-analysis of 8 RCTs comparing high-flow nasal cannula with other noninvasive methods of oxygen delivery after extubation in critically ill adults found that HFNO compared with conventional oxygen therapy decreased reintubation (relative risk, 0.46; 95% CI, 0.30–0.70; moderate certainty) and postextubation respiratory failure, but had no effect on mortality (relative risk, 0.93; 95% CI, 0.57–1.52; moderate certainty), or ICU length of stay (mean difference, 0.05 days fewer;

95% CI, 0.83 days fewer to 0.73 days more; high certainty).[41] In this population, HFNO compared with NIV had no effect on reintubation, mortality, or postextubation respiratory failure.[41]

A systematic review and network meta-analysis that included 25 RCTs and 3804 patients with AHRF owing to causes other than COVID-19 found lower mortality risk associated with face-mask NIV (risk ratio, 0.83; credible interval, 0.68–0.99) and helmet NIV (risk ratio, 0.40; credible interval, 0.24–0.63) compared with conventional oxygen therapy.[42] The benefit of helmet NIV but not face-mask NIV was maintained after excluding patients with chronic obstructive pulmonary disease exacerbation or cardiogenic pulmonary edema.[42] Face-mask NIV, helmet NIV, and HFNO were associated with lower risk of endotracheal intubation.[42]

Evidence from Observational Data in Patients with COVID-19

A simulation model projected that a scenario in which HFNO is available would result in 10,000 to 40,000 fewer deaths in the United States compared with a scenario in which HFNO was unavailable and in fewer days without available ventilators.[43] A retrospective study evaluated 379 consecutive patients with COVID-19 admitted to 4 ICUs for AHRF in Paris, France, between February 21 and April 24, 2020. The 146 (39%) patients who received HFNO within the first 24 hours after ICU admission were compared with the 233 patients who did not. Propensity-score adjusted analysis showed that HFNO was associated with fewer patients requiring invasive mechanical ventilation by day 28 (55% vs 72%; $P < .0001$) with similar 28-day mortality (21% in the HFNO group vs 22% in the other group).[44] Other studies on the outcomes associated with HFNO in patients with COVID-19 are summarized in **Table 1**.

There are multiple observational studies that evaluated NIV in the management of COVID-19 in different settings that vary between ICU and wards, mostly owing to unavailability of ICU beds (see **Table 1**).[36] One multicenter retrospective observational study found that patients treated with NIV had significantly lower mortality (171/534; 32.0%) than those who received invasive mechanical ventilation (128/154; 83.1%). Although the multivariable regression attempted to address bias inherent in this nonrandomized study, it is not clear whether the higher mortality in this study reflects severity of illness in those intubated or a true cause and effect.[45] In patients with confirmed COVID-19 treated in respiratory units outside the ICU with either HFNO (n = 163, 24.3%) or CPAP/NIV (n = 507, 75.7%), the intubation rate was similar in the 2 groups, but the mortality was lower in the HFNO group.[36] In an interim analysis of the international, multicenter HOPE COVID-19 cohort (1933 patients), 390 (20%) patients were treated with NIV, 44.4% of whom had the composite outcome of death or need for intubation.[46] Other studies on the outcomes associated with NIV in patients with COVID-19 are summarized in **Table 1**.

Evidence from Randomized Controlled Trials in Patients with COVID-19

A recent RCT conducted in patients with COVID-19 admitted to 4 Italian ICUs with moderate to severe AHRF found that helmet NIV did not result in significantly fewer days of respiratory support at 28 days (primary outcome) as compared with HFNO alone (mean difference, 2 days; 95% CI, −2 to 6; $P = .26$).[47] However, the helmet NIV group had a lower intubation rate (30% vs 51%; $P = .03$) and more days free of invasive mechanical ventilation within 28 days (median of 28 vs 25 days; $P = .04$).[47] The hospital mortality was 24% in the helmet NIV group and 25% in the HFNO group.[47] In the RECOVERY-Respiratory Support multicenter RCT, 1272 hospitalized patients with acute respiratory failure owing to COVID-19 were randomized to CPAP (n = 380; 29.9%), HFNO (n = 417;

32.8%), or conventional oxygen therapy (n = 475; 37.3%).[48] The composite outcome (tracheal intubation or mortality within 30 days) was lower in the CPAP group compared with conventional oxygen therapy (CPAP group, 36.3%; conventional oxygen therapy, 44.4%; unadjusted odds ratio, 0.72; 95% CI, 0.53–0.96; $P = .03$), but similar in the HFNO and conventional oxygen therapy groups (HFNO, 44.4%; vs conventional oxygen therapy, 45.1%; unadjusted odds ratio, 0.97; 95% CI, 0.73–1.29; $P = .85$).[48] There are no data from RCTs that compare CPAP with pressure support mode.

PRONE POSITIONING WITH HIGH-FLOW NASAL OXYGEN AND NONINVASIVE VENTILATION

Awake prone positioning can easily be performed in patients receiving HFNO. In a pilot study of 9 patients with COVID-19 and AHRF requiring HFNO for greater than 2 days, prone positioning led to an increase in blood oxygen saturation (Sao_2) from 90% ± 2% to 96% ± 3% ($P<.001$) and in blood oxygen partial pressure (Pao_2) from 69 ± 10 to 108 ± 14 mm Hg ($P<.001$).[49]

Awake prone positioning has also been used in patients with COVID-19 while receiving NIV, but data are limited. Small observational studies have shown that NIV in the prone position is feasible and is probably safe, even outside the ICU.[50,51] In an a priori collaborative metatrial of 6 RCTs, adults who required respiratory support with high-flow nasal cannula for AHRF owing to COVID-19 (n = 1126) were randomly assigned to awake prone positioning or standard care.[52] The primary composite outcome was treatment failure (intubation or death within 28 days), which was lower with awake prone positioning compared with standard care (40% vs 46%; relative risk, 0.86; 95% CI, 0.75–0.98).[52]

MONITORING OF PATIENTS DURING HIGH-FLOW NASAL OXYGEN AND NONINVASIVE VENTILATION

The success of the new modalities of noninvasive respiratory support starts with ensuring availability, having the needed infrastructure and resources, and establishing programs that train HCWs as well as creating protocols, policies, and procedures on their use (see **Fig. 1**). Close monitoring and short-interval assessments for worsening of respiratory failure are critical for patients receiving noninvasive respiratory support (see **Fig. 1**).[53] Monitoring during HFNO and NIV should encompass monitoring the inspiratory effort, respiratory rate, tidal volume, Fio_2, and oxygenation parameters (Sao_2/Fio_2 or Pao_2/Fio_2 ratio), as these variables may indicate HFNO or NIV failure and the need for intubation.[15] A small retrospective study evaluated 17 patients with ARDS secondary to COVID-19 who were managed with HFNO.[54] The HFNO failure rate, defined by the need of NIV or intubation as rescue therapy, was 0% (0/6) in patients with Pao_2/Fio_2 greater than 200 mm Hg versus 63% (7/11) in those with $Pao_2/Fio_2 \leq 200$ mm Hg ($P = .04$).[54] The ROX ([Spo_2/Fio_2]/respiratory rate) index has been validated to predict the success of HFNO in non-COVID-19 patients. A 2-year multicenter prospective cohort study validated the ability of the ROX index to predict intubation in 191 patients with non-COVID-19 pneumonia treated with HFNO.[55] ROX $\geq$ 4.88 at 2 hours (hazard ratio [HR], 0.434; 95% CI, 0.264–0.715), 6 hours (HR, 0.304; 95% CI, 0.182–0.509), or 12 hours (HR, 0.291; 95% CI, 0.161–0.524) after HFNO initiation was associated with a lower intubation risk. An ROX less than 2.85 at 2 hours, less than 3.47 at 6 hours, and less than 3.85 at 12 hours predicted HFNO failure (specificities 98%–99%).[55] A single-center retrospective study of 196 patients with ARDS secondary to COVID-19 observed that 40 patients were treated with HFNO.[56] The ROX index was significantly higher in the group that did not require intubation

Table 2
Randomized controlled trials (recruiting or nonrecruiting) evaluating noninvasive respiratory support (high-flow nasal oxygen or noninvasive ventilation) in patients with COVID-19 and acute hypoxemic respiratory failure

Trial	Identifier/Status	Country	Design	Population	Sample Size	Intervention	Primary Outcome
Comparison of HFNO, face-mask NIV and helmet NIV in COVID-19 ARDS patients (NIV COVID-19)	ClinicalTrials.gov Identifier: NCT04715243 Recruiting	Oman	Multicenter RCT	Patients with confirmed COVID-19 in the emergency department, the ward, high dependency, or ICU with ARDS requiring NIV	360	Patients assigned to 1 of 3 arms: HFNO, face-mask NIV, or helmet NIV	Rate of endotracheal intubation
Helmet noninvasive ventilation for COVID-19 patients (Helmet-COVID)	ClinicalTrials.gov Identifier: NCT04477668 Recruiting	Saudi Arabia	Multicenter RCT	COVID-19 with AHRF	320	Pragmatic parallel RCT that will compare helmet NIV with standard of care to standard of care alone in 1:1 ratio. The trial will be implemented in multiple centers	28-d all-cause mortality
Early CPAP in COVID-19 patients with respiratory failure (EC-COVID-RCT)	ClinicalTrials.gov Identifier: NCT04326075	Italy	Single-center RCT	Patients in the emergency department with confirmed or suspected COVID-19 and $Spo_2 < 95\%$ with PF ratio > 200	900	Early helmet CPAP vs usual care	Death or need of intubation
High-flow nasal oxygen vs CPAP helmet in COVID-19 pneumonia (COVIDNOCHE)	ClinicalTrials.gov Identifier: NCT04381923 Not recruiting (by August 26, 2021)	USA	Single-center RCT	Patients with COVID-19 and refractory hypoxemia ($Spo_2 \leq 92\%$ on $O_2 \geq 6$ L/min by nasal cannula)	200	Advanced respiratory units will be assigned to use 1 of 2 default interventions (helmet CPAP vs HFNO) as the first-line treatment	Ventilator-free days within 28 d

| High-flow nasal therapy vs conventional oxygen therapy in COVID-19 (COVID-HIGH) | ClinicalTrials.gov Identifier: NCT04465638 Recruiting | Italy | Multicenter RCT (Europe) | Patients with confirmed COVID-19-related AHRF in any hospital ward caring for COVID-19 patients | 364 | HFNO vs conventional oxygen therapy | Proportion of patients needing escalation of treatment (ie, NIV, including CPAP, or intubation) by 28 d |

The search was performed on August 26, 2021, in ClinicalTrials.gov, using the following terms: adults ($\geq$18 y), COVID, interventional studies, all countries, recruiting or nonrecruiting, and each of the following: noninvasive ventilation (yielded 167 studies) OR high-flow nasal oxygen (yielded 26 studies) OR continuous positive airway pressure (yielded 15 studies). Only 5 studies were RCTs as reported. Additional search on September 15, 2021, in International Clinical Trials Registry Platform and ISRCTN registry, did not yield any additional studies.

(5.0 $\pm$ 1.6 vs 4.0 $\pm$ 1.0 for those who required intubation; $P = .02$).[56] An ROX index less than 4.94 measured 2 to 6 hours after the start of therapy was associated with increased risk of intubation (HR, 4.03; 95% CI, 1.18–13.7).[56] A multicenter retrospective study of 272 patients with COVID-19 managed with HFNO found that ROX index greater than 3.0 at 2, 6, and 12 hours after initiation of HFNO was 85.3% sensitive for identifying subsequent HFNO success. Another study found that at 6 hours ROX score $\geq$ 3.7 was 80% predictive of successful weaning, whereas ROX $\leq$ 2.2 was 74% predictive of failure. A systematic review that included 8 cohort studies (n = 1301 patients) showed that ROX index had a sensitivity of 0.70 (95% CI, 0.59–0.80) and specificity of 0.79 (95% CI, 0.67–0.88) for predicting HNFC failure, resulting in a good discriminatory value, with a summary area under the curve of 0.81 (95% CI, 0.77–0.84).[57]

There is evidence that the ROX index may also predict the success of NIV to avoid delay in intubation.[58] Another index, the HACOR scale, which incorporates heart rate, acidosis, consciousness, oxygenation, and respiratory rate, may also predict NIV failure.[59]

FUTURE DIRECTIONS

Multiple RCTs on noninvasive respiratory support in patients with COVID-19 are ongoing (**Table 2**).[60] These trials are addressing the effectiveness of HFNO, facemask NIV, and helmet NIV. Other studies are needed to evaluate the safety and effectiveness of noninvasive respiratory support outside of the ICU setting and validate the predictors of success or failure of HFNO and NIV.

SUMMARY

HFNO and NIV are used as first-line respiratory support in most patients with AHRF owing to COVID-19. The increasing use during the pandemic was associated with a reduction in the need for invasive mechanical ventilation and mortality, although causal inferences cannot be made. Results from ongoing RCTs are awaited to answer questions regarding the effects of HFNO and NIV on patient-centered outcomes.

CLINICS CARE POINTS

- Both NIV and HFNO are associated with better survival than invasive ventilation in COVID-19. It is not clear if this is cause and effect or merely a reflection of lesser severity of illness.
- Early intubation (<48 hours) seems to result in better outcomes in those who fail NIV and HFNO.
- In one trial, continuous positive airway pressure (CPAP), but not HFNO, resulted in a lower composite endpoint of tracheal intubation or mortality compared to conventional oxygen therapy.
- Data on the effectiveness of helmet NIV compared to mask NIV or HFNO in COVID-19 are limited.
- The risk of nosocomial transmission of COVID-19 is low with NIV or HFNO.

ACKNOWLEDGMENTS

Dr. Arabi would like to acknowledge King Abdullah International Medical Research Center, Riyadh, Saudi Arabia, for funding the Helmet COVID trial (NCT04477668).

REFERENCES

1. World Health Organization. WHO coronavirus (COVID-19) dashboard. Available at: https://covid19.who.int/. Accessed January 22, 2022.
2. Grasselli G, Zangrillo A, Zanella A, et al. Baseline characteristics and outcomes of 1591 patients infected with SARS-CoV-2 admitted to ICUs of the Lombardy Region, Italy. JAMA 2020;323(16):1574–81.
3. Schenck EJ, Hoffman K, Goyal P, et al. Respiratory mechanics and gas exchange in COVID-19–associated respiratory failure. Ann Am Thorac Soc 2020;17(9):1158–61.
4. Grasselli G, Tonetti T, Protti A, et al. Pathophysiology of COVID-19-associated acute respiratory distress syndrome: a multicentre prospective observational study. Lancet Respir Med 2020;8(12):1201–8.
5. Baillie JK, Baruch J, Beane A, et al. ISARIC COVID-19 Clinical Data Report issued: 15 December 2021. medRxiv 2021. https://doi.org/10.1101/2020.07.17.20155218.
6. Guan W-J, Ni Z-y, Hu Y, et al. Clinical characteristics of coronavirus disease 2019 in China. N Engl J Med 2020;382(18):1708–20.
7. Ñamendys-Silva SA. Respiratory support for patients with COVID-19 infection. Lancet Respir Med 2020;8(4):e18.
8. Richardson S, Hirsch JS, Narasimhan M, et al. Presenting characteristics, comorbidities, and outcomes among 5700 patients hospitalized with COVID-19 in the New York city area. JAMA 2020;323(20):2052–9.
9. Wang D, Hu B, Hu C, et al. Clinical characteristics of 138 hospitalized patients with 2019 novel coronavirus-infected pneumonia in Wuhan, China. JAMA 2020;323(11):1061–9.
10. World Health Organization. Clinical management of COVID-19: interim guidance. Geneva: World Health Organization; 2020.
11. Karagiannidis C, Hentschker C, Westhoff M, et al. Observational study of changes in utilization and outcomes in mechanical ventilation in COVID-19. PLoS ONE 2022;17(1):e0262315. https://doi.org/10.1371/journal.pone.0262315.
12. Dysart K, Miller TL, Wolfson MR, et al. Research in high flow therapy: mechanisms of action. Respir Med 2009;103(10):1400–5.
13. Parke RL, Eccleston ML, McGuinness SP. The effects of flow on airway pressure during nasal high-flow oxygen therapy. Respir Care 2011;56(8):1151–5.
14. Brambilla AM, Aliberti S, Prina E, et al. Helmet CPAP vs. oxygen therapy in severe hypoxemic respiratory failure due to pneumonia. Intensive Care Med 2014;40(7):942–9.
15. Grieco DL, Maggiore SM, Roca O, et al. Non-invasive ventilatory support and high-flow nasal oxygen as first-line treatment of acute hypoxemic respiratory failure and ARDS. Intensive Care Med 2021;47(8):851–66.
16. Marini JJ, Rocco PR, Gattinoni L. Static and dynamic contributors to ventilator-induced lung injury in clinical practice. Pressure, energy, and power. Am J Respir Crit Care Med 2020;201(7):767–74.
17. Repesse X, Charron C, Vieillard-Baron A. Right ventricular failure in acute lung injury and acute respiratory distress syndrome. Minerva anestesiologica 2012;78(8):941–8.
18. Arulkumaran N, Brealey D, Howell D, et al. Use of non-invasive ventilation for patients with COVID-19: a cause for concern? Lancet Respir Med 2020;8(6):e45.
19. Marini J, Gattinoni L. Management of COVID-19 respiratory distress. JAMA 2020;323(22):2329–30.

20. Brochard L, Slutsky A, Pesenti A. Mechanical ventilation to minimize progression of lung injury in acute respiratory failure. Am J Respir Crit Care Med 2017; 195(4):438.

21. Guan L, Zhou L, Le Grange JM, et al. Non-invasive ventilation in the treatment of early hypoxemic respiratory failure caused by COVID-19: considering nasal CPAP as the first choice. Crit Care 2020;24(1):1–2.

22. Morais CC, Koyama Y, Yoshida T, et al. High positive end-expiratory pressure renders spontaneous effort noninjurious. Am J Respir Crit Care Med 2018;197(10): 1285–96.

23. Kang BJ, Koh Y, Lim C-M, et al. Failure of high-flow nasal cannula therapy may delay intubation and increase mortality. Intensive Care Med 2015;41(4):623–32.

24. Chandel A, Patolia S, Brown AW, et al. High-flow nasal cannula in COVID-19: outcomes of application and examination of the ROX index to predict success. Respir Care 2021;66(6):909–19.

25. Hui DS, Chow BK, Lo T, et al. Exhaled air dispersion during high-flow nasal cannula therapy versus CPAP via different masks. Eur Respir J 2019;53(4):1802339.

26. Ip M, Tang JW, Hui DS, et al. Airflow and droplet spreading around oxygen masks: a simulation model for infection control research. Am J Infect Control 2007;35(10):684–9.

27. Hui DS, Chow BK, Chu L, et al. Exhaled air dispersion during coughing with and without wearing a surgical or N95 mask. PLoS One 2012;7(12):e50845.

28. Loh N-HW, Tan Y, Taculod J, et al. The impact of high-flow nasal cannula (HFNC) on coughing distance: implications on its use during the novel coronavirus disease outbreak. Can J Anesth 2020;67(7):893–4.

29. Avari H, Hiebert RJ, Ryzynski AA, et al. Quantitative assessment of viral dispersion associated with respiratory support devices in a simulated critical care environment. Am J Respir Crit Care Med 2021;203(9):1112–8.

30. Hui DS, Chow BK, Ng SS, et al. Exhaled air dispersion distances during noninvasive ventilation via different Respironics face masks. Chest 2009;136(4): 998–1005.

31. Aziz S, Arabi YM, Alhazzani W, et al. Managing ICU surge during the COVID-19 crisis: rapid guidelines. Intensive Care Med 2020;46(7):1303–25.

32. Gaeckle NT, Lee J, Park Y, et al. Aerosol generation from the respiratory tract with various modes of oxygen delivery. Am J Respir Crit Care Med 2020;202(8): 1115–24.

33. Harding H, Broom A, Broom J. Aerosol-generating procedures and infective risk to healthcare workers from SARS-CoV-2: the limits of the evidence. J Hosp Infect 2020;105(4):717–25.

34. Vianello A, Arcaro G, Molena B, et al. High-flow nasal cannula oxygen therapy to treat patients with hypoxemic acute respiratory failure consequent to SARS-CoV-2 infection. Thorax 2020;75(11):998–1000.

35. Guy T, Créac'Hcadec A, Ricordel C, et al. High-flow nasal oxygen: a safe, efficient treatment for COVID-19 patients not in an ICU. Eur Respir J 2020;56(5): 2001154.

36. Franco C, Facciolongo N, Tonelli R, et al. Feasibility and clinical impact of out-of-ICU noninvasive respiratory support in patients with COVID-19-related pneumonia. Eur Respir J 2020;56(5):2002130.

37. Faraone A, Beltrame C, Crociani A, et al. Effectiveness and safety of noninvasive positive pressure ventilation in the treatment of COVID-19-associated acute hypoxemic respiratory failure: a single center, non-ICU setting experience. Intern Emerg Med 2021;16(5):1183–90.

38. Haymet A, Bassi GL, Fraser JF. Airborne spread of SARS-CoV-2 while using high-flow nasal cannula oxygen therapy: myth or reality? Intensive Care Med 2020; 46(12):2248–51.
39. Simioli F, Annunziata A, Polistina GE, et al. The role of high flow nasal cannula in COVID-19 associated pneumomediastinum and pneumothorax. Healthcare (Basel, Switzerland) 2021;9(6):620.
40. Rochwerg B, Granton D, Wang D, et al. High flow nasal cannula compared with conventional oxygen therapy for acute hypoxemic respiratory failure: a systematic review and meta-analysis. Intensive Care Med 2019;45(5):563–72.
41. Granton D, Chaudhuri D, Wang D, et al. High-flow nasal cannula compared with conventional oxygen therapy or noninvasive ventilation immediately postextubation: a systematic review and meta-analysis. Crit Care Med 2020;48(11): e1129–36.
42. Ferreyro BL, Angriman F, Munshi L, et al. Association of noninvasive oxygenation strategies with all-cause mortality in adults with acute hypoxemic respiratory failure: a systematic review and meta-analysis. JAMA 2020;324(1):57–67.
43. Gershengorn HB, Hu Y, Chen J-T, et al. The impact of high-flow nasal cannula use on patient mortality and the availability of mechanical ventilators in COVID-19. Ann Am Thorac Soc 2021;18(4):623–31.
44. Demoule A, Vieillard Baron A, Darmon M, et al. High-flow nasal cannula in critically ill patients with severe COVID-19. Am J Respir Crit Care Med 2020; 202(7):1039–42.
45. Forrest IS, Jaladanki SK, Paranjpe I, et al. Non-invasive ventilation versus mechanical ventilation in hypoxemic patients with COVID-19. Infection 2021;49(5): 989–97.
46. Bertaina M, Nuñez-Gil IJ, Franchin L, et al. Non-invasive ventilation for SARS-CoV-2 acute respiratory failure: a subanalysis from the HOPE COVID-19 registry. Emerg Med J 2021;38(5):359–65.
47. Grieco DL, Menga LS, Cesarano M, et al. Effect of helmet noninvasive ventilation vs high-flow nasal oxygen on days free of respiratory support in patients with COVID-19 and moderate to severe hypoxemic respiratory failure: the HENIVOT randomized clinical trial. JAMA 2021;325(17):1731–43.
48. Perkins GD, Ji C, Connolly BA, et al. An adaptive randomized controlled trial of non-invasive respiratory strategies in acute respiratory failure patients with COVID-19. medRxiv 2021. https://doi.org/10.1101/2021.08.02.21261379.
49. Tu G-W, Liao Y-X, Li Q-Y, et al. Prone positioning in high-flow nasal cannula for COVID-19 patients with severe hypoxemia: a pilot study. Ann Transl Med 2020; 8(9):598.
50. Sartini C, Tresoldi M, Scarpellini P, et al. Respiratory parameters in patients with COVID-19 after using noninvasive ventilation in the prone position outside the intensive care unit. JAMA 2020;323(22):2338–40.
51. Burton-Papp HC, Jackson AI, Beecham R, et al. Conscious prone positioning during non-invasive ventilation in COVID-19 patients: experience from a single centre. F1000Research 2020;9:859.
52. Ehrmann S, Li J, Ibarra-Estrada M, et al. Awake prone positioning for COVID-19 acute hypoxaemic respiratory failure: a randomised, controlled, multinational, open-label meta-trial. Lancet Respir Med 2021;9(12):1387–95.
53. Alhazzani W, Evans L, Alshamsi F, et al. Surviving sepsis campaign guidelines on the management of adults with coronavirus disease 2019 (COVID-19) in the ICU: first update. Crit Care Med 2021;49(3):e219–34.

54. Wang K, Zhao W, Li J, et al. The experience of high-flow nasal cannula in hospitalized patients with 2019 novel coronavirus-infected pneumonia in two hospitals of Chongqing, China. Ann Intensive Care 2020;10(1):1–5.

55. Roca O, Caralt B, Messika J, et al. An index combining respiratory rate and oxygenation to predict outcome of nasal high-flow therapy. Am J Respir Crit Care Med 2019;199(11):1368–76.

56. Panadero C, Abad-Fernández A, Rio-Ramirez MT, et al. High-flow nasal cannula for acute respiratory distress syndrome (ARDS) due to COVID-19. Multidisciplinary Respir Med 2020;15(1):693.

57. Prakash J, Bhattacharya PK, Yadav AK, et al. ROX index as a good predictor of high flow nasal cannula failure in COVID-19 patients with acute hypoxemic respiratory failure: a systematic review and meta-analysis. J Crit Care 2021;66:102–8.

58. Zaboli A, Ausserhofer D, Pfeifer N, et al. The ROX index can be a useful tool for the triage evaluation of COVID-19 patients with dyspnoea. J Adv Nurs 2021; 77(8):3361–9.

59. Duan J, Han X, Bai L, et al. Assessment of heart rate, acidosis, consciousness, oxygenation, and respiratory rate to predict noninvasive ventilation failure in hypoxemic patients. Intensive Care Med 2017;43(2):192–9.

60. Arabi YM, Tlayjeh H, Aldekhyl S, et al. : Helmet non-invasive ventilation for COVID-19 patients (Helmet-COVID): study protocol for a multicentre randomised controlled trial. BMJ Open 2021;11(8):e052169.

61. Chen Q, Zheng Z, Zhang C, et al. Clinical characteristics of 145 patients with corona virus disease 2019 (COVID-19) in Taizhou, Zhejiang, China. Infection 2020;48(4):543–51.

62. Lagi F, Piccica M, Graziani L, et al. Early experience of an infectious and tropical diseases unit during the coronavirus disease (COVID-19) pandemic, Florence, Italy, February to March 2020. Eurosurveillance 2020;25(17):2000556.

63. Calligaro GL, Lalla U, Audley G, et al. The utility of high-flow nasal oxygen for severe COVID-19 pneumonia in a resource-constrained setting: a multi-centre prospective observational study. EClinicalMedicine 2020;28:100570.

64. Zhou F, Yu T, Du R, et al. Clinical course and risk factors for mortality of adult inpatients with COVID-19 in Wuhan, China: a retrospective cohort study. The lancet 2020;395(10229):1054–62.

65. Yang X, Yu Y, Xu J, et al. Clinical course and outcomes of critically ill patients with SARS-CoV-2 pneumonia in Wuhan, China: a single-centered, retrospective, observational study. Lancet Respir Med 2020;8(5):475–81.

66. Avdeev SN, Yaroshetskiy AI, Tsareva NA, et al. Noninvasive ventilation for acute hypoxemic respiratory failure in patients with COVID-19. Am J Emerg Med 2021; 39:154–7.

67. Bellani G, Grasselli G, Cecconi M, et al. Noninvasive ventilatory support of patients with COVID-19 outside the intensive care units (WARd-COVID). Ann Am Thorac Soc 2021;18(6):1020–6.

68. Menga LS, Delle Cese L, Bongiovanni F, et al. High failure rate of noninvasive oxygenation strategies in critically ill subjects with acute hypoxemic respiratory failure due to COVID-19. Respir Care 2021;66(5):705–14.

69. Burns GP, Lane ND, Tedd HM, et al. Improved survival following ward-based non-invasive pressure support for severe hypoxia in a cohort of frail patients with COVID-19: retrospective analysis from a UK teaching hospital. BMJ Open Respir Res 2020;7(1):e000621.

70. Xie J, Wu W, Li S, et al. Clinical characteristics and outcomes of critically ill patients with novel coronavirus infectious disease (COVID-19) in China: a retrospective multicenter study. Intensive Care Med 2020;46(10):1863–72.

71. Garcia PDW, Fumeaux T, Guerci P, et al, Investigators R–I. Prognostic factors associated with mortality risk and disease progression in 639 critically ill patients with COVID-19 in Europe: initial report of the international RISC-19-ICU prospective observational cohort. EClinicalMedicine 2020;25:100449.

72. Elhadi M, Alsoufi A, Abusalama A, et al. Epidemiology, outcomes, and utilization of intensive care unit resources for critically ill COVID-19 patients in Libya: a prospective multi-center cohort study. PLoS One 2021;16(4):e0251085.

73. Rahim F, Amin S, Noor M, et al. Mortality of patients with severe COVID-19 in the intensive care unit: an observational study from a major COVID-19 receiving hospital. Cureus 2020;12(10):e10906.

74. Carpagnano GE, Buonamico E, Migliore G, et al. Bilevel and continuous positive airway pressure and factors linked to all-cause mortality in COVID-19 patients in an intermediate respiratory intensive care unit in Italy. Expert Rev Respir Med 2021;15(6):853–7.

75. Rodríguez A, Ruiz-Botella M, Martín-Loeches I, et al. Deploying unsupervised clustering analysis to derive clinical phenotypes and risk factors associated with mortality risk in 2022 critically ill patients with COVID-19 in Spain. Crit Care 2021;25(1):1–15.

76. Roomi S, Shah SO, Ullah W, et al. Declining intensive care unit mortality of COVID-19: a multi-center study. J Clin Med Res 2021;13(3):184.

77. Grosgurin O, Leidi A, Farhoumand PD, et al. Role of intermediate care unit admission and noninvasive respiratory support during the COVID-19 pandemic: a retrospective cohort study. Respiration 2021;100(8):786–93.

Critical Care Response During the COVID-19 Pandemic

Samuel Rednor, DO[a],*, Lewis A. Eisen, MD[b],
J. Perren Cobb, MD, FCCM[c,d], Laura Evans, MD, FCCM[e],
Craig M. Coopersmith, MD[f]

KEYWORDS

• COVID 19 • Critical care organization • sURGE LOGISItics • Health equity

KEY POINTS

- Critical care organizations play a central role in surge logistics for a hospital system.
- Critical care organizations, using the principles of the Four S's (space, staff, supplies, and systems), can best coordinate the response to health disasters, such as the COVID-19 pandemic.
- Critical care organizations can play a pivotal role in promoting health equity.

INTRODUCTION

The ongoing COVID-19 pandemic, which has led to the deaths of millions of people worldwide, serves to highlight the essential role critical care organizations (CCOs) plays in responding to a public health emergency. A CCO is an organization that integrates the business and operations of critical care, focusing on patient care, safety, and quality programs.[1] CCOs can be found in Academic Medical Centers (AMCs), non-AMCs, and across health care systems—in which case, the CCO serves multiple hospitals simultaneously. In ideal scenarios, a CCO will provide a common organizational structure and chain of command for critical care divisions and departments with

[a] Division of Critical Care Medicine, Albert Einstein College of Medicine, Jack D. Weiler Hospital, 1825 Eastchester Road, 4th Floor, Bronx, NY 10461, USA; [b] Division of Critical Care, Department of Medicine, Montefiore Medical Center, Albert Einstein College of Medicine, 201 East 87th Street, Apartment 15c, Bronx, NY 10467, USA; [c] Surgical Critical Care, Department of Surgery, Critical Care Institute, Keck Medicine of USC, Health Care Consultation Center, 1510 San Pablo Street #514, Los Angeles, CA 90033, USA; [d] Surgical Critical Care, Department of Anesthesiology, Critical Care Institute, Keck Medicine of USC, Health Care Consultation Center, 1510 San Pablo Street #514, Los Angeles, CA 90033, USA; [e] Pulmonary, Critical Care and Sleep Medicine, University of Washington, University of Washington Medical Center, 1959 NE Pacific Street, Seattle, WA 98195, USA; [f] Department of Surgery, Emory Critical Care Center, 101 Woodruff Circle Suite WMB 5105, Atlanta, GA 30322, USA
* Corresponding author.
E-mail address: srednor@montefiore.org

Crit Care Clin 38 (2022) 623–637
https://doi.org/10.1016/j.ccc.2022.01.007
0749-0704/22/© 2022 Elsevier Inc. All rights reserved.

criticalcare.theclinics.com

the intention of enhancing throughput, instilling quality control, creating uniformity of care, and integrating critical care within the broader framework of the hospital or health care system.[2,3]

A CCO differs from the traditional critical care model in several key details. Within the traditional critical care model, critical care is decentralized across various ICUs, which are staffed by physicians of different specialties (eg, anesthesia, surgery, medicine). Additionally, ICUs under the traditional critical care model function under their own leadership and have differing command structures, protocols, policies, and expertise with triage and admission of patients, dependent on the bed availability of the individual ICU.

Hospitals and health care systems with active CCOs (or other organizational bodies seeking to provide an organized response to the pandemic) were likely better positioned to address heightened demands during the ongoing COVID-19 pandemic for a variety of reasons. During COVID-19, hospitals and health care systems experienced unprecedented patient surges. When surges occurred, the unification of ICU services became especially important, as there was an enhanced need to rapidly triage patients, sustain communication across disciplines, and optimize care coordination when ad hoc ICUs were created to accommodate the patient influx. Further, during the ongoing COVID-19 pandemic, coordination from the national and state level to the hospital and health care system level was inconsistent, and so, in the absence of consistent government oversight, organizations like the CCO became more vital, as they were uniquely equipped to enact organizing and standardizing measures.

Before addressing what future steps might be taken by CCOs to encourage improved outcomes in the management of the COVID-19 pandemic (and future health emergencies), it is first necessary to examine recent experiences with pandemic response, both the triumphs and challenges, to learn from recent history. Throughout the COVID-19 pandemic, health care providers witnessed shortfalls in preparedness, on the one hand, and moments of success and innovation, on the other. Early in the pandemic, there was a dearth of personal protective equipment for front-line workers and a lack of available COVID-19 testing. As the COVID-19 pandemic progressed, the stark disparities rooted in race and ethnicity that exist within the United States were brought to the forefront of our consciousness, as we witnessed the outsized effect the pandemic had on Black, Indigenous, and People of Color (BIPOC). It is equally important to acknowledge the heroic efforts of nurses, respiratory therapists, physical therapists, and ancillary staff as well as the rapid response of governments, scientists, and the pharmaceutical industry. The latter allowed for the creation of a vaccine in a historically short period of time, as well as the performance of clinical trials (also conducted in record-time), which yielded multiple pharmacologic therapies that improved patient outcomes, summarized in the NIH guidelines for the treatment of COVID-19[4]

Extrapolating from these examples; mass coordination, cooperation, and organization are at the heart of the successful outcomes related to the pandemic response. It follows that a coordinated, cooperative, and organized critical care response is also of the utmost necessity. Moving forward, CCOs are uniquely positioned to enact meaningful change in this regard.

The purpose of this review is to identify the role the CCO plays in a pandemic response; to highlight which measures were effective and which were ineffective; and to make recommendations for what can be done differently in future scenarios to yield more favorable outcomes. This review will also serve as an after-action report of which preparatory measures were successful and which preparatory measures need improvement. Finally, this review will underscore the importance of both the material needs of a health care system and the human cost of practicing medicine during an ongoing pandemic.

Pre–COVID-19 PANDEMIC GUIDANCE AND THE CRITICAL CARE ORGANIZATIONS

In 2009, with the advent of H1N1 influenza, many medical centers and medical organizations began developing pandemic response plans. Before COVID-19, pandemic response guidelines were issued by the Society of Critical Care Medicine (SCCM), Institute of Medicine/National Academy of Medicine (IOM/NAM), Assistant Secretary for Preparedness and Response Technical Resources Assistance Center and Information Exchange (ASPR TRACIE), the American College of CHEST Physicians (CHEST).[5–8] It is useful to review these early guidelines through the prism of the COVID-19 pandemic to understand how they are applicable and how they might also be expanded or qualified by CCOs in the future. Typically, these guidelines address 4 fundamental principles of disaster relief, known colloquially as the "Four S's": space, staff, supplies, and systems.

Ultimately, CCOs should be at the center of coordinating the "Four S's" to ensure that the needs of each category are being met, and that the "Four S's" are working in concert, as each category has bearing on the others. This is illustrated in **Fig. 1**. We will review how pre–COVID-19 guidelines measured up to the actual experience of COVID-19.

Space

With the advent of patient surges during a pandemic, space becomes a highly valuable resource. CHEST's early guidelines, pre–COVID-19, point to the importance of using "deployable critical care assets," or "field hospitals," which have historically been implemented by the military and have only more recently been considered for civilian applications.

In New York City, The United States Naval Ship Comfort, treated 182 patients, while the Javits Convention Center treated more than 1000 patients.[9] Additional field hospitals were established, with varying success at the United States Tennis Association U.S.T.A. Billie Jean King National Tennis Center and in Central Park. The former treated a total of 79 patients and cost 52 million dollars, while the latter had only 68 beds but was able to treat 315 patients.[10,11] In London, the UK National Health Service (HS) established the Nightingale Hospital of London (NHL), a large capacity field hospital that could admit up to 4000 ventilated patients. This facility was constructed in an event space in 9 days. By the end of the first wave, the NHL had admitted a total of 54 patients.[12]

As these figures demonstrate, the use of deployable critical care assets was ultimate of limited utility. In the instances of the Naval Ship Comfort and the Javits Center, both deployable critical care assets initially only accepted patients with non–COVID-

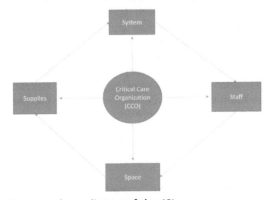

Fig. 1. The CCO as the central coordinator of the 4S's.

19, as their intended function was to ensure that care could still be administered in New York City to patients with non–COVID-19, while freeing up space in legacy New York City hospitals for patients with COVID-19.[13,14] But during the COVID-19 pandemic, New York City experienced a reduction in patients seeking treatment of non–COVID-19 related reasons. Faced with this reality, both The Comfort and the Javits Center rethought their original plans and implemented new ones. The Comfort decided to accept patients with COVID-19, but required reconfiguration to effectively isolate patients with COVID-19 from patients with non–COVID-19.[13] By the time the reconfiguration of the infrastructure was complete, the Comfort's expanded bed capacity was no longer needed, due to the decline in the number of patients with COVID-19 at that point. The Javits center also redesignated beds for patients with COVID-19 after a similar structural reconfiguration, but the strict criteria for admission limited the use of the 2500 beds made available.[14] The strict criteria for admission stemmed from a concern that patients with COVID-19 who required surgery or ICU level care would not be able to receive adequate care at the Javits center, due to the nature of the facility.

In sum, the reduction in common clinical ailments for which New York City residents sought treatment during the 1st wave of COVID-19 and the fact that The Comfort and Javits Center was initially designed to accommodate patients with non–COVID-19 resulted in the limited utility of these deployable critical care assets.

Staff

The need to deliver a high level of care to an influx of critical care patients requires the services of highly trained staff, which predominantly consists of critical care nursing and respiratory therapists, working with advanced practice providers, hospitalists, residents, and intensivists. Moreover, an effective team approach can be achieved when medical staff from across specialties is working in concert to treat patients: whether it is the incorporation of physical therapists into a proning team or a pharmacist's insight into potential medication scarcity (and the pharmacist's recommendations for alternative regimens).[15] Without this team approach, hospitals are unlikely to be able to offer the highest level of critical care to as many affected patients as possible. A CCO with long-standing working relationships with all intensive care ancillary specialties would be well-placed to rapidly deploy these staff to areas they are most needed. Ideally, CCO's would regularly convene interdisciplinary meetings to optimize preparedness so that the hospital is ready "the day before it's needed." For example, noncritical care providers, deployed to the critical care service in the event of a pandemic-related patient surge, require early or on-the-ground education on the nuances of providing support with devices with which they are unfamiliar.

While the expansion of the critical care team to include noncritical care personnel was an effective means of load-leveling, it allowed for the delivery of care, but not necessarily the highest level of care achievable in nonpandemic times. During the pandemic, the ratio of patients to nurse, respiratory therapist, advanced care provider, physical therapists, and physicians were higher than desirable. Many hospitals expanded the care team by having a critical care nurse oversee a medical/surgical nurse, allowing for a team approach to nursing care. In some cases, a CCO can ensure that this is uniformly done throughout the critical care system while providing just-in-time education and adhering to the scope of practice of each individual nurse.[16]

Supplies

The critical care surge medical workers experienced during the onset of the COVID-19 pandemic demonstrated firsthand that the stockpiling of equipment is paramount, as is the inclusion of the hospital's various services (eg, pharmacy, laboratory, respiratory, and so forth) in the planning for a mass critical care incident.

As indicated in the stockpiling equipment guidelines, the targeting of specific supplies, which are usually on low par, may need to be adjusted and their acquisition should be increased before an anticipated event, as was seen during the outbreak of H1N1.[17,18] Additionally, as suggested, "local" efforts can be augmented by a consortium of regional hospitals that can better provide and be prepared for a large scale, persistent event, such as COVID-19.[19]

Moving forward, emphasis should be placed on adhering to equipment stockpiling guidelines, while preevent planning should also consider the physical areas of a hospital that can store this equipment safely, accommodate patients on ventilators, and the need for oxygen delivery to those areas. Further, when accounting for supplies, ventilator supplies, transport ventilators, noninvasive machines, and anesthesia machines should all be accounted for. It would be additionally beneficial for central supply, or the equipment ordering entity for the hospital or health care system, to be included in any discussion of the stockpiling of equipment, as the lack of venous access devices, endotracheal tubes, stylets, and other critical devices is detrimental to patient outcomes.

Systems

Pre–COVID-19 guidelines regarding "systems" mostly focus on the issue of triage. Before the beginning of the 1st surge of COVID-19, the triage of the chronically critically ill out of the ICU allowed for the placement of the incoming sick into the ICU. As an example, at Montefiore Medical Center, (Bronx, NY), the critical care medicine service/CCO tasked the rapid response teams with the role of triage while having a centralized command center with whom to discuss triage decisions. This centralized command center was both an entity that would offer a second opinion and one that had the ability to track bed availability across the health care system and could thus facilitate transfers among the hospitals. The deescalation of non–COVID-19 services, the cancellation of elective procedures, and the conversion of outpatient care to telemedicine allowed for additional resources and providers to assist with the increased patient care demands. The critical care rapid response team and command center were also responsible for allocating noninvasive ventilation (NIV) and high flow nasal cannula (HFNC) to those in need of an elevated delivery of oxygen.[20]

Indisputably, the COVID-19 pandemic laid bare the stark disparity in health equity that exists within the United States, with COVID-19 cases being 10% higher in Blacks and 30% higher among Latinx individuals when compared with White patients. An additional and critical statistical to note is that People of Color were three times more likely to be hospitalized, compared with their white counterparts.[21] These differences extend to vaccination rates, as well. The Bronx can be viewed as a microcosm of the United States, wherein 50% of the population of the Bronx is vaccinated, but when looking at the racial breakdown, only 33% of Black people and 46% of Hispanic people had received the full vaccine as of 9/6/2021.[22]

CCOs can play a crucial role in helping to combat racial disparity in access to health care, especially during a health disaster, such as COVID-19. During a pandemic, it is often the patients without privilege and access to resources whose health is impacted most severely, while patients with privilege tend to be impacted less severely but are also the ones with the greatest access to resources. Having a CCO at the helm can allow for the equitable distribution of resources to the patients most in need. The CCO can maintain an operational and a bird's eye view of all the resources available, redirecting patients as needed to sites that can accommodate them, especially during a patient surge, as was experienced during the COVID-19 pandemic.

Fig. 2 is a flow chart, demonstrating the core role that CCOs can play in providing standardization and organization during a pandemic, such as COVID-19.

PANDEMIC GUIDELINES ISSUED DURING COVID-19: A BRIEF REVIEW

As the COVID-19 pandemic progressed and evolved, additional guidelines, rooted in real-world pandemic experience, were released by many medical organizations, such as the NIH.[4] For this review, we will focus on the guidelines issued by the Task Force for Mass Critical Care (TFMCC), but the reader is invited to compare with other organization's guidelines.[23]

The TFMCC is a collection of experts from the fields of bioethics, critical care, disaster preparedness and response, emergency medical services, emergency medicine, infectious disease, hospital medicine, law, military medicine, nursing, pharmacy, respiratory care, and local, state, and federal government planning and response. This coalition of experts from various fields was then overseen by a steering committee comprised of representatives from the organizational members of the Critical Care Collaborative (CCC), as well as North American disaster experts, unaffiliated with CCC.[24] The TFMCC's additional suggestions built on their initial guidelines released in 2014. Their additional guidelines also incorporated modified versions of several existing sources, including: the World Health Organization's established rapid guideline methodologies and the Guidelines International Network-McMaster Guideline Development Checklist.[24–27] Finally, the TFMCC's additional suggestions considered experiential evidence, peer-reviewed papers, and evidence from lay media sources.[23]

It is helpful to review the TFMCC's additional guidelines as we contemplate ways CCOs can play an even more prominent role in pandemic response. The guidelines issued by the TFMCC can be found in **Table 1**.

Extrapolating from these guidelines, it is essential to acknowledge that it is optimal for the CCO to maintain adequate throughput, while also assisting in other areas of the

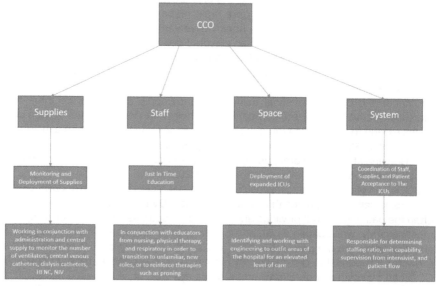

Fig. 2. The CCO coordinating in real time with various services to optimize, supplies, staff, system, and space.

Table 1
10 suggestions with 10 operational strategies for the 4 categories of staffing, load balancing, communication, and technology

Suggestions	Operational Strategy	Category
Suggestion 1: We suggest graded staff-to-patient ratios with consideration to experience level, resources, and patient acuity to optimize contingency care and avoid crisis care.	Three staffing models are presented to effectively scale up surge staffing to maintain contingency level care.	Staffing
Suggestion 2: We suggest limiting overtime to <50% above normal for all HCWs to minimize the risk of burn-out and exhaustion.	Limit overtime to <50% above normal for all staff to minimize the risk of burnout	Staffing
Suggestion 3: We suggest that the mental health needs of all HCWs are priorities for maintaining an effective response and staffing capacity.	Identify HCWs at risk for moral injury or exhaustion, address necessary preventative changes IN clinical care, and promote an informed supportive culture	Staffing
Suggestion 4: During surge, we suggest minimizing redundant clinical documentation requirements to focus on core elements directly relevant to bedside care.	Responsibly streamline documentation requirements	Staffing
Suggestion 5: We suggest that resource strain level be actively monitored and determined by front line clinical leaders based on the assessment of available resources and conditions.	Clinical leaders, ICU directors, and service chiefs should be empowered to determine local resources including strain indicators as being conventional, contingency, or at crisis levels	Load-Balancing
Suggestion 6: We suggest there is a transition zone toward the limits of contingency care when increasingly scarce resources are modified beyond routine standards of care to preserve life. This critical clinical prioritization level precedes triage of scarce resources and is a powerful indicator for needed resources to maintain contingency level care.	Educate clinicians to recognize critical prioritization to request resources or patient transfers; prepare decision support for potential crisis scenarios; prioritize communication systems for rapid access to ethical, legal, administrative counsel when triage of scarce resources is encountered	Load-Balancing
Suggestion 7: We suggest that early transfer of patients before a hospital is overwhelmed promotes the effective conservation of resources and less deviation from routine care standards.	Transfer(load-balance) patients early before a hospital are overwhelmed to maintain contingency level care	Load-Balancing

(*continued on next page*)

Table 1 (continued)		
Suggestions	**Operational Strategy**	**Category**
Suggestion 8: We suggest earlier utilization of regional transfer centers for load-balancing during surge for patient transfers and placement. We also suggest having intensivist or hospitalist availability to help prioritize transfers and provide support to bedside clinicians when transfers are delayed.	Implement regional transfer centers to improve bed access and assure efficient ICU bed use through active management and load-balancing of admissions across all hospitals in a state or region. On-call Intensivists or hospitalist support should be available as a resource	Load-Balancing
Suggestion 9: We reemphasize that designated clinicians who are actively engaged in clinical work (especially intensivists and hospitalists) actively participate in hospital incident command structure; this group should provide updates to clinical staff for improving situational awareness, ensuring bidirectional communication.	Establish formal communication structures between incident command and front-line clinicians, such as PCSS/team to ensure bidirectional communication and situational awareness	Communication
Suggestion 10: We suggest hospitals apply telemedicine technology to augment critical care early and in the broadest sense possible.	Use telemedicine technology to support bedside critical care and connect specialty clinicians to distant sites and support visitation needs of families	Technology

From Dichter JR, Devereaux AV, Sprung CL, et al. Mass Critical Care Surge Response During COVID-19: Implementation of Contingency Strategies - A Preliminary Report of Findings From the Task Force for Mass Critical Care [published online ahead of print, 2021 Sep 6]. Chest. 2021;S0012-3692(21)03845-9. https://doi.org/10.1016/j.chest.2021.08.072; with permission.

hospital. Quaternary Care Centers are typically the de facto centers of specialty excellence for surrounding area hospitals, which often send their most complex patients from satellite campuses. Given this reality, health care systems need to have the ability to flexibly increase a fixed number of beds to accommodate an expanding patient pool. This is illustrated in **Fig. 2**. To ensure this process unfolds smoothly, regular exercises (simulated events) with the involvement of the CCO are essential, especially as the regionalization of health care and resources are still being established.

Furthermore, the provisioning of beds across a health care system is best orchestrated by the CCO working in conjunction with an intensivist, who can advise on whereby to properly triage patients, and, if those patients are delayed in their arrival to the hospital, assist with the management of those patients via telemedicine.[28] Involving an intensivist in this process also allows for the early recognition of a crisis, as well as the optimization of care and capacity to implement appropriate strategies to cope with the influx of patients. If ultimately necessary, the intensivist can also assist with the implementation of a standardized triage system.[29] This is demonstrated in **Fig. 3**.

In addition to focusing on patients, it is paramount to focus on the health and mental health of medical workers, per recommendation #3 of the TFMCC's guidelines. With increasing shortages of nurses, respiratory therapists, and intensivists, the need to provide preventative care to staff and to address moral injury or risk factors for burnout

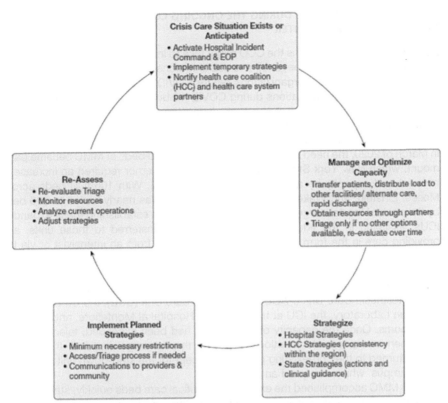

Fig. 3. Process for crisis care integration with incident command. (*From* Maves RC, Downar J, Dichter JR, et al. Triage of Scarce Critical Care Resources in COVID-19 An Implementation Guide for Regional Allocation: An Expert Panel Report of the Task Force for Mass Critical Care and the American College of Chest Physicians. Chest. 2020;158(1):212 to 225. https://doi.org/10.1016/j.chest.2020.03.063; with permission)

and exhaustion requires early recognition. Early recognition of burnout or moral injury cannot be achieved without first establishing open communication among the team. Incorporating a regular staff check-in, or at the very least issue a daily reminder of the psychological resources available to all staff members, helps to foster an environment of safety and lessens the risk of moral injury. A CCO can make sure these resources are distributed appropriately.

Though not specifically addressed in the guidelines circulated by TFMCC, the guidelines implicitly acknowledge the importance of a team approach and team learning. One of the many lessons the COVID-19 pandemic taught us is the importance of academic work during a crisis, and a CCO is uniquely positioned to ensure that this academic work is carried out. An optimal CCO will incorporate education and research as part of its core mission, which is critical to achieving up-to-date patient care. Ultimately, this academic integration facilitates a culture of patient safety and excellence of care through a thoroughly backed and supported quality improvement program. With appropriate funding and international reach, the research done by an academically integrated CCO allows for the rapid transmission of information to the world at large, which in turn, results in the cessation of ineffective treatments and the widespread adoption of optimal treatments.[2]

CRITICAL CARE EXPERIENCE DURING THE ONGOING COVID-19 PANDEMIC AT MONTEFIORE MEDICAL CENTER

As we consider future actions the CCO might take to improve care during the ongoing COVID-19 pandemic (and beyond), it is useful to consider not only the guidelines issued by various medical organizations before COVID-19 and the guidelines issued by various medical organizations during COVID-19 but also the measures individual hospitals and health care systems took during the pandemic to respond to their pandemic experiences in real-time.

Montefiore Medical Center (MMC), serves as an example: when the 1st surge began in March of 2020, the need to increase the number of ICU beds at MMC became paramount, which New York State reinforced when the governor required an increase of hospital bed capacity by a minimum of 50% to 100%. With 106 ICU beds across Moses, Einstein, and Wakefield, the number of beds was nearly tripled to 306 beds by the peak of the 1st surge.[15] The CCO was involved in establishing these expanded ICUs, assisting in the education of nurses being transferred to those units, and providing care in the form of either direct patient care from an intensivist or via the E-ICU that had been established in the command center. These beds were created in areas of the hospital whereby the transition to delivery of advanced critical care would be most easily accomplished. These areas included: the step-down units, the Post-Anesthesia Care Unit (PACU), the Cardiac Care Unit (CCU), the Cardiac Catheterization Laboratory, the ICU at the Children's Hospital at Montefiore, and the operating rooms. Once the capacity of these areas had been exceeded, telemetry units were then converted into functional ICUs. As the 1st surge receded, these areas were returned to their preexisting purposes, except for the step-down unit at the Einstein campus, which remained an ICU.[15]

While MMC accomplished the expansion of critical care beds quickly, staffing these expanded units was a challenge. To cope with the expanded needs of these units, Certified Nurse Anesthetists, OR and PACU nurses, Nurse Practitioners, and ICU nurses were deployed. The CCO coordinated whereby these staff would be allocated and in what capacity. To staff, these units with providers, Head and Neck, General Surgeons, Cardiothoracic surgeons, Neurologists, Anesthesiologists, and critical care hospitalists were installed in the role of critical care attending. To assist with these expanded roles for the expanded provider base, the command center was outfitted with live monitoring as well as with critical care attending available 24 hours a day, 7 days a week. With the expanded need for renal replacement therapy across an increased number of units, perfusionists were cross-trained in managing CRRT.[15]

In terms of training, the original nursing staff for these units were given a boot camp in how to manage patients with COVID-19 facilitated by the CCO. They underwent briefing sessions that included primers on what to look for if their patient was decompensating; the medications with which they would need to become familiar (eg, sedatives and paralytics); and what their role would be during intubation. Additionally, they were given instruction in how to prone patients. To this end, the physical therapists and occupational therapists were deployed as a proning team to help with the sheer number of patients who required proning throughout the hospital. The ICU nurses who were deployed to these units also became the head of a nursing team, which would consist of nurses from that unit, outpatient nurses, or telemetry nurses. This organizational structure is illustrated in **Fig. 4**.

As new COVID units were being created at MMC, the volume of patients the critical care rapid response team was treating increased in tandem, which lead to the deployment of multiple rapid response teams to each campus coordinated by the command

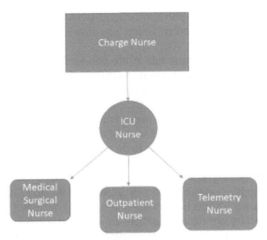

Fig. 4. Nursing team based around a critical care nurse.

center. These expanded rapid response teams were staffed by cardiology fellows at the Wakefield campus; critical care locum tenens and Nurse Practitioner volunteers at Einstein; and across all 3 campuses Certified Registered Nurse Anesthetists (CRNAs). These expanded critical care teams allowed for the rapid delivery of critical care to all areas of the hospital. They were also able to assist with the increased need for intubations, with up to 25 emergent intubations on patients with COVID being done per day.[15] A solitary rapid response team was not enough to address the increased demand so additional teams were added. The rapid response team was also able to assist in the expanded ICUs, when needed, and was the action arm of the command center.

The establishment of a critical care command center allowed for the centralization of the available critical care resources. The command center consisted of 6 socially distanced workspaces, as well as remote access to the telemetry and waveforms of all the various critical care units. Once the command center was established, it helped to triage patients across multiple campuses, as the physician in charge of the command center not only knew whereby beds were available but also beds were already assigned. This alleviated the pressure on the rapid response teams and allowed them to focus on providing direct patient care, knowing that the patients accepted to the ICU would be sent to an open bed in either a legacy unit or one of the newly created ICUs. The command center also functioned as a hotline for the hospital at large, answering general critical care questions and assisting with the weaning of HFNC, ventilators, and NIPPV.

Load-leveling was a strategy that was used by some hospitals and health care systems, as well as entire cities, such as Detroit, throughout the pandemic to accommodate patient surges. At Montefiore Medical Center, patients deemed stable for transfer were moved to available beds across the 3 main campuses of Montefiore (Moses, Einstein, and Wakefield), as a means of using resources across multiple campuses, The transport ranged from ACLS transport in an ambulance to a medically capable bus that would bring patients from Einstein to Moses and vice versa. All transfers both within and without the hospital center were centrally handled by the CCO in the command center, with the goal of effectively balancing the patient load.

While the load-leveling system established at Montefiore was specific to their health care system, load-leveling occurred more widely throughout the pandemic and took various forms. For instance, Detroit applied load-leveling across the city, using a Medical Operation Coordination Center, which was able to leverage all available beds to those in need.[6]

E-consult also played a central role in the pandemic response. Due to the highly infective nature of COVID-19, and limitations in PPE, E-consult allowed for the conservation of PPE, while still adequately maintaining expert consultation. To ensure uniformity across all areas of critical care, the CCO should make uniform guidelines for when E-consults from other specialties are acceptable and when in-person care should be done. Also, through telemedicine, E-consults for critical care services could be increased to allow critical care services to be more timely when stretched thin. Finally, it is interesting to note that a body of literature exists, pointing to the efficacy of E-ICU beyond the pandemic experience.[28]

When discussing the realities of practicing medicine during COVID-19, it is essential to acknowledge the toll it has had on providers, which has been well-documented in surveys conducted by physician-scientists as well as in wide-ranging discussions in the media, with upwards of 45.8% of physicians reporting symptoms of burnout.[30] To alleviate burnout at MMC, and to establish a safe space in which to discuss what MMC providers were seeing and feeling during their rounds, clinicians from psychiatry met with the critical care team weekly. They also made themselves readily available to support physicians who wished to discuss their experiences in a more private setting. Internally, the critical care department developed a daily email, "the daily note of positivity," which would include positive anecdotes from throughout the day (eg, a patient who was extubated, a heartwarming patient interaction, an example of effective multidisciplinary teamwork, or to highlight a new innovation in the care of patients with COVID-19).[15]

CONCLUSION: LESSONS LEARNED

The CCO is uniquely positioned to implement further changes that will help us manage the ongoing COVID-19 pandemic, as well as to apply the knowledge we've gained from this real-world experience to future pandemics. The implementation of international guidelines assisted in the care of patients and laid an important framework that was able to scale up as the need arose, but there are several additional initiatives that can now be implemented by the CCO to improve outcomes as we look toward the years ahead.

The first is the need for an increased critical care workforce and additional advanced practice providers. During a post 1st surge feedback session conducted at MMC, many of the nurses, critical care providers, and respiratory staff remarked on the deficit of critical care physicians during the 1st surge and the subsequent need for additional staffing. Second: while the COVID-19 pandemic was (and continues to be) an evolving situation, clarity in the form of recommended personal protective equipment early on in the pandemic would have gone a long way in fostering trust between staff, providers, and administration. The lack of PPE, due to increased demand and supply constraints, was predicted, but the impact on morale and the perception that those working bedsides were undervalued, and to an extent unseen, is something to be avoided in the future. **Box 1** has a list of risk factors for health care worker burnout and moral injury. Third: As previously discussed in this review, the COVID-19 pandemic further revealed the racial disparities in access to health care and health care resources that exist within the United States. CCOs can play a vital role in achieving greater health care equality by redistributing resources and directing patients with limited resources to health care sites that can best care for them. In

---

Box 1
Risk factors for health care workers developing burnout and or moral injury

WORK ENVIRONMENT
  Inadequate access to personal protective equipment or essential supplies
  High perception of personal risk for infection
  Inability to rest
  Prolonged working times
  Excessive workload
  Working in a high-risk environment
  Involuntary deployment
  Perceived inadequate training
  Lack of sufficient communication and updated information
  Regret about restricted visitation policies
  Witnessing hasty end of life decisions
  Inadequate organizational support, insurance, or compensation

SOCIAL FACTORS
  Fear of being infected
  Fear of spreading the illness to family and friends
  Inability to care for one's family
  Struggling with difficult emotions
  being quarantined
  Social rejection or isolation
  Moral distress
  Lack of social support

From Dichter JR, Devereaux AV, Sprung CL, et al. Mass Critical Care Surge Response During COVID-19: Implementation of Contingency Strategies - A Preliminary Report of Findings From the Task Force for Mass Critical Care [published online ahead of print, 2021 Sep 6]. Chest. 2021;S0012-3692(21)03845-9. https://doi.org/10.1016/j.chest.2021.08.072 with permission.

---

conclusion, the CCO's unification of ICU units before the onset of the COVID-19 Pandemic, and the resulting standardization of care and integration of critical care within the larger structure of the hospital, positioned the hospital to be better equipped to adapt to the demands of the pandemic. CCOs should continue to make changes, based on the real experience of COVID-19 that would lead to improved care during the ongoing pandemic, and beyond.

CLINICS CARE POINTS

- The Four S's (space, staff, supplies, and systems) work as a foundational framework from which CCOs can build their response to a disaster.
- CCOs play a central role in a response to a disaster or pandemic.
- COVID-19 has highlighted the importance of health equity at every level of care.

DISCLOSURE

The authors have nothing to disclose.

REFERENCES

1. Leung S, Gregg SR, Coopersmithet CM. Critical care organizations: business of critical care and value/performance building. Crit Care Med 2018;46(1):1–11.

2. Moore JE, Oropello JM, Stoltzfus D. Critical care organizations: building and integrating academic programs. Crit Care Med 2018;46(4):e334–41.

3. Dichter DA JR, Sprung CL, Mukherjee V, et al. Task Force for mass critical care writing group. Mass critical care surge response during COVID-19: implementation of contingency strategies a preliminary report of findings from the Task Force for mass critical care. Chest; 2021.

4. Coronavirus disease 2019 (COVID-19) treatment guidelines. 2021. Available at: https://www.covid19treatmentguidelines.nih.gov/.

5. COVID-19 pandemic lessons. 2021. Available at: https://www.sccm.org/getattachment/bad71d50-653a-4128-b406-cf4ba24064dd/COVID-19-Pandemic-Lessons-Infographic.

6. National Academies of Sciences, E. And medicine, rapid expert Consultation on staffing Considerations for crisis Standards of care for the COVID-19 pandemic16. Washington, DC: The National Academies Press; 2020.

7. ASPR/TRACIE. 2021. Available at: https://asprtracie.hhs.gov/.

8. Einav S, Hick JL, Hanfling D. Surge capacity logistics: care of the critically ill and injured during pandemics and disasters: CHEST consensus statement. Chest 2014;146(4 Suppl):e17S–43S.

9. Schwirtz M. The 1,000-bed Comfort was Supposed to Aid New York. It has 20 patients. 2021. Available at: https://www.nytimes.com/2020/04/02/nyregion/ny-coronavirus-usns-comfort.html.

10. LINTON C. Field hospital that treated coronavirus patients in Central Park to close. 2021. Available at: https://www.cbsnews.com/news/field-hospital-that-treated-coronavirus-patients-in-central-park-to-close/.

11. Rosenthal BM. This hospital cost $52 million. It treated 79 Virus patients. 2021. Available at: https://www.nytimes.com/2020/07/21/nyregion/coronavirus-hospital-usta-queens.html.

12. Collins GB, Ahluwalia N, Arrol L. Lessons in cognitive unloading, skills mixing, flattened hierarchy and organisational agility from the Nightingale Hospital London during the first wave of the pandemic 2021;10(3):e001415.

13. Simkins JD. Hospital ship Comfort departs NYC, having treated fewer than 200 patients. 2020. Available at: https://www.navytimes.com/news/your-navy/2020/04/30/hospital-ship-comfort-departs-nyc-having-treated-fewer-than-200-patients/.

14. Abby Narishkin , S.C., and Libertina Brandt. Why NYC's largest emergency hospital is pretty much empty. 2020.

15. Keene AB, Shiloh AL, Eisen L. Critical care surge during the COVID-19 pandemic: implementation and feedback from Frontline providers. J Intensive Care Med 2021;36(2):233–40.

16. Anderson BR, Ivascu NS, Brodie. Breaking Silos: the team-based approach to coronavirus disease 2019 pandemic staffing. Crit Care Explor 2020;2(11):e0265.

17. Baekkeskov E. Pandemic preparedness and responses to the 2009 H1N1 influenza: crisis management and public policy insights. UK: Oxford University Press; 2020.

18. Fineberg HV. Pandemic preparedness and response — lessons from the H1N1 influenza of 2009. N Engl J Med 2014;370(14):1335–42.

19. Coleman CN, Hrdina C, Casagrande R. User-managed inventory: an approach to forward-deployment of urgently needed medical countermeasures for mass-casualty and terrorism incidents. Disaster Med Public Health Prep 2012;6(4):408–14.

20. Sprung CL, Joynt GM, Christian MD. Adult ICU triage during the coronavirus disease 2019 pandemic: who will live and who will Die? Recommendations to improve Survival. Crit Care Med 2020;48(8):1196–202.
21. Baker DW. Breaking Links in the chain of racial disparities for COVID-19. JAMA Netw Open 2021;4(6):e2112879.
22. NYC vaccine Data. 2021. Available at: https://www1.nyc.gov/site/doh/covid/covid-19-data-vaccines.page#people.
23. Dichter JR, Devereaux AV, Sprung CL. Mass critical care surge response during COVID-19: implementation of Contingency strategies A Preliminary report of findings from the Task Force for mass critical care. Chest 2021.
24. Devereaux A, Christian MD, Dichter JR. Summary of suggestions from the Task Force for mass critical care summit. Chest 2008;133(Suppl 5):S1–7.
25. GIN-McMaster guideline development Checklist. 2021. Available at: https://cebgrade.mcmaster.ca/guidecheck.html.
26. WHO handbook for guideline development. 2021. Available at: https://apps.who.int/iris/bitstream/handle/10665/75146/9789241548441_eng.pdf;jsessionid=579702B307D1F8B00AF936592C76EE4F?sequence=1.
27. Garritty CM, Norris SL, Moher D. Developing WHO rapid advice guidelines in the setting of a public health emergency. J Clin Epidemiol 2017;82:47–60.
28. Vranas KC, Slatore CG, Kerlin MP. Telemedicine Coverage of intensive care Units: a Narrative review. Ann Am Thorac Soc 2018;15(11):1256–64.
29. Maves RC, Downar J, Dichter JR. Triage of Scarce critical care resources in COVID-19 an implementation Guide for regional allocation: an expert Panel report of the Task Force for mass critical care and the American College of chest physicians. Chest 2020;158(1):212–25.
30. Shanafelt TD, Boone S, Tan L. Burnout and satisfaction with work-life balance among US physicians relative to the general US population. Arch Intern Med 2012;172(18):1377–85.